Psychiatric and Mental Health Essentials in Primary Care

Psychiatric and Mental Health Essentials in Primary Care addresses key mental health concepts and strategies for time-pressured practitioners in various healthcare settings serving diverse populations. It offers theoretically sound and succinct guidelines for compassionate, efficient, and effective service to people in emotional and physical pain and distress, capturing the essentials of mental healthcare delivered by primary care providers.

The text provides a theoretical overview, discussing mental health assessment, crisis care basics, alternative therapies, and vulnerable groups such as children, adolescents, and older people. It includes chapters that focus on the following topics in primary care practice:

- suicide and violence
- anxiety
- mood disorders
- schizophrenia
- substance abuse
- chronic illness and mental health.

This invaluable text is designed for primary care providers in either graduate student or practice roles across a range of primary care practice, including nurse practitioners and physician assistants.

Lee Ann Hoff is a nurse-anthropologist and mental health professional with extensive clinical, management, teaching, research, and consulting experience in crisis and mental healthcare, women's health, and sociocultural issues affecting health. She is Adjunct Professor in the Faculty of Health Sciences, University of Ottawa, Canada, and Visiting Professor at the Institute for Applied Psychology (ISPA) Lisbon, Portugal.

Betty D. Morgan is Associate Professor at the University of Massachusetts Lowell, USA, where she is the coordinator for the Adult Psychiatric Mental Health nursing graduate program, and the post-Master's Adult Psychiatric Mental Health nursing certificate program.

Psychiatric and Mental Health Essentials in Primary Care

Lee Ann Hoff and Betty D. Morgan

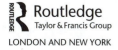

Routledge
Taylor & Francis Group

LONDON AND NEW YORK

First published 2011
by Routledge
2 Park Square, Milton Park, Abingdon, Oxon, OX14 4RN

Simultaneously published in the USA and Canada
by Routledge
270 Madison Avenue, New York, NY 10016

Routledge is an imprint of the Taylor & Francis Group, an informa business

Typeset in Times New Roman by Keystroke, Station Road, Codsall, Wolverhampton
Printed and bound in Great Britain by CPI Antony Rowe, Chippenham, Wiltshire

British Library Cataloguing in Publication Data
A catalogue record for this book is available from the British Library

Library of Congress Cataloging in Publication Data
Hoff, Lee Ann.
Psychiatric and mental health essentials in primary care / Lee Ann Hoff and Betty Morgan.
p. ; cm.
Includes bibliographical references.
1. Psychiatric nursing. 2. Primary care (Medicine) 3. Nurse practitioners. I. Morgan, Betty, 1947–
II. Title.
[DNLM: 1. Psychiatric Nursing. 2. Mental Disorders–nursing. 3. Mental Health. 4. Nurse Practitioners.
5. Primary Health Care. WY 160 H698p 2011]
RC440.H58 2011
616.89'0231–dc22
2010019469

ISBN13: 978–0–415–78090–2 (hbk)
ISBN13: 978–0–415–78091–9 (pbk)
ISBN13: 978–0–203–84022–1 (ebk)

To primary care providers worldwide,
and the people they care for

Contents

Figures

Tables

Boxes

About the Authors

Lee Ann Hoff, PhD, MSN, is a psychiatric/mental health nursing clinical specialist, with an interdisciplinary doctorate including social anthropology, medical sociology, and women's health. She holds a graduate certificate in crisis and suicidology, and is founding director of the Life Crisis Institute based in Boston. Dr. Hoff has extensive national and international experience as an educator, consultant, clinician, and crisis services manager. Acknowledging her outstanding work in initiating and developing national standards for crisis programs, the American Association of Suicidology bestowed on her its first national service award in 1985. In 2000 she received an Honorary Recognition Award from the American Nurses Association for her work on violence issues. As a professor at the University of Massachusetts Lowell, she developed and coordinated the psychiatric/mental health Masters program, which included faculty collaboration around integration of psychiatric mental health nursing in the Nurse Practitioner curriculum. Her major publications include the award-winning book, *People in Crisis: Clinical and Diversity Perspectives*, 6th Ed. (2009, Routledge); *Violence and Abuse Issues: Cross-cultural Perspectives for Health and Social Services (*2010, Routledge); and *Battered Women As Survivors* (1990, Routledge). Currently, Dr. Hoff is Adjunct Professor, University of Ottawa, Faculty of Health Sciences; Visiting Professor, ISPA (Institute for Applied Psychology), Lisbon, Portugal; and Consultant at the International Institute, Boston, and Vida Health Communications, Inc., Cambridge, Massachusetts.

Betty D. Morgan, PhD, PMHCNS, BC, is a psychiatric clinical nurse specialist. She completed a post-graduate certificate in Alcoholism and Drug Abuse and is a trainer in the End of Life Nursing Education Consortium (ELENC). Dr. Morgan is currently an Associate Professor at the University of Massachusetts Lowell and coordinates the Adult Psychiatric Mental Health Nursing graduate program and post-Master's certificate program. She has worked with a variety of medically ill patients over the past 25 years, including people with HIV/AIDS. She maintains a small clinical practice providing therapy to HIV-infected persons who have substance abuse and mental health problems. Dr. Morgan also provides support and consultation to groups of nurses and other healthcare providers who work with "difficult," underserved, and disenfranchised patients. She received the Association of Nurses in AIDS Care (ANAC) 2008 Richard L. Sowell Award for Outstanding Article in the *Journal of Association of Nurses in AIDS Care* (JANAC). In 2006 she received the Research in Addictions Nursing Award from The International Nurses Society on Addictions. Her publications include articles in a variety of nursing journals and co-authorship of several book chapters.

About the Contributors

Lisa Brown, MS, APRN, BC, is a psychiatric/mental health nurse practitioner at Bridgewell Counseling Services in Lowell, Massachusetts. She also works as a psychiatric consultant at Lowell General Hospital, and as a clinical instructor in psychiatric nursing at Salem State College. She is co-author of the chapter, "Comprehensive Mental Health Assessment: An Integrated Approach," in *Geropsychiatric and Mental Health Nursing*. Her professional interests include addiction, chronic illness, and diversity issues in healthcare.

Mary Linda O'Reilly, MS, APRN, BC, a nurse practitioner, is a primary care provider, psychotherapist, and coordinator at the HIV Clinic of the University of Massachusetts Memorial Health Center in Worcester, MA. She holds a post-graduate certificate in psychiatric/mental health nursing. She is also a consultant for the HIV service of Fitchburg Community Health Connections, and serves as Adjunct Faculty at the University of Massachusetts at Worcester. Her publications include "Spirituality and Mental Health Clients," and as co-author, "Crisis Intervention," for an e-course: Mental Health in Primary Care, a university consortium in Ontario, Canada. Her professional interests include: HIV management and post-exposure prophylaxis, psychopharmacology, and trauma intervention.

Valerie Grdisa, RN, MS, PhD, is an advanced practice nurse specializing in child and adolescent psychiatry. Her experience includes an array of health and social service roles in clinical practice, management, research, policy, education, and consulting. As director of the Nurse Practitioner Programs at the University of Toronto, she was active in national and provincial policy making to advance the educational standards and role of nurse practitioners in Canada. Currently, she is a part-time faculty member at McMaster University, School of Nursing, in Hamilton, Ontario, and is a Senior Manager at KPMG, Advisory Services, Healthcare Practice. Her dissertation research used diverse methodological approaches to evaluate service integration among 93 child and youth service providers representing six distinct sectors. Dr. Grdisa's publications include peer-reviewed journal articles and presentations on children with chronic conditions, interprofessional education, and health and human services integration. Her professional interests are health and human services transformation, child and youth mental health service delivery, and community governance.

Jane Bindley, BA, BS, EdM, is a licensed physical therapist at Boston Medical Center. Over the years she has obtained several certificates for integrating Eastern healing arts into her physical therapy practice. These include, for example, extensive training in Zero Balancing, Process Acupressure, BioSynchronistics®, muscle energy, Jones strain/counterstrain, structural strategies, visceral manipulation, and myofacial release. Her typical clients are persons whose histories range from serious orthopedic injuries and war trauma to childhood sexual abuse. These patients cite their limited success with traditional surgery, psychotherapy, and medication regimens. This experience has led to Ms. Bindley's strong belief in the therapeutic value of carefully applied techniques from both Western and Eastern traditions in rehabilitation medicine.

Preface

Our fascination with the mysteries of mind, body, and spirit laid the foundation for this book. Increasingly, the general public and healthcare providers accept and expect attention to mind/body connections in health matters. Yet, doing justice to holistic practice is often constrained by the Cartesian mind/body split influencing our cultural legacy. Also, time and the easy availability of providers can profoundly influence outcomes for clients presenting in general medical settings with mental health problems or serious psychiatric illness.

Over the years we grew to appreciate the special challenges of caring for those patients historically out of sight in mainstream medical and nursing arenas. But just as most psychiatric patients lived out their lives in largely segregated facilities until recently, the rewards of working with them are typically less visible and tangible than dramatic surgical cures, for instance. Our vision for this book is to share our insights beyond the typically few psychiatry lectures for primary care graduate students.

In our early consultation and psychiatric liaison work, the national and international "golden era" of community-based mental healthcare had not yet arrived. Unfortunately, the ideal model of integrating medical and psychiatric/mental health services in a single comprehensive entity is still unrealized in many communities. We know from experience that a brief encounter and meaningful exchange with a patient can be the basis of a long-term professional relationship that brings satisfaction to both the patient and provider. The need for an integrated model of care will be a continued focus in the U.S. as health insurance expands and mental health parity becomes a reality in our healthcare system.

We see a natural affinity between primary care and mental health. Complementing social psychiatry, primary care providers—especially family physicians (GPs) and nurse practitioners—serve individual patients in the context of family, jobs, ethnicity and other factors affecting health status. Yet, a dearth of easy-to-use resources often shortchanges these practitioners in the mental health essentials required in busy practice arenas. Our aim is to provide key mental health concepts and strategies for such time-pressured practitioners—keeping in mind the "essentials" in the book's title—and to build strong and supportive bridges between primary care providers and mental health specialists.

Defining Features of This Book

Theory–Practice Integration and Illustration

Primary care providers will readily recognize the typical scenarios we present from various practice arenas. Each clinical-focused chapter (a) includes a brief overview of the medical/psychiatric condition or life-threatening crises drawn from current psychiatric/mental health theory; and (b) features inter-related medical and psychosocial issues, psychopharmacology, and the essential knowledge, attitudes, and skills demanded for an effective and healing response.

Generalist-Psychiatric Specialist Teamwork

Another feature is our selection of those conditions—gleaned from teachers and practitioners—most commonly presenting in primary care settings. We avoid in-depth coverage of the dozens of psychiatric diagnoses already addressed in psychiatric texts, while noting important criteria for referral to mental health specialists. Instead, we offer basic principles and strategies relevant across a range of mental health/medical scenarios, guidelines for teamwork with specialists and for closing health system loopholes that can hinder coordinated treatment planning, and references for further study.

Diversity Issues

While keenly aware of our personal history, education, and other factors affecting professional practice, and the value of cross-cultural exchange, we do not assume "competence" in cultures other than our own in the multicultural milieu of the United States—this despite some of our education, teaching, and research experience across cultures.

Throughout the book are examples of the varied manifestations of mental health phenomena among diverse clientele. Since no single practitioner can fully grasp the nuances of social norms and values among their multicultural clientele, we emphasize the importance of this *key question*: What *meanings* do different people attach to illness and how to respond to pain and suffering within their society and its ritual and belief system? We are also keenly aware of the importance of examining books like ours for sensitivity to both *commonalities* and *differences* across cultures. For example, ethnographic research reveals that "schizophrenia" occurs cross-culturally but may not be called that in some cultures; nor is it treated primarily with psychotropic drugs, as in the West. To our international and other readers: We welcome your critique as you consider how the concepts and strategies we present may be applied in your particular cultural milieu, and in possible future editions of the book. We also invite accounts of success with family and community-focused approaches such as "open-dialog therapy" in Scandanavian countries and the more selective and limited use of medications in reducing life-long disability among persons experiencing psychosis.

Accessible Language and Time Sensitivity

While avoiding both a simplistic approach and obscure psychiatric language, we recognize the reality of time pressures in most primary care settings. The book offers mental health basics in accessible language and relevant practice strategies to enhance treatment outcomes—not the in-depth skills of mental health specialists, but those within reach of primary care providers' repertoire of already established skills. We have deliberately avoided an encyclopedic tome in favor of a brief theoretical overview, succinct assessment and treatment guidelines, and case illustrations for compassionate and efficient service by primary care providers.

We know from experience and the general literature that most primary care providers care deeply about the overall needs of their clients, though many lack easy-to-use resources to address the psychosocial needs of diverse clients in busy healthcare arenas. Sometimes, *less is more,* especially when offered in the context of a caring provider/client relationship and community supports. For example: A sincere and succinctly expressed concern in a 10–15 minute session with an acutely distressed client can be life-saving. People who are acutely upset and in physical and emotional pain don't expect miracles, but they should expect empathic response, life-saving information, at-home strategies for dealing with the emotional and social toll of chronic medical and psychiatric conditions, and appropriate follow-up regardless of busy schedules.

Audience

The book's major audience is graduate students in programs preparing for primary care practice across a range of healthcare settings: nurse practitioners (NP) medical practitioners (MD) physician assistants (PA), including, for example, adult, family, pediatric, geriatric, and women's health clientele.

We believe it would be appropriate either as a *required* text or as a supplement to the large clinical texts which typically include only *a chapter or two addressing mental health issues*. If introduced early in the curriculum, students would find it a useful resource over the course of clinical rotations across practice arenas.

Other readers may include:

- The large number of *already practicing primary care providers* (medicine, nursing, and physician assistants) who have Continuing Education requirements, or whose graduate curricula did not adequately prepare them for the mental health practice issues they currently face.
- The many psychologists, advanced practice psychiatric nurse specialists, and clinical social workers often called on for consultation by primary care providers—physicians, NPs, and PAs. The challenge in some of these consultative relationships is providing *enough* but *not too much* information: that is, paring down vast psychiatric specialty knowledge to a level both understandable and useable in time-pressured primary care settings.
- In the global health arena, health sciences curricula worldwide. While in many practice settings cross-culturally, life-and-death medical needs by necessity command front-burner attention, e.g., in refugee camps, among disaster survivors, etc. Yet, the psychosocial sequelae of catastrophic loss, crippling diseases, homelessness, violence, and violent deaths of loved ones can also be addressed by primary care providers who feel secure in offering emotional support when time is short, and who have confidence in applying the essentials presented in this book.
- Undergraduate nursing and medical students. Increasingly in nursing, the curricula for these students have seen a shrinkage of time allotted to psychiatric/mental health issues. The large psychiatric tomes addressed to this audience are simply beyond the capacity of crowded undergraduate nursing curriculum requirements. This book might serve as the main, more manageable text, with the large text a designated additional resource.
- Health sciences libraries worldwide.
- Lay readers who may wish to learn more about psychiatric/mental health issues—their own, or among their family members and friends.

Acknowledgments

Many people have contributed directly or indirectly to the life of this book. Through guest lectures, workshops, university courses, and our liaison work over the years, we have been affirmed time and again by hundreds of students' and colleagues' enthusiastic response to the importance of psychiatric and mental health concepts in general healthcare practice. You know who you are, and we thank you.

Our deepest gratitude also goes to our own teachers, clinical supervisors and supportive colleagues whose wisdom, deep knowledge, and clinical skills have been the foundation and continuous anchor in the challenging journey that inspired this book. We cannot name them all, but most recently our teaching colleague, Dr. Margaret Edmands, at the University of Massachusetts Lowell has been the best cheerleader any author could wish for. We also thank Department Chairs, Dr. May Futrell and Dr. Karen Devereau Melillo, gerontology specialists, for their keen appreciation of mental health content in NP curricula. To Pauline Beaulieu: Only you can imagine the shape of our final manuscript minus your technical assistance so graciously delivered. We thank you deeply. At the University of Massachusetts Boston, College of Nursing and Health Sciences, Dr. Margaret McAllister is a pioneer who advocated and obtained federal funding for introducing a required mental health course in the Family Nurse Practitioner curriculum she coordinates, with hundreds benefiting from the course. Her conviction of its importance for best practice in primary care has been an inspiration for beginning and completing this book. We thank you, Maggie, and hope others emulate your example.

Most immediately and profoundly, we thank our contributors to several of the book's chapters: Lisa Brown (Chapter 2), Linda O'Reilly (Chapter 8), Valerie Grdisa (Chapter 11), and Jane Bindley (Chapter 13). Without their knowledge and clinical expertise at current front lines of practice—not to mention their patience and endurance over the challenging phases of production—this most certainly would be a lesser book. Besides specific chapter content, they offered valuable critique and support of the entire manuscript. It has been our distinct pleasure to work with you on this book (see contributors' information for a fuller description of their background).

We also thank our colleagues, Dr. Rosemary Theroux and Dr. Ruth Remington, NP faculty members at the University of Massachusetts Medical Center and University of Massachusetts Lowell, Department of Nursing, for manuscript critiques. Their help in integrating mental health and primary care content has made this a better book. We are also grateful to Cathy Miller and Alaine Duncan, at www.CrossingsHealingworks.org, and volunteers at Walter Reed Army Medical Center who work with traumatized war veterans, and to Dr. Ricardo Bianco, a psychologist at Boston Behavioral Medicine. These bridge-builders helped us with their specialty knowledge of Complementary and Alternative Medicine, Chapter 13. We are also deeply grateful for the helpful suggestions of the anonymous reviewers solicited by the publisher.

Our deep gratitude goes to Grace McInnes, our editor at Routledge for her belief in this book, her consistent and gracious support and guidance, and her astute suggestions for fine-tuning the manuscript. But without editorial assistant, Khanam Virjee, and her timely and accurate attention to production detail, who knows what the final product might have looked like! We also thank the army of behind-the-scenes workers at Routledge who, while publicly invisible, are essential to every book seeing the light of day. And for any unintended omissions of contributors or content errors, we offer our apologies.

Last but not least, we thank our family and friends for their patience and support through the many phases of seeing this book through to publication. You are a firm testament to this key concept—the necessity of people who believe in us during very stressful times, contribute to our mental health, and stand ready to celebrate the positive results of a challenging life event!

1   Theoretical Overview and Generalist/Specialist Roles

- Mind–Body–Spirit Connections
- Key Mental Health and Psychiatric Concepts Relevant to Primary Care
- Palliative Care Essentials and Mental Illness
- Diversity Perspectives in Primary Care
- Comprehensive Treatment and Inter-professional Collaboration
- References

Mind–Body–Spirit Connections

Centuries ago, father of medicine Hippocrates said: It is better to know the man who has the disease than the disease the man has. Of course this is not an either/or proposition, but rather, the fact that both apply. A psychiatrist illustrated this practice scenario with the following statement: If I treated a person with anti-psychotic medication on the assumption that the troubling hallucinations were a symptom of schizophrenia, and he/she subsequently died from complications of a malignant brain tumor, I would never forgive myself for the failure to have made a differential diagnosis before beginning treatment.

Similarly, primary care providers (PCPs) are faced with multiple situations where patients present with physical health symptoms that may mask mental and emotional problems. For example, besides the risks of the serious physical illness itself, inattention to impending despair on learning of life-threatening cancer or heart disease could result in a preventable death by suicide. Or, a presenting symptom of delirium needs differentiation between its medical and/or psychiatric origins as a basis for treatment—whether from cognitive decline, delusions from psychosis, or a multiplicity of factors that influence brain functioning. We thus recognize the intrinsic connection between mind and body in contemporary healthcare practice, and therefore the importance of treating the whole person a diseased or bruised body, a grieving soul, and the mind and emotions of a distressed and suffering person.

A potentially dangerous vacuum is left when primary care providers feel unprepared in the psychosocial realm of practice. This problem arises when the provider is challenged with addressing multiple medical and psychosocial issues simultaneously in a very limited amount of time. The challenge presented is to routinely incorporate essential mental health strategies into tight schedules. Although not commonplace, some patients will present with the life-threatening situation of harm to themselves or others—for example, in response to learning about a serious medical illness. It is commonplace for a depressed person to neglect ordinary hygiene or routines such as exercise and proper diet. Such situations sandwiched between a diabetic patient with a glucose level over 500 and a sore throat awaiting treatment can claim an inordinate amount of time and provoke extreme anxiety for the provider, who may also lack confidence to address them appropriately.

Keeping in mind Hippocrates' wisdom and ideals with respect to our understanding and treatment of the whole person, let us consider these examples.

CASE EXAMPLES: UNDERSTANDING THE WHOLE PERSON

Case Example 1: Mr. Richard Ebbers

Mr. Ebbers, age 76 and recently widowed, is the father of three children, two daughters and one son. One daughter, Karen, lives with her husband and two children in the same small town as her father. Her sister Joan and brother David live with their families an hour's drive from their father's home. Until age 62, Richard worked as an electrical engineer in a prominent high technology company. The chief reason for his early retirement was his wife Louise's diagnosis of leukemia which entailed a series of chemotherapy sessions over an eight-year period. During this time, Richard assumed major responsibility for his wife's medical appointments and home-based care-taking needs, as well as routine housekeeping and cooking tasks that his wife could no longer handle. He also had to work in appointments for his own injury-related knee problems for which he had joint replacement surgery four years ago, and for routine checks on his blood sugar levels given his family history of diabetes. On his father's side, there is a genetic risk of Alzheimer's disease.

Following the death and burial of his wife, Richard felt some relief from the 24/7, eight-year strain of his care-taking role which left little time for personal interests. But after years of a very happy marriage and successful career, he is now aware of an "emptiness" in his life. He has begun using alcohol as a way to drown out the loneliness of long evenings alone, and has been deviating from his long-standing adherence to diet and exercise as preventive measures to avoid diabetes. Richard's daughter Karen has noted the change in her father, including his over-indulgence in alcohol and sweets at family dinners—this, a distinct departure from his lifelong self-care habits. All three siblings have observed some "forget-fulness" in their father, and hope this is not a sign of early Alzheimer's. Karen has urged Richard to see his primary care provider, and perhaps a counselor to help him through a difficult period of serious changes.

This scenario and similar mind/body challenges to maintaining health and well-being over the life-span are played out for many families in North America (including immigrants) where children don't live geographically close to their parents. In a situation such as Richard's the primary care provider indeed may be the *only* one who can zero in and follow up on the changes noticed by his children. The PCP response to a client like Richard—what to ask and what to do—is addressed in detail in Chapter 2, "Assessment," especially ascertaining Richard's suicide risk level around his use of alcohol in response to loneliness, and his long-term risk of cognitive impairment.

Case Example 2: Ms. Denise Evans

Denise Evans, age 35, is the mother of three children ages 15, 12, and 8. She is employed as an administrative assistant in a biotechnology laboratory. Denise has been seeing a family nurse practitioner for the past three years, usually for sleep disturbance, chronic fatigue, and periodic intestinal pain. She confided her concerns about her marriage and expectation by her husband to continue working full-time, and his failure to ease her workload through help with the children's homework and after-school activities. Although Denise has considered divorce, she has decided to stick with the marriage primarily out of financial concerns for herself and her children. After referral to a gastroenterologist, she was diagnosed with irritable bowel syndrome. Despite stress-reduction activities like exercise and meditation, her symptoms continued, and she expressed concern about her need to rely increasingly on medication to get a good night's sleep. One day Denise came to the NP's office after referral from a nearby emergency department where she was treated for bruises and a broken arm from assault by her husband. During the NP's intake interview, Denise revealed that she had been suffering verbal abuse and threats of divorce from her husband over three years, but did not think it would escalate to violence, since he held a prestigious position in a local corporate office. Complicating the situation, the couple's children overheard many of their parents' arguments, and the youngest one witnessed the physical assault.

Together, these two cases illustrate a pivotal point in primary care practice: Understanding who the whole person is—not just a patient's presenting symptoms—lays the foundation for next steps in the assessment and treatment process, of which ascertaining immediate risk to life is paramount (discussed in Chapter 2). Healthcare providers' responses to these clients can make the difference between positive or negative outcomes—for example, empathic listening, risk assessment, crisis intervention, and referral for follow-up counseling or therapy vs. a message of disinterest and lack of time that can hasten a person's downward spiral toward substance abuse, suicide, or violence toward others in response to acute distress. Major mental health concepts that aid PCPs' understanding of clients and their families are discussed next.

Key Mental Health and Psychiatric Concepts Relevant to Primary Care

Increasingly, the general public and healthcare providers accept and expect attention to mind/body connections in health matters. Yet, doing justice to holistic practice remains challenging—not only because of the Cartesian mind/body split influencing our cultural legacy, but also because time and financial constraints confound the continuing bias against those with emotional/mental problems. It takes knowledge of behavioral, psychosocial, addictive, psychosomatic, and mental disorders for an effective holistic response to clients' medical needs and attendant emotional responses—in essence, mental health and psychiatric basics are fundamental to primary care practice.

A summary of key mental health and psychiatric concepts relevant to primary care practice are presented with recognition that it is mental health specialists who are expected to master the complexities and multiplicities of this body of knowledge. These theoretical underpinnings are drawn from nursing, psychiatry and community mental health, psychosomatic medicine, psychology (especially developmental theory, ego psychology, and client-centered therapy), and socio-cultural theory applied to mental health. Among the multi-disciplinary concepts affecting primary care and psychiatric specialty practice today, three discoveries that evolved into movements over the past century are significant for their lasting influence on the health provider–client relationship and quality of care, regardless of one's discipline or the presenting clinical problems:

1. Freud's discovery of the impact that repressed emotions (the unconscious facet of personality) can have on one's physical and mental health;
2. the discovery of psychotropic drugs in the 1950s that rivaled Pinel's work a century earlier by releasing the mentally ill from the "chains of demonology" (Dossey & Guzzetta, 1994);

3.   the launching of crisis theory and its public health premise of early detection and preventive intervention.

An overview of these and complementary concepts relevant to primary care practice includes brief reference to the cases of Richard Ebbers and Denise Evans. This will lay the foundation for Chapter 2 in which mental health assessment in primary care will be discussed and illustrated with examples.

Primary Healthcare and Community Mental Health

The World Health Organization's (WHO) 1978 Alma Atta Declaration, and national and international agencies increasingly recognize the fundamental place of primary healthcare in the health status of a nation's people (U.S. Department of Health and Human Services, 2010). WHO's original focus was on immunization, sanitation, nutrition, maternal and child health, and the economic, occupational, and educational underpinnings of health status. Currently, health planners and policymakers acknowledge that mental health status is also tied to socioeconomic and cultural factors among various population groups. Clinicians as well increasingly recognize that the physical health status of people with mental illness is significantly poorer than that of persons without mental illness (Ustan, 1999). The detrimental impact of cognitive and emotional impairment affects one's capacity for self-care behaviors that enhance physical health status, as well as a person's economic stability through successful work performance. Policy statements throughout the globe state that *there is no health without mental health*.

In the United States, the foundation for systematic inclusion of mental health services in primary care and local community settings was laid by the Congressional Committee on Mental Illness and Health, published as *Action for Mental Health* (1961). This document revealed that for *any* problem, people typically went *first* to either their physician or clergy person for help—a help-seeking pattern relevant today in underscoring the pivotal role of primary care providers (physicians, nurse practitioners, physician assistants) as a first contact for people in distress. It also resulted in a federally sponsored and generously funded sharp twist away from lengthy psychiatric stays at large state-run institutions. Mental healthcare was to be provided in community health centers allowing patients to remain in their own environment. This change from institutionalization to community-based care also addressed the significant need for preventive mental health and 24/7 crisis care that had been lacking (Hoff, 1993; Levine, 1981; Paykel, 1990).

Supporting this de-institutionalization process is the principle of providing care and treatment in the "least restrictive environment," an admirable practice embedded in the basic human right to be free of unnecessary constraint—a right complicated in the case of seriously mentally ill people who refuse psychotropic medication (Hoff, 1993; Johnson, 1990).

Unfortunately, despite the fact that 24/7 institutional care is more costly than preventive and community-based services for the mentally ill, various policies and related factors have resulted in serious under-funding and therefore shortchanging the promise of more humane approaches to treating persons with serious mental illness. One of the more tragic and common examples of these failed goals is that significant numbers of homeless people are discharged mental patients who lack economic and other supports. Staff of a shelter for the homeless in one large U.S. city refer to their agency as the state's "largest mental institution." Prisons are also cited as contemporary substitutes for closed psychiatric institutions, but without the necessary mental health professionals to treat seriously mentally ill people with a criminal record (Earley, 2006). Meanwhile, physicians and nurses of some hospitals have set up clinics just to serve the special needs of homeless people, which brings us back to the role of primary care providers in regular clinics whose clientele include any number of people who, in another era, would have been treated in mental institutions. In both the United States and Canada a *housing first* model is being implemented. For example, the Canadian Federal government allocated $110 million to the Mental Health Commission of Canada to find ways to help the growing number of homeless people who have a mental illness. Projects are being implemented in five different cities and include evaluation designs.

These set-backs in mental health services can be traced in part to several themes and policy issues:

1. The mind/body split in health practice (Edmands, Hoff, Kaylor, Mower & Sorrell, 1999).
2. An individual versus population-based focus in health service delivery (Fee & Brown, 2000), especially in the United States where a culture of individualism sometimes overrides larger community concerns (Bellah, Madsen, Sullivan, Swidler & Tipton, 1985).
3. A continuing bias against and disparity in insurance coverage for those with mental or emotional illness.
4. The increasing "caretaker burden" on family members with major home-based respon-sibility for seriously ill, disabled, or dying relatives over extended periods of time. Economic factors, inadequate health insurance, and lack of respite services have been associated with increased morbidity and mortality rates among family caretakers.

Principles of Psychosocial Care in Primary Care Settings

While the generalized bias against acknowledging and publicly funding mental health services on a parity basis with physical health problems is gradually fading, the fact of primary care as an entry point for *any* problem—physical or psychosocial—is undisputed. Worldwide, fiscal constraints have forced even greater attention to the centrality and cost-effectiveness of primary care in a nation's healthcare system. Box 1.1 summarizes the basic principles for providing such necessary psychosocial services in community-based primary care settings conveniently available to diverse population groups.

BOX 1.1 Principles for Providing Psychosocial Care in a Primary Care Setting

- Development of Therapeutic Relationship

- Active Listening

- Empathic Recognition of the Problem

- Assessment of Safety

- Assessment of Social Support System

- Attention to Diversity Issues

- Scheduling of Return Visit for Review of Medical Problems

- Referral for Mental Health Counseling when Appropriate

Public Health and Preventive Mental Healthcare

Among the essential elements of comprehensive mental health services, illustrated in Figure 1.1, the least costly in both human and financial terms are Consultation/Education, and 24/7 access to Crisis Care, while hospital or other institution-based care is the most expensive financially and in constraints on the basic human need of mastery, and control of one's own life. In Parson's (1951) classic work on the "sick role," it is clearly in a seriously ill patient's best interest to forfeit independence and decision-making to the knowledge and skill of one's health provider, but this does not preclude a healthy provider/patient collaboration for predicting most desirable treatment outcomes. The following overview of public health principles of primary, secondary, and tertiary prevention and attention to health promotion—with specific reference to mental health—lays the foundation for succeeding Chapters' illustration among specific population groups appearing in primary care settings.

Primary Prevention and Enhancement   Primary prevention includes education, consultation, and crisis intervention and is designed to reduce the occurrence of mental disability and promote growth, development, and resistance to emotional/mental health breakdown among community members. There are several means of doing this:

1. Eliminate or modify the hazardous situation: For example, eliminate substandard housing for vulnerable older people or those disadvantaged by poverty; sponsor school and public forums on the signs of suicidal or homicidal danger.
2. Reduce exposure to hazardous situations: For example, advise and screen young people entering the potentially stressful situation of college, or suggest healthy self-care in demanding jobs like policing, nursing, or fire fighting.
3. Reduce vulnerability by increasing coping ability: In the psychosocial sphere, older people, the poor, and refugees are most often exposed to the risk of urban or homeland dislocation. Connecting them to physical resources, social services, and community supports can counter the negative social and emotional effects of hazardous situations like ethnic conflict in a housing complex. New parents will feel less vulnerable and less prone to abuse or neglect of children if they are prepared for the special challenges of child-rearing.

The success of anticipatory preventive measures depends largely on a person's openness to learning, cultural values, previous problem-solving success, and the educational skills and enthusiasm of primary care providers convinced of the importance of prevention in avoiding later more serious problems.

Secondary Prevention   This term implies that some form of mental or emotional disability has already occurred—either because of the absence of primary prevention, or because a distressed person was unable to benefit from preventive activities. The aim of secondary prevention is to shorten the duration of disability through sustained support and easy access to crisis services. Psychiatric hospitalization and the potentially disabling effect of institutional treatment can often be avoided for emotionally and mentally disturbed people if readily accessible and comprehensive community-based care and treatment are available. Such service is also vital to avoid recidivism (repeated hospitalization) among the seriously mentally ill, especially in instances of premature discharge on financial grounds (i.e., disparity in insurance coverage) rather than on clinical readiness criteria.

Tertiary Prevention   This level of prevention assumes existence of a mental disorder with the aim of reducing its disabling long-term effects. Social and rehabilitation programs, often in concert with psychotropic drug treatment are central to helping people return whenever possible to social and occupational roles or learn new ones (Paykel, 1990). Or, if an irreversible brain disorder such as Alzheimer's disease or other dementia is already evident, mobilizing all available resources to reduce the negative effects for both patient and family is also important. Ready access to crisis care is also important for the same reasons noted in Secondary Prevention.

The Pivotal Role of Preventive Psychiatry

As illustrated in Figure 1.1, the cost of short-changing preventive mental health services is enormous in financial, social, and client independence terms. The work of several pioneers has been pivotal in demonstrating the role of preventive psychiatry and its intersection with primary healthcare. Eric Lindemann (1944) studied the survivors of the Cocoanut Grove Melody Lounge fire that killed 492 people. Findings of this classic study revealed the serious psychopathologies of survivors who lacked support in the normal grieving process following such a serious loss. Lindemann's work constitutes an important foundation of contemporary crisis theory and later work by psychiatrists Gerald Caplan (1964), Norris Hansell (1976), and Paul Polak (1971).

Most important in this discussion is the blending of social and preventive psychiatry principles with the judicious use of psychotropic drugs for the emotionally and mentally disturbed. It is unfortunate and very short-sighted that in too many instances psychotropic drug treatment is the *only* treatment received by some of these patients—this, despite 50-plus years of data documenting that the most effective outcomes of psychotropic drug treatment are when used in *combination* with counseling and/or social rehabilitation therapies. This topic is discussed further in Chapter 13, while the critical role of primary care providers in addressing the issue is illustrated throughout the book A preview on this topic follows in the next section, including the centrality of *listening* to patients—in this case, to complaints of very unpleasant side effects of some psychotropic drugs that are the primary reason some patients stop taking their medication, even in the face of relapse to psychotic symptoms, for example, the hallucinations that may accompany schizophrenia.

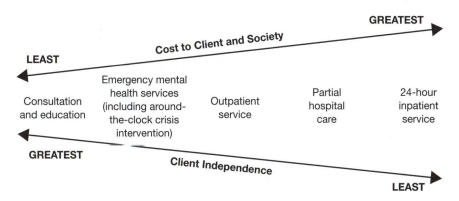

Figure 1.1 Continuum of Mental Health Services: Cost and Client Independence. Assisting distressed people in their natural social roles (homemaker, paid worker, student) through consultation, education, and crisis services is the *least* costly means of service and allows the *greatest* client independence; institution-based care is the *most* costly means and allows the *least* client independence.

Psychoanalytic and Personality Theories—Relevance to Primary Care Practice

Freud's pioneering work over a century ago emphasizes the role of early childhood conflicts in the development of neurotic symptoms in later life—an approach now widely criticized as "determinism." While not dismissing the importance of traumatic childhood experiences, the amazing *human capacity for resilience and growth in the face of great odds* should never be discounted—keeping in mind that social support is a key factor in any person's ability to heal from various injuries. Freud's psychoanalytic technique of listening is a mainstay of the contemporary therapeutic relationship.

In the primary care setting, distressed clients like Richard and Denise do not expect to consume the equivalent of the 50-minute therapeutic hour of time. But the provider's "listening attitude" and belief in people's ability to move beyond their immediate trauma and distress—even in a 15-minute appointment!—will readily be detected by clients. When the provider intuits from triage and assessment questions (illustrated in Chapter 2) that a client is burdened with tumultuous feelings but time does not permit exploration, a simple statement like this can make the difference between a client feeling listened to or dismissed: "Mr. Ebbers, I sense that you're feeling pretty down since your wife's death, but we've got only a short time today, so I'd like to set up another time to see you very soon . . . How does that sound?" In Denise's case, we can assume the NP's "listening attitude" from the client's revelation of abuse history. With this listening foundation, the nurse practitioner might say: "Denise, I'd like to see you again in the next week or so to follow up with your GE and sleeping problems. But meanwhile, besides what you're going through, would you be willing to see someone in our counseling department who specializes in family violence issues— including child witnesses?"

While attentive listening is basic to any health provider–client relationship, probing around unconscious conflicts a client may be burdened with is *not* appropriate in busy primary care settings, where 15 to 20 minute appointment times may be the norm. Even if a distressed client volunteers or hints at deep unresolved emotional conflicts, and it is apparent that deep-seated issues are affecting the client's overall health status, rather than probing for more detail, the most appropriate response from the PC provider is an empathic recognition of the issue, for example: "You seem very troubled by some painful experiences in your past. . ." and then, "You might find it helpful to see one of our counselors . . . We know that stress and unresolved problems from one's past have a subtle but definite way of eating away at a person's general health over time." Thus, Denise's irritable bowel problems may be exacerbated by the stress of a troubled marriage and fear for her own and her children's safety. The general principle, then, is to listen and acknowledge the realities of mind–body stress factors, but not probe into and open old wounds for which there is insufficient time or psychotherapeutic skill in responding to deep-seated emotional problems. The *next important principle* is offering a referral to specialty mental health services, and following up with the same during the next primary care visit.

Psychiatrist Harry Stack Sullivan (1892–1949) modified Freud's ideas and emphasized more developmental theories of human behavior. Sullivan was strongly influenced by sociology and focused on the importance of interpersonal relations, including the role of close friendships in maintaining mental health. He moved beyond Freud's biological determinism to emphasize social factors in personality development. His interpersonal theory of psychiatry is central to the inclusion of family and environmental issues in the diagnosis and treatment of distressed or mentally ill people. Ego psychologists Erich Fromm (1941), Erik Erikson (1963), and Abraham Maslow (1970) emphasized a key developmental concept—a person's ability to learn and grow throughout life. Thus, with social support—and in some cases, professional counseling—people like Richard Ebbers and Denise Evans can avoid the psychological hazards and potentially life-threatening dangers of the problems they currently face. Of particular relevance here is Maslow's five-leveled Hierarchy of Needs, a model widely used to explain human behavior. In this pyramid of basic needs, if *physical safety and shelter*, from the elements or dangerous people, are not met, people cannot attend to higher level needs such as for love and fulfillment of one's sense of life purpose. Applied to Denise, so long as she fears for her life and the safety of her children, she is not likely to focus on a long-term social need of life with a supportive, non-abusive partner.

Juxtaposed to this view is the concept of existential despair and danger of suicide. Thus, if someone like Richard Ebbers can see little purpose in life without his wife and his caretaker role, he may give up. For example, he may feel some relief after his wife's death, but also guilt for feeling that way. Dealing with such conflicted feelings requires empathy, timely support, and Mr. Ebbers' "sense of coherence" (Antonovsky, 1980, 1988) regarding his stressful situation. Put another way, the meaning one attaches to stressful life events is pivotal in the person's ability to find and accept available support and heal from various psychological wounds (discussed further in the section on diversity and resilience, and in the chapters on crisis, suicide, and violence).

Palliative Care Essentials and Mental Illness

Palliative care is "specialized, interdisciplinary care for patients with serious, life-limiting or chronic debilitating illnesses" (Doran & Geary, 2005). The hallmark of palliative care is management of the physical, psychosocial, and spiritual needs of patients, with a goal of symptom management to maximize quality of life. Palliative care can occur at any age or any point in the illness trajectory if the illness is life-limiting or chronically debilitating. This differs from hospice care, which may be a part of palliative care, but is focused on care of the dying patient and one's family.

Characteristics of Palliative Care

Psychologist Stephen Connor (2009) cites the essential components of palliative care programs that apply to a broad population of patients with life-limiting conditions and accompanying symptoms. He notes "humanism" as the philosophical underpinning of palliative care and its reverence for the universal human experience of search for life's meaning and preparing for death (Frankl, 1963). We briefly summarize palliative care principles here (Connor, 2009, pp. 7–9).

- The patient and family are the unit of care, and often the family's needs are equal to or greater than the dying person's.
- Care is provided in the home and/or in inpatient facilities, depending on the patient's wishes.
- Symptom management—not curing the disease—is the focus of treatment.
- Palliative care treats the whole person, addressing the patient's physical, social, psychological, spiritual, and practical needs.
- Services are available 24 hours a day, 7 days a week.
- Palliative care is interdisciplinary, with the team including physicians, nurses, social workers, chaplains, volunteers, and others.
- Palliative care is physician-directed, in that the attending physician determines an incurable condition and must order the palliative care to be delivered.
- Volunteers are an integral part of palliative and hospice care.

- Palliative care is community-based and provided without regard to ability to pay.
- Bereavement services are provided as needed by families.

Palliative Care Issues with Psychiatric Patients

Patients enter healthcare systems in great distress, and palliative care settings are no exception. For patients with mental illness and/or developmental disabilities, the distress may be even greater than in the general population, since they may have inadequate coping resources and are more prone to a crisis state when dealing with a life-threatening illness (see Chapter 3).

People with Serious Mental Illness (SMI) reportedly die 20–25 years earlier than the general population worldwide (Parks, Svendsen, Singer, & Foti, 2006). The increase in mortality has been associated with issues such as suicide, homicide, and accidental death as well as hypertension, cardiac disease, diabetes, and other metabolic conditions, respiratory illnesses, obesity, renal disease, cerebrovascular disease, cancer, and HIV/AIDS (Baker, 2005; Hiroeh, Appleby, Mortensen, & Dunn, 2001).

People with mental illness often seek care later in the course of the disease which can exacerbate their complex care needs. Typically, inadequate support systems may affect their ability to access medical care and navigate the complex health system. Difficulties with adherence, homelessness, and lack of transportation as well as inadequate finances may complicate a mentally ill person's ability to receive timely care or treatment. Stigma can affect communication about all aspects of care and can have an impact on assessment, diagnosis, and treatment of the person with mental illness (Morgan, 2010). (See Chapter 2 for assessment of mental competency for decisions regarding end of life care, and Chapter 12 on the necessity of primary care and neuropsychiatric specialist collaboration around treatment of cognitively impaired older persons.)

Diversity Perspectives in Primary Care

In its broadest sense, diversity includes much more than its frequent reference point to culture and ethnicity. It encompasses identity markers and our responses to them among people "different" from ourselves—gender, race, class, language, ethnicity, sexual identity, age, values, religion, citizenship status. Across cultures, these markers take on varied meanings for particular individuals, for the larger societies in which they dwell, and for health professionals providing service to a diverse clientele. For example, some Asian cultures do not have "language" for mental health issues, or respond differently to psychotropic medications.

Discourse in the field of applied anthropology includes questions about the concept of culture and its explanatory value regarding issues of human and ethnic diversity (Kuper, 1999; Chambers, 2009, p. 376). The following vignettes illustrate diversity issues—race, ethnicity, and class differences—and concepts not only in respect to patients, but also their relevance to inter-professional collaboration.

A psychiatric clinical nurse specialist is doing consultation in a primary care section of a healthcare facility on a U.S. Indian reservation—the facility under jurisdiction of the U.S. Public Health Service and Bureau of Indian Affairs. On one occasion a registered nurse (from a poor working class Caucasian background) expresses to the nurse consultant her "disgust" with some of her Indian patients with this remark: "If I could manage to get my R.N. diploma, what's wrong with some of these people living like they do and neglecting their health"—a reflection of the deeply embedded value of individualism in American culture that crosses class and ethnic boundaries: "I've pulled myself up by my bootstraps . . . Why can't they?"

An African-American psychiatrist devotes himself to ending "black-on-black" violence, putting his analysis and efforts into the historical context of slavery and economic, social, and cultural oppression. The American Medical Association has only in 2008 apologized to the African-American community for its systematic exclusion of black physicians from the AMA.

A Caucasian nurse practitioner says that both the "worst" and "best" of her professional experiences have been at the hands of her fellow nurses—as in worker-on-worker abuse and oppressed group behavior.

Key Concepts Regarding Diversity

Ethnicity is tied to the notion of shared origin and culture. In multicultural societies such as the United States, UK, and Canada, for example, ethnic identities can shift and change based on power distribution and factors like language, skin color, religion, or country of origin, while some groups may define themselves as *bicultural* within a dominant culture of a particular society (Loustaunau & Sobo, 1997). In a national public radio interview, an internationally renowned cellist, YoYoMa said in 2008 about his tri-cultural identity (French, Chinese, and American): "I explore what I don't understand." This point might serve as a mantra of sorts for a PCP who meets a client whose identity and beliefs about life and illness may diverge widely from one's own—a divergence that forms the *context* for health assessment and intervention. But despite such "diversity" between client and provider, PCPs can count on certain universals among their clientele, for example, a desire for pain relief, or grief over loss of a loved one.

Ethnocentrism is the emotional attitude that one's own ethnic group, nation, or culture is superior to that of others. Exaggerated ethnocentrism can lead to prejudice, bias, and discrimination toward others based on their ethnic identity, e.g., racial, ethnic, or homophobic slurs hurled at people different from oneself.

Stereotyping refers to an unvarying pattern of thinking and pigeonholing a person or group in a box that disallows for individuality, critical judgment, and basic respect for people different from ourselves. Together with ethnocentrism, stereotyping can have a powerful negative influence on communication, client empowerment, and positive healthcare outcomes.

Cultural relativism is a more complex concept. It requires that instead of pre-judging others, we consider various actions, beliefs or traits within their cultural *context* in order to better understand them. Cultural relativism presents difficulties, however, especially in healthcare practice, in that some cultural practices may be harmful to physical and emotional health and welfare. It allows outsiders to ignore, explain, or excuse certain human rights violations such as woman-battering as "that's just part of their culture." This fact underscores the importance of inquiring of patients how various symptoms are interpreted for their meaning in particular cultures.

"Cultural Competence": Re-assessment of its Meaning

While navigating the complex terrain of diversity issues in primary care, many employ the currently popular "cultural competence" required of healthcare providers working in multicultural societies like the UK, Canada, and the United States. Such recommended "competency" presents a daunting challenge for many providers who face a multitude of languages and belief systems among their clients. Even if we are well traveled globally, or are fluent in more than one's native language, most people will never completely understand or be comfortable except in their own ancestral culture with its values, beliefs, etc.

Instead of "cultural competence," we therefore suggest for health providers the phrase "cultural awareness and sensitivity" to diversity issues. But regardless of terminology, most important for providers is to recognize the wisdom and clinical relevance of this *key principle*: Whatever our ethnic or other identity, we should never assume that, even with extensive study and exposure, we can ever be fully knowledgeable about people whose culture and beliefs are different from our own. Such sensitivity might include, for example, providers learning basic courtesy phrases and translations of common medical terms in practice areas where clients include immigrants with a minimal grasp of the host country's dominant language.

Most major metropolitan cities where the majority of such refugees seek safety from abuse, sexual slavery, and financial exploitation have access to multi-language translators. PCPs must readily enlist such services to facilitate action on the basic principle of healthcare as a basic human right within cultural meaning systems, while allowing time for refugees to learn the host country's language.

Commonalities and Cross-cultural Differences in Primary Care

Despite ethnocentrism and one's natural tendency to accept and adhere to one's own cultural heritage (good and not so good), alongside the *distinctions* among different groups, PCPs must sensitively balance cultural *differences* with what is *common* among people experiencing physical pain and/or psychological distress, and the real or perceived origins of their suffering.

In doing so, careful attention must be paid to varying *meanings* attached to pain (e.g., fate, as in, "It just happened . . . that's life . . .", a message from God, deserved punishment, another person's evil behavior), and the socio-cultural norms that guide both the client's and provider's response to the pain or psychological upheaval. In short, this involves a twofold task: (1) Uncovering what is *unique* about each person's explanation of the presenting problem*;* and (2) without over-generalizing, ascertaining what the client has *in common* with others worldwide who have suffered a serious life-threatening illness, and/or a catastrophic event such as torture or disaster. It also involves clarity about a "disease" that is verifiable from *objective* laboratory and other data, and "illness" which includes the person's *subjective* response to observable injury and the disease process, e.g. advanced cancer or HIV/AIDS.

CASE EXAMPLE: TRADITIONAL PERCEPTION OF MENTAL ILLNESS

Within traditional Chinese culture, mental illness is perceived as something mythical like possession by some evil spirit. In Buddhist thinking, one's suffering is the consequence of previous misdeeds. Thus, mental illness may be perceived as punishment of misdeeds done by clients themselves or their family members. Within this orientation, mental illness is a shameful label for mentally afflicted persons and their family members. It implies that a related family member may have done something immoral or mischievous in this life or the previous life. In Buddhism, one has three lives, the previous, the present and future. One is a man in this life but may become an animal in the next life because of his misdeeds. Accordingly, family members of clients with mental illness, especially those in traditional rural areas, may feel reluctant to disclose or even admit their relatives' mental illness. The following self-narration told by a Chinese farmer illustrates the influence of traditional superstition on family members of clients with mental illness:

> Oh heaven, what misdeeds I have done in my previous life that deserve that kind of punishment. I cast all my hope on my son. I spent all my money for his schooling but he was crazy just because the leaving of girlfriend. He talked to himself frequently saying that he was the God of heaven that attracted beautiful girls. Everybody in the village knew that he was crazy. It was a terrible shame to our whole family. My neighbors gossiped around me thinking that my son's madness was a consequence of my misdeeds done in my present and previous life. In fact, I have done nothing immoral in my life. I tried to be kind hearted to everybody. The only misdeed I had done so far was killing of my cow that had worked for me for fifteen years, but it was so sick and painful. My wife blamed me that my son's craziness was due to my misbehaviors toward our god in our village temple. Last year I refused to go the temple and attended the annual ceremony for our god's birthday.
>
> http://www.psychosocial.com/IJPR_10/Family_Caregiving_in_China2_Yip.html

Resilience, its Variability, and Diverse Perceptions of Healers

History is replete with heroic life stories of people who faced torture, war, human trafficking, but who effectively rebounded from psychological terror, physical injury and illness, and massive losses, but went on to productive, even celebrated lives. Resilience refers to one's ability to recover quickly following setbacks or a serious upset; it is a dynamic process of "bouncing back" in the context of significant adversity. Resilience research builds on the pioneering work of giants in social psychology, philosophy, holocaust and disaster studies (Hoff, Hallisey, & Hoff , 2009; Sanders, 2008). Such resiliency is facilitated by personal, family, community, and political advocacy (Collishawa, *et al.*, 2005).

From his cross-cultural research on concentration camp survivors and women in menopause, sociologist Antonovsky (1980) proposes the concept of "resistance resources" (pp. 99–100), including social network support and a "sense of coherence" (SOC), as intervening variables in stressful situations. SOC includes the person's perception of events as *comprehensible, manageable*, and *meaningful* in socio-cultural context. It is highly compatible with resilience and protective factors that aid suffering people in their response to disease, traumatic events, and their consequences. Accordingly, a person with a strong SOC will define social stressors as *social* rather than assuming blame for trouble that did not originate from oneself, and can make the difference between one's positive or negative responses to stressful events or life-threatening experiences. Individual responses to pain and suffering are influenced by socio-cultural norms; for example, expected stoicism or open emotional expression, seeking help from a traditional healer or clerical authority, or requesting medication from primary care providers trained in contemporary medical practice (Dobkin de Rios, 2002; Fadiman, 1997; Freire, 1989; Loustanunau & Sobo, 1997; Kleinman, 1988.) Overall, variable resilience bolsters the importance of focusing on prevention rather than on "fixing" people after the damage is done.

CASE EXAMPLE: DIVERSITY AND GENDER ROLES

Mr. Mahadi is a 45-year-old married man from Pakistan who was admitted to the hospital section of a comprehensive health agency with pneumonia related to his HIV disease. On admission he was withdrawn, spoke English fluently, but was minimally responsive to questions, and appeared depressed. Following a workup for depression that included ruling out underlying medical problems as well as HIV dementia, and treatment for pneumonia, a psychiatric consultation was arranged, which included Mr. Mahadi's wife who visited daily and was able to provide a description of increased agitation and despondency at home, as well as increased difficulties in their relationship. On intake assessment, the cause or precipitant to these feelings was unclear. The initial treatment plan included use of antidepressant medication as well as brief counseling with the psychiatric clinical nurse specialist (CNS).

Mr. Mahadi was reluctant to take the antidepressant medication and would not give a clear explanation about his concerns. In his meetings with the CNS, Mr. Mahadi talked freely of his past history in Pakistan, love for his family and country of origin, and acknowledged no previous difficulties with mental health issues. He did acknowledge past drug use, but was reluctant to share details about his drug use. Although he was very respectful and graciously thanked all his providers, he was quite guarded in offering health-related information and often did not follow through on treatment recommendations.

His care team consisted of all female providers (physician, nurse practitioner, social worker, and psychiatric clinical nurse specialist—CNS) with the exception of the male psychiatrist. After three unsuccessful attempts to meet with Mr. Mahadi for further assessment, the CNS arranged for a joint meeting with the psychiatrist. There was an immediate dramatic difference in the interaction and Mr. Mahadi offered information freely to the psychiatrist that he had previously not divulged to any other providers. He acknowledged symptoms of severe depression, sadness, and guilt over past behavior (including infecting his wife with HIV) and acknowledged the extreme difficulties that had surfaced in his marriage over the prior month. He agreed to take the antidepressants and was eager to meet with the psychiatrist again.

The example of Mr. Mahadi dramatically illustrates clients' diversity in gender role expectations among male and female health providers. In Western cultures, despite growing parity between male and female health providers generally, in medicine the majority of surgeons are male and the majority of pediatricians are female, while in nursing the very lopsided majority are female—mirroring traditional gender roles vis-à-vis caretaking and perceived male authority in male-dominated specialties, such as orthopedic surgery for treating sports injuries. Parallel gender role issues are evident in attendance at childbirth where, in traditional cultures virtually untouched by Western medical practice, midwives and female relatives were and still are the cultural norm for assisting mothers in the delivery of children. The case also calls attention to providers' willingness to *openly discuss* such issues in team collaboration sessions to avoid power struggles and their potential negative impact on patient care and treatment outcomes. Failure to do so has particular implications in treating victims/survivors of abuse which, at its most basic, represents the *abuse of power and control* across cultures and wide swaths of interpersonal behavior. In these instances, health providers should *model* collaboration and teamwork which can serve as an antidote to violence as a conflict resolution tactic. (See Chapters 7 and 10 on depression, and chronic pain.)

Comprehensive Treatment and Inter-professional Collaboration

The previous example of successful referral to a counselor or mental health specialist assumes a carefully planned and operational network of players in a comprehensive healthcare institution. Stories from both clients and healthcare providers document that being caught in a "systems problem" can be more frustrating and exhausting than the original health issue for which one sought help. It is commonly understood and expected in complex health service agencies that no one provider or specialist can meet the varied and inter-related problems presented by a single client and his or her family. But as complex as some systems can be, mechanisms should be in place to assure that no individual client feels lost or "caught" in the system.

CASE EXAMPLE: PRIMARY CARE IN A COMPLEX SYSTEM

Robert, an 80-year-old man with orthopedic and heart problems cited his anxiety and exasperation trying to find someone who would interpret the results of an MRI he had done on his spine. His primary care provider seemed "too busy" to talk to him about it. He also didn't particularly like this provider, and was trying—unsuccessfully thus far—to find someone else who would be more interested. He said: "Maybe I should talk to the cardiologist; he's easy to talk to and seems to have time for me." His daughter, a nurse, advised that this was not the role of a cardiologist, but rather, the PCP who ordered the MRI. She promised to help him find a new PC provider.

The Challenges and Rewards of Primary Care

This example brings into stark relief the principles discussed above, and the pivotal role of the PCP to coordinate the results of various specialty consults, and communicate the outcomes and next steps in a language the client understands. Unfortunately, there is a shortage of primary care providers. Nevertheless, PCPs are pivotal in delivering holistic care crossing physical, emotional, and mental health domains.

In contrast to medical specialists, primary care providers must know the essentials across the wide range of physical and mental health disorders. It is also useful to remember that the *vast majority of health problems do not require the services of a specialist.* But a well-prepared primary care provider also recognizes when referrals to medical, surgical, or other specialists are indicated. And of course this includes knowledge of mental health "basics" to be delivered by PCPs, and when to refer to mental health specialists. Thus, while the primary care role is very demanding, its rewards outweigh the demands—especially that of getting to know the whole person and keeping the pivotal aspects of treatment running smoothly in a sometimes chaotic and understaffed situation. From the perspective of many patients, the rewards are even greater, as in "Someone really understands me . . . who I am, not just my heart or knee problem [or other ailment]."

The importance of the primary care provider's coordinating function cannot be overstated, especially in an era of increased specialization that can compromise the end results of treatment. It also highlights the ideals of community-based mental health services that should be smoothly and efficiently linked in geographic proximity to general medical services. In the U.S., the community health center model, begun some decades ago to address access to services by inner-city and often poor residents, typically includes basic counseling services on the same premises.

Principles and Healthcare Goals in Inter-professional Collaboration

Inter-professional collaboration is rooted in the basic principles of community-based health services. In this book, it also assumes a perspective of healthcare as one of the *major domains* of all societies worldwide: Family organization; an economic system; political structure;

value and belief systems (religion); the arts; and health—treatment and care of the sick and needy. These domains vary across cultures, but overall, they intersect in pivotal ways with a nation's health. Thus, even in the event of a nuclear holocaust including destruction of medical systems, by human nature, survivors would care for the sick and dying.

While the term "health" should denote the whole person—body, mind, and spirit— unfortunately we must still specify "mental health" as an integral facet of health, most vividly revealed in the United States in the existing disparities between general medical and mental health insurance coverage. Yet, preventive care such as 24/7 crisis intervention comparable to emergency "medical" treatment is still a more distant prospect for many. A further ideal in the 1960s and 1970s was to organize delivery of mental health treatment in *close synchrony and proximity with general medical services*, preferably in interdisciplinary and inter-departmental services organized under a single administrative umbrella. Such a model would not only better serve clients but also curtail costs through elimination of duplicative administrative structures.

Today in the United States, such integrated models exist—not because of a national comprehensive model designed and financially supported for all (as we have, for instance, in fire and clean water protection)—but primarily because of the vision and concerted efforts of many providers and consumer advocates. These advocates know that segmented services are a disservice to needy clients. And they have also observed that uncoordinated care consumes an inordinate amount of public monies that could be better spent in actual delivery of services—this instead of spending valuable professional time trying to navigate the byzantine network of private insurance companies and government programs to find appropriate service for their clients.

A current illustration of this visionary effort is called the "Medical Home" approach launched by the Tufts Medical Center in Boston and the New England Quality Alliance, one of a number of approaches nationwide initiated as a response to the current segmented system, and involving thousands of primary care physicians. This model moves beyond the typical 15-minute session treating a single "episode" or disease to caring for the *whole* person in a long-term relationship with the primary care provider. It might include time to discuss, for example, why a diabetic patient might be misusing insulin as a slow form of self-destruction from burnout after years of caring for a spouse with Alzheimer's and limited social supports in a small community, and how the PCP could use widely recognized medical power to address such a situation.

CASE EXAMPLE: ASIAN HUMAN SERVICES—CHICAGO, ILLINOIS

Asian Human Services (AHS) began three decades ago primarily to address the social/mental health needs of Asian immigrants and their families. We present here its evolution toward integration with a family health clinic that encompasses general health services for individuals and entire families. As an ideal rooted in the principles of comprehensive community health, this example underscores the best of an integrated approach to healthcare. That is, general medical, and related emotional, social, and psychiatric facets of healthy functioning as whole individuals and families, should be readily available to all as a basic human right, regardless of ability to pay or other disadvantages.

Asian Human Services was established by leaders from the Japanese, Chinese, Filipino, Korean, Asian Indian, and Vietnamese communities to meet the critical human service and healthcare needs of the growing ethnic Asian immigrant and refugee population and other minorities in the Chicago metropolitan area. Programming is directed at every age group from children and adolescents to seniors. Its goal is to increase integration across all programs providing a broad selection of services for underserved or underprivileged clients speaking English, Spanish, and 10 different Asian languages.

For example, a client met with a primary care physician, and reported that he was experiencing marital stress, financial difficulties, and immigration issues which were causing him to feel depressed and hopeless. Consultation with a behavioral health counselor resulted in a referral for counseling. Also provided was education about his immigration status, links to financial support that he did not know he was entitled to, and medication for depression. Currently the client is living independently, has an active social life, and is currently free from depressive symptoms. He continues to come to Asian Human Services Family Health Center for both his physical and mental health needs.

Providers' Response to an Integrated Practice Model

Most certainly, other idealistic models such as Asian Human Services exist throughout the United States, Canada, and elsewhere. Here are some of the responses of AHS staff interviewed about their work. Praise of the agency dominated discussion, and staff enthusiasm was almost palpable among interviewees.

Most Satisfying Aspect of Work:

I can spend more time with patients [vs. administration] and have easy access to multilingual mental health professionals on the premises . . . Treatment is holistic, not piecemeal . . . There are a lot more easily accessible resources for consultation and referral, so when new problems surface during intake, it's convenient and saves time [in obtaining needed services].

We're like a mini-UN, very diverse. A formal survey revealed our satisfied clients from 100 zip codes (clinic director). Our staff turnover rate is just 8%. We're all behind the goal of best client outcomes . . . This is the richest experience of my entire career.

(Administrators)

Most Challenging or Difficult Aspect of Work:

Although we're generally on the same page, occasionally there's a breakdown in communicating.

We're very big on client needs assessment, for example, medical care, job, school, and ESL (English as Second Language), and on follow-up to prevent "the revolving door" of readmission. As in any agency, there's politics and some divisive challenges at times, but not frequently. Some new people just move on, but most staff are very passionate about their work here.

Suggestions for Improvement/Additional Comments:

Developing new collaborations and connections with the community is challenging . . . Our CEO is a good role model on social change and advocacy. As a supervisor, it's a pleasure to support the learning and growing of staff.

In conclusion, we hope that PCPs and others with a vision about collaboration between primary care and mental health service providers will be inspired to reserve a fraction of their time in efforts to bring integrated practice models to the forefront as a central issue in comprehensive healthcare for all. With the professional and personal rewards of primary care practice in the examples discussed here, the U.S. shortage of primary care providers may even be alleviated.

References

Antonovsky, A. (1980). *Health, stress, and coping*. San Francisco, CA: Jossey-Bass.

Antonovsky, A. (1988). Unraveling the mystery of health: How people manage stress and stay well. San Francisco, CA: Jossey-Bass.

Baker, A. (2005). Palliative and end-of-life care in the serious and persistently mentally ill population. *Journal of the American Psychiatric Nurses Association*, 11(5), 298–303.

Bellah, R.N., Madsen, R., Sullivan, W.M., Swidler, A., & Tipton, S.M. (1985). *Habits of the heart: Individualism and commitment in American life*. Berkeley, CA: University of California Press.

Caplan, G. (1964). *Principles of preventive psychiatry*. New York: Basic Books.

Chambers, E. (2009). In both our possibilities: Anthropology on the margins. *Human Organization*, 68(4), 374–379.

Collishawa, S., Pickles, A., Messer, J., Rutter, M., Shearer, C., & Maughana, B. (2005). Resilience to adult psychopathology following childhood maltreatment: Evidence from a community sample. *Child Abuse & Neglect*, 31, 211–229.

Congressional Commission on Mental Illness and Health. (1961). *Action for mental health*. New York: Basic Books.

Connor, S.R. (2009). *Hospice and palliative care: The essential guide*. (2nd ed.) London & New York: Routledge.

Dobkin de Rios, M. (2002). What we can learn from shamanic healing: Brief psychotherapy with Latino immigrants. *American Journal of Public Health*, 92(10), 1576–1578.

Doran, M. & Geary, K. (2005). End of life. In K.D. Melillo & S.C. Houde, *Geropsychiatric and mental health nursing* (pp. 347–362*)*. Boston: Jones and Bartlett Publishers.

Dossey, B.M., & Guzzetta, C.E. (1994). Implications for vio-psycho-social-spiritual concerns in cardiovascular nursing. *Journal of Cardiovascular Nursing*, 8, 72–88.

Earley, P. (2006). *Crazy: A father's search through America's mental health madness*. New York: G.P. Putnam's Sons.

Edmands, M.S., Hoff, L.A., Kaylor, L., Mower, L., & Sorrell, S. (1999). Bridging gaps between mind, body and spirit: Healing the whole person. *Journal of Psychosocial Nursing*, 37(10), 1–7.

Erikson, E. (1963). *Childhood and society* (2nd ed.). New York: Norton.

Fadiman, A. (1997). *The spirit catches you and you fall down*. New York: The Noonday Press, Farrar, Straus and Giroux.

Fee, E., & Brown, T.M. (2000). The past and future of public health practice. *American Journal of Public Health*, 90(5), 690–691.

Frankl, V. (1963). *Man's search for meaning*. New York: Washington Square Press: Simon & Shuster.

Freire, P. (1989). *Pedagogy of the oppressed*. New York: Continuum.

Fromm, E. (1941). *Escape from freedom*. Austin, TX: Holt, Rinehart and Winston.

Hansell, N. (1976). *The person in distress*. New York: Human Sciences Press.

Hiroeh, U., Appleby, L., Mortensen, P.B. & Dunn, G. (2001). Death by homicide, suicide and other unnatural causes in people with mental illness: A population-based study. *Lancet*, 358(9299), 2110–2112.

Hoff, L.A. (1993). Review essay: Health policy and the plight of the mentally ill. *Psychiatry*, 56(4), 400–419.

Hoff, L.A., Hallisey, B.J., & Hoff, M. (2009). *People in crisis: Clinical and diversity perspectives* (6th ed.). New York: Routledge.

Johnson, A.B. (1990). *Out of bedlam: The truth about deinstitutionalization*. New York: Basic Books.

Kleinman, A. (1988). *The illness narratives: Suffering, healing, and the human condition*. New York: Basic Books.

Kuper, A. (1999). *Culture: The anthropologists' account*. Cambridge, MA: Harvard University Press.

Levine, M. (1981). *The history and politics of community mental health*. New York: Oxford University Press.

Lindemann, E. (1944). Symptomatology and management of acute grief. *American Journal of Psychiatry*, 101–148.

Loustaunau, M.O., & Sobo, E.J. (1997). *The cultural context of health, illness, and healing*. Westport, CT: Bergin & Garvey.

Maslow, A. (1970). *Motivation and personality* (2nd ed.). New York: HarperCollins.

Morgan, B. (2010). End of life care for patients with mental illness and personality disorders. In Ferrell, B. & Coyle, N. (Eds.) *Textbook of palliative care nursing (3rd Ed.)* New York: Oxford University Press.

Parks, J., Svendsen, D., Singer, P., & Foti, M. (2006). Morbidity and mortality in people with serious mental illness. National Association of State Mental Health Program Directors. Alexandria, VA: (NASMHPD) Medical Directors Council. http://www.nasmphd.org (accessed on 14 July 2010).

Parsons, T. (1951). Social structure and the dynamic process: case of modern medical practice. In T. Parsons (ed.) *The social system* (pp. 428–479). New York: Free Press.

Paykel, E. (1990). Innovations in mental health care in the primary care system. In I.M. Marks & R. Scott (Eds.), *Mental health care delivery: Innovations, impediments and implementation* (pp. 69–83). Cambridge: Cambridge University Press.

Polak, P. (1971). Social systems intervention. *Archives of General Psychiatry*, 25, 110–117.

Sanders,S. (2008). *Understanding resilience*. New York: Routledge.

U.S. Department of Health and Human Services. (2010). *Healthy people 2010: Understanding and improving health*. Washington, DC: Author.

Ustan, T.B. (1999). The global burden of mental disorders. *American Journal of Public Health*, 89(9), 1315–1321.

2 Mental Health Assessment and Service Planning

With Lisa Brown

- Overview of Assessment Methods
- *Diagnostic and statistical manual of mental disorders* (DSM-IV TR)
- The Global Mental Health Assessment Tool—Primary Care Version (GMHAT/PC)
- Triage Tool: Assessing for Immediate Risk of Harm to Self and/or Others
- A Comprehensive Mental Health Assessment Tool (CMHA)
- CMHA and McHugh's "Essentials": Description and Commonalities
- Appendix
- References

The first chapter in this book addressed the essential issue of the mind–body connection. Primary care providers (PCPs) face the challenge of providing holistic care for their patients and acknowledge that separating the body and mind is contrary to their practice. They are not afforded the opportunity to say "that's not my area"—everything is their "area." Chapter 2 addresses key facets of mental health assessment and collaborative practice among PCPs and psychiatric professionals. In theory, it would be ideal to have mental health specialists readily available and even more wonderful if all patients with emotional needs were willing to seek specialized mental health services. Primary care providers know it is not that simple. This chapter offers a conceptual framework and tools to aid the PCP in assessing the urgency of mental health concerns, and provides language to help ease the transition of mental health services to a specialist when necessary.

In the physical realm, providers can rely on a variety of technological and other objective assessment and diagnostic tools. Although mental health assessment tools exist, they will never be as accurate as those utilized in diagnosing physical phenomena. The difference lies in the *subjectivity* of people's emotional, cognitive, and spiritual response(s) to life events. To illustrate: The indifferent attitude of a provider ordering laboratory tests for diagnosing a physical problem will not affect the *objective* laboratory results, although it may exacerbate a patient's distress, whereas an indifferent attitude of a provider aiming to ascertain a depressed person's risk for suicide may result in denial of suicidal plans and failure to obtain other data for assessing suicide risk. This means that in addition to structured assessment guides, the *provider–patient relationship* and the provider's *communication skills* constitute the most essential "tools" in the psychiatric/mental health assessment process (Peplau, 1993).

Overview of Assessment Methods

Varied assessment tools are available to health and mental health providers. Most are specific to symptoms, such as mania scales, depression scales, etc. Many of these were designed as research tools and therefore are not always suitable for clinical practice. This is especially true in primary care settings or in high-risk situations where time is of the essence. The universal goal of thorough assessment is further challenged by the significant amount of work to be done in primary care—usually in a very limited time period.

In our overview and critique of assessment methods, we present six sources relevant to primary care practice: the *Diagnostic and Statistical Manual of Mental Health Disorders* (DSM); the International Classification of Diseases (ICD); the Global Mental Health Assessment Tool—Primary Care version (GMHAT-PC); a 5-question Triage/Risk assessment tool; the Comprehensive Mental Health Assessment (CMHA) tool; and psychiatrist Dr. Paul McHugh's "essentials" approach to psychiatric diagnosis (at Johns Hopkins Medical School, an alternative to the DSM). The "essentials" framework is highly complementary to the CMHA and its emphasis on holism and basic life functions, and their disruptions by physical illness and/or psychiatric disorders. We illustrate use of the CMHA and service planning with a case example in primary care, thus laying the foundation for its use in subsequent chapter topics.

Diagnostic and statistical manual of mental disorders (DSM-IV TR)

The *Diagnostic and statistical manual of mental disorders* (DSM) is currently published in its fourth edition with revisions (DSM-IV TR). *Diagnostic and statistical manual*, 5th Edition (DSM-V) is expected to be released in the year 2012. The DSM was originally intended for psychiatrists, and later, for advanced practice psychiatric nurses, social workers, and psychologists as a guide for diagnosing mental disorders. But (as noted in Chapter 1), today in the U.S. and other countries the bulk of treatment (including psychotropic drug monitoring) of patients discharged from in-patient psychiatric care is done by primary care providers in general medical settings. Further, in the U.S., a DSM diagnosis is required as a basis for insurance reimbursement for mental health services. It is therefore important for primary care providers to be familiar with the DSM, including its benefits and limitations in practice.

The DSM was first published in 1952 and was a compilation of diagnostic categories with a description of each. The word *reaction* was utilized with each description, reflecting the influence of Adolf Meyer's psychobiologic approach and his belief that each disorder was a *reaction* to psychological, social, or biological factors, or a combination thereof. The DSM-II eliminated the word *reaction*, thereby removing discussion of "cause" and ultimately the mind–body connection.

In 1980, the DSM-III was published. This edition included explicit diagnostic criteria, a multiaxial system and a "descriptive approach that attempted to be neutral with respect to theories of etiology" (American Psychiatric Association, 2000, p. 26). One of the primary goals in creating this edition was to provide a medical nomenclature for researchers and clinical providers in psychiatry. The DSM-IV was published in 1994, the fourth edition with text revisions in 2000.

Healthcare analysts and social scientists have noted that each edition of the DSM contains new psychiatric "disorders," while also dropping, for example, the diagnosis of "homosexuality" from its nomenclature in response to growing concern about attaching a psychiatric label to a phenomenon—in this case, sexual identity—that is *not* mental illness (see Caplan, 1995; Cooksey & Brown, 1998 regarding the social construction of mental illness). The DSM –IV-TR contains 943 pages (hundreds more since its first edition), with 10.5 pages of codes.

We might well ask: Does this represent an evidence-based increase in mental illness, or perhaps the "social construction" of mental illness (Hoff, Hallisey, & Hoff, 2009, pp. 71–77) —overall, a lot to master, especially for PCPs without specialty psychiatric training.

The DSM-IV has been widely accepted in clinical and research settings. Significant controversy surrounded the development of the DSM-III and the revised text (Caplan, 1995; Cooksey & Brown, 1998; Luhrmann, 2000). The controversy appears to have abated with the fourth edition with text revision (APA, DSM-IV-TR, 2000) and although there is dialogue in the medical literature regarding the upcoming DSM-V, there is very little thought provoking discourse.

In a 2007 article, Regier, vice-chair of the task force to develop DSM-V describes the DSM as "a dictionary of mental disorder diagnoses that describes the characteristics of each mental disorder diagnosis" (p.1). He states the DSM-V will pay greater attention to "measurement based care" (p. 2). Regier emphasizes the need for this tool in research, reminding us that although the DSM is used in clinical practice, the DSM-III, IV and IV-TR were all primarily designed with research in mind. Another important goal of the DSM-V is to attempt to be more congruent with the International Classification of Diseases (ICD).

The International Classification of Diseases is currently published in its 9th edition with the 10th edition due for publication in 2014. The ICD is published by the World Health Organization and used worldwide for morbidity and mortality statistics, as well as in reimbursement systems. This system is designed to promote international comparability in the collection, classification, and presentation of disorder.

The ICD includes a section classifying mental and behavioral disorders. This has been developed alongside the *Diagnostic and statistical manual of mental disorders* and the two manuals seek to use the same codes. According to Regier (2007), the goal is to achieve close to 90% congruence between the DSM-V and the ICD 10th edition. Currently there are significant differences; for example, the ICD includes personality disorders on the same axis as other mental disorders whereas the DSM lists personality disorders on a separate axis/category. According to Mezzich (2002, p. 75) "A recent international survey across 66 countries has found ICD-10 more frequently used for clinical diagnosis and training, and DSM-IV more used for research."

The five axes of the multiaxis systems of the DSM-IV-TR are as follows:

- Axis I: Clinical disorders, such as major depression and schizophrenia. Other conditions, such as alcohol dependence, that may be a focus of clinical attention.
- Axis II: Personality disorders and mental retardation.
- Axis III: General medical conditions, for example: HIV infection may cause dementia (Axis I), or alcohol dependence (Axis I) may cause cirrhosis (Axis III).
- Axis IV: Psychosocial and environmental problems—includes events and stressors that may precipitate, result from, and/or affect mental status and treatment outcomes.
- Axis V: Global assessment of functioning scale. This axis indicates the patient's overall level of function, including psychologic, social, and occupational well-being. The scale ranges from 0–100 with the higher number correlating with higher functioning (APA, 2000, p. 27; O'Brien, Kennedy, & Ballard, 1999, pp. 64–65).

The Comprehensive Mental Health Assessment tool (CMHA) also assesses for all the above with a more extensive focus on overall functionality and its effect on activities of daily living. Axis V correlates most closely with the CMHA, but its "global" score does not discriminate between low, moderate, and high functioning levels in particular life areas such as family relations, financial stability, problem solving ability, etc.—significant factors affecting mental and emotional health. Another advantage of the CMHA rating scale (in contrast to

Axis V global score) is its use for charting a client's progress from admission to discharge in assessed areas of concern (see Appendix in this chapter).

The broad acceptance of the DSM-IV, often referred to as the "bible" of psychiatry, is evident in the paucity of literature discussing its use, benefits and limitations (Cooksey & Brown, 1998, p. 526). Despite its questionable value based on scientific evidence, it is widely used worldwide. Ethan Watters (2010) cites its role in marketing diseases as well as pharmaceutical profit in Hong Kong, the island of Zanzibar, Sri Lanka, and Japan and in "homogenizing" the diversity of "madness" as defined across cultures.

Its controversial status is most obvious in the areas of nursing and the social sciences. A limited amount of discussion and objective evaluation can be found in the medical literature and among psychiatric practitioners. Many clinicians simply accept the DSM at face value without critique, or with resignation: "That's all there is."

This stance signifies a growing acceptance of "pathologizing" (i.e., diagnosing and therefore "treating") more and more aspects of everyday life, its *normal* challenges, and problems (see Brownlee, 2007). To paraphrase social psychologist Anton Antonovsky (1988) vis-à-vis preventive care: Our assessments should include more often the question "What keeps people healthy?" rather than focusing excessively on what makes them sick. Or, as a medical gerontologist noted to PCPs in a workshop on mental health: Would you please do a *functional* assessment, and not send an 80-year-old to his/her grave with a psychiatric diagnosis? That is, what supports (and perhaps which sleep aid) does such a patient need while mourning the loss of a spouse and facing alone the twilight of life?

This is not meant to minimize the fact of the real, deep, and long-lasting psychic pain of depression and/or a brain disease like schizophrenia (formerly attributed to dysfunctional mothering) that require specialized psychiatric treatment. But not every psychosocial problem merits a DSM diagnosis. For example: But for the activism of women psychiatrists and psychologists at the DSM revision proceedings, the criminal act of rape would have been added to the DSM with the diagnosis, "rapism." In short, designating a DSM diagnosis is a reality in primary care practice today in the U.S., but caution should be used in the context of the age-old legacy of social bias against those carrying the label of a psychiatric diagnosis, when support and counseling for psychosocial problems may suffice.

Cooksey and Brown (1998) note nurses' criticism of the DSM in its inadequacy in providing information regarding the patient's individual experience. This is an important concept for a PCP to ponder: in contrast to having a standard of care for a patient with a diagnosis of diabetes, there is no "standard of care" for the patient with both diabetes and bipolar I disorder, for example. The diagnosis of bipolar I may or may not have a significant impact on the same patient's diabetes, but conversely, the question remains: "What impact does a diagnosis of bipolar I disorder have on your ability to manage your diabetes?" It can be assumed that laboratory work for diabetes will be required. What cannot be assumed is the impact of the mental health diagnosis on the overall health of the individual patient. As a group, however, it is clear that persons with severe mental illness endure more physical health hazards as a result of their cognitive and emotional impairment and related sequelae such as poverty and self-care deficits (Ustan, 1999).

The Global Mental Health Assessment Tool: Primary Care Version (GMHAT/PC)

This computerized assessment tool was developed to detect psychiatric disorders in patients served by general practitioners in the UK who—as in the U.S., Canada, and other countries—increasingly are seen in primary care settings (Sharma, *et al.*, 2004). It focuses on identifying the most common as well as more serious psychiatric conditions. Several computer screens offer a series of questions appearing in a tree-branch structure with one or two questions for each disorder.

This tool also allows for rating the severity of symptoms—a clear advantage over the DSM that has no rating scales. It includes risk of self-harm assessment and drug misuse, and automatically produces a referral letter to psychiatric services. Its design draws on the ICD-10 (2004), the international classification system in general medicine that reveals interrelated clinical disorders that affect fundamental body functions as in the vascular, gastrointestinal, and musculoskeletal systems. It thus complements the "essentials perspective" vs. an "appearance-driven" (i.e., symptoms) approach to diagnosis that McHugh and Clark (2006) propose as an alternative to the DSM. This tool is also complementary to the CMHA tool's focus on assessing and rating basic life functions such as family and occupational stability which typically are interrelated to mental illness and histories of violence and/or sexual abuse.

At this point, we expect the reader may be thinking "Yes! But how can I now be expected to do a mental health assessment too?" In reality you are always doing a mental health assessment whether it is acknowledged or not. As you interview and examine your patient, you unknowingly are establishing the person's level of orientation, mood, affect, and ability to comprehend. It is also well known that most patients come to their PCP *first* with their mental health concerns—whether directly with complaints of change in mood or indirectly with somatic complaints.

Triage Tool: Assessing for Immediate Risk of Harm to Self and/or Others

This area of questioning may or may not be comfortable for you. Often providers are reluctant to ask these questions out of the misguided fear that inquiring about risk of suicide or violence will "put the idea into their head." Or you may be concerned about "opening up a can of worms that I don't have time or expertise to deal with" (see Sugg & Inui, 1992; and Chapters 3, 4, and 5 of this book).

Discussing thoughts of suicide, risk of harm by a partner, or fantasies of harming someone else do not influence the person to commit the act. Conversely, it opens up dialogue that more likely will prevent an act of harm toward self or others. PCPs are generally given "carte blanche" by patients to ask about their most intimate experiences including sexual practices and bodily functioning; assessing for one's safety is not any more intrusive or less important to holistic care.

Safety assessment, if not part of a routine visit or complete physical examination, should be incorporated into basic intake protocols in order to address any serious concerns immediately. The question can simply be framed from observation, e.g. "Ms. Green, I'm concerned about the bruises on your upper arms, how did they occur?" or, to Mr. Brady, "I sense from your symptoms and what you said on the admission form, that you may be depressed. I want to talk more about that, but first I want to talk about your safety."

This risk assessment presumes an initial contact information form, administered either by telephone, or on arrival at the primary care setting.

Initial Contact Form

Today's Date: _____2/5/2008_____   ID#: _____

Name: ___Bob Brady___

Age: 47 Relationship Status: Married __X__   __Single__

Other

Address: 23 Any Street, Anytown, USA

Telephone: 887-532-4563___

Have you talked with anyone about your problem? No X   Yes

If yes, who? Date of last contact

Significant other (name & phone): Sue Brady—wife –same information

Are you taking any medication now? No X   If yes,

What?

Crisis rating: 1   2   **(3)**   4   5

                    Not urgent   Very urgent

Probability of engaging for follow-up treatment & counseling (1= high; 5= low)

1 2 **(3)** 4 5

Summary of Presenting Situation or Problem and Help-seeking Goal:

My wife thinks I need psychiatric help. Maybe I do, I know I haven't felt like myself in some time.

Date of next contact/appointment: _____

Signature (intake/triage person): _____   Date: _____

Figure 2.1 Initial Contact Form

BOX 2.1   Essential Triage Questions

The following five triage questions draw on research with abused women using the CMHA tool (Hoff, 1990) and are adapted from research by Hoff & Rosenbaum (1994). They provide the PCP with a sample tool that illustrates a safety assessment of Mr. Brady.

1.   Have you been troubled or injured by any kind of abuse or violence? (e.g., hit by partner, forced sex)

     Yes __X_____   No_____   Not sure_____   Refused_____

     If yes, check one: By someone in your family_____ By an acquaintance or stranger _____ Describe: *Beaten by father as a kid*_____

2. If yes: Has something like this ever happened before?

Yes _____ No__X__ If yes, when?_____. Describe_____

3. Do you have anyone you can turn to or rely on now to protect you from possible further injury?

Yes__X_____ No_____ If yes, who? _*Wife, Sue*_

4. Do you feel so badly now that you have thought of hurting yourself/suicide?

Yes_*Vaguely*_____ No_____,

If yes: What have you thought about doing? *Not sure*_____.

If yes: Have you ever hurt yourself in the past?

Yes_____ No____X_____

5. Are you so angry about what's happened that you have considered hurting someone else?

Yes_____ No__X_____

If yes: have you ever threatened or hurt someone in the past?

If a risk of danger is assessed, an immediate referral to the local crisis service is required. Referral to a hospital emergency department is appropriate *only* if the department staff includes on-site or on-call mental health specialists. It is important to note that self injurious behavior such as excessive alcohol consumption is not necessarily an indication of suicide risk. Based on Triage assessment, in the case of Mr. Brady, an *immediate* referral to mental health is not indicated. Mr. Brady is given information about mental health services, and strongly recommended to make an appointment soon with a counselor to consider his and his wife's concerns beyond what the PCP can provide. Mr. Brady states he is not willing to go see a counselor and would like to "just see you." We will return to discussing Mr. Brady after further review of the CMHA.

A Comprehensive Mental Health Assessment Tool (CMHA)

The Comprehensive Mental Health Assessment Tool (CMHA) was developed and tested in the 1970s in the Erie County Mental Health System, Buffalo, NH (see Hoff, Hallisey, & Hoff, 2009, pp. 97–104). A major impetus for this tool came from the New York State government's need for a record system to track the incidence of mental disorders, as well as the effectiveness of community-based services for a range of people in distress and crisis, or with serious mental illness. The tool's origin coincided with a nationwide development of the community mental health system following Congressional legislation in 1963 and 1965.

The entire CMHA record system consists of ten forms. Our goal is to provide an easy-to-use tool that PCPs can use for initial psychosocial and psychiatric screening as a foundation and linkage to follow-up mental health specialty services that may be needed. After further review of the CMHA, its purpose, and its relevance to primary care, we illustrate its use with the case example of Mr. Brady.

The CMHA forms provide a structured guide to the intake interview, assessment, and service planning process with patients. Their intended use is within a health service system that recognizes the intrinsic relationship between physical, emotional, and sociocultural factors affecting the mental health status of individuals. The underlying philosophy of this record system emphasizes three key assumptions:

1. The person in distress or crisis is a member of a social network.
2. The stability of a person's social attachments and gratification of basic human needs strongly influences his or her physical, emotional, and mental health, and one's related ability to function within the community.
3. The provision of crisis prevention, early intervention, and social support services will conserve costly healthcare dollars by restoring and maintaining people in non-institutional settings and preventing readmission to psychiatric facilities whenever possible.

The current CMHA version builds on Hoff's (1990) research with abused women, in which the tool was used to assess mental heath sequelae of violence and victimization. Its updated edition was developed and pilot-tested by Lee Ann Hoff and psychiatric nursing graduate students at the University of Massachusetts Lowell (Hoff, Hallisey, & Hoff, 2009). Clinicians in this pilot study were from an emergency medical department in Boston and a community-based crisis service in Ontario, Canada.

The CMHA assessment and planning tool emphasizes client-centered, goal-oriented treatment. It utilizes a five-point Likert-like scale (1=excellent/very high functioning, 3=fair; 5= very poor/very low functioning) to ascertain client stress level in 21 areas of biopsychosocial functioning, through active collaboration with the client and significant others. It also allows for systematic evaluation of treatment outcomes and follow-up planning.

The CMHA tool is designed to assist in the achievement of several mental health service objectives:

1. To provide health/mental health providers, clients, and collaborating agencies a standardized framework for gathering data, while including subjective, narrative-style information from the client and significant others that is relevant to mental health across the life cycle.
2. To organize this information in a way that sharply defines their client's level of functioning (emotional, cognitive, and behavioral) and life-threatening risk, and outlines complementary treatment goals and methods to evaluate progress toward desired outcomes in specified functional areas.
3. To assist in fostering continuity between service during acute crisis states and the longer-term mental health treatment needed by some clients. (This objective is especially relevant vis-à-vis the issue of "socially constructed suicidality" that is sometimes used as the only "ticket" to psychiatric in-patient admission when health system economic factors supersede client need in clinical decision making.)
4. To provide supervisory staff with the information necessary to monitor service and assure quality and continuity of client care.
5. To provide administrative staff with information for monitoring and evaluating achievement of crisis intervention, counseling or psychotherapy, and related services for individual clients and cumulative data revealing service outcomes in relation to agency objectives.

In an era of providing cost-effective healthcare—without compromising the quality of care—this assessment and planning tool is especially relevant in its focus on client-centered, goal-oriented treatment and systematic evaluation of service outcomes. Its design depicting a person's functional level also avoids the negative effects of psychiatric labeling. Data from the CMHA concerning a client's "Basic Life Attachments" and "Signals of Distress" (Hansell, 1976) offer a structured, holistic, humanistic framework for addressing a range of human experience and functioning, affected by various life events and traumas and the emotional/mental illness or disabilities that may follow.

The 21 assessment items in the CMHA, with ratings from high to low functioning, can serve as a checklist to assure that a thorough evaluation has been done. Of the 21 items, three are contingent on injury from violence and current dangers to a victimized client and children. The scaled items evaluate a person's physical, mental, emotional, behavioral, spiritual, and social concerns, allowing for prioritizing issues for action to assure crisis and follow-up mental health services. The tool can facilitate meeting the demands of cost-effective service delivery emphasis on community-based treatment, client empowerment, and evaluation of observable treatment outcomes as manifested by the functional level of the client and his/her quality of life.

The CMHA allows for varying techniques in collecting data and exemplifies the importance of obtaining collateral information from other healthcare providers as well as significant others. Depending on the clinical situation, cultural concerns, and/or language proficiency, the Client Self-Assessment Worksheet can be given to and completed by the client before formal interview or used as an interview guide. But in no case should it simply be used without in-person discussion between the client and PCP. Either way, it serves to reinforce the idea of the client's active involvement in the assessment process. The complete assessment protocol includes data collection from a significant other (or others) on the same 21 items.

The structured five-point Likert-like scale allows for formal comparative assessment at (1) initial, (2) interim, and (3) termination phases of counseling or treatment. Besides prioritizing problems, immediate risks, and goals, it presents visually the potential progress in a client's strengths, functional level, and/or stress reduction. The scales and descriptive comments also assist both client and mental health provider to keep focused and to chart progress toward meeting treatment goals. Finally, the tool is a guide for additional interventions or referrals that might follow from the crisis intervention and/or counseling process. (See Appendix of this chapter for the complete CMHA protocol. Descriptions and operational definitions of two of the scales are found in Chapters 4 and 5. Operational definitions of remaining items and information about ongoing evaluation of this tool can be found online at www.crisisprograms.org.)

CMHA and McHugh's "Essentials": Description and Commonalities

Elements of the CMHA are complementary to the work of Dr. Paul McHugh of Johns Hopkins University. In his critique of psychiatric assessment tools, McHugh states:

> At Johns Hopkins Department of Psychiatry we have long held that psychiatry needs a new conceptual structure that ties the mental disorders we treat to mental life as psychological science understands it today. Such a structure would insist on defining mental disorders by their essential natures rather than by their appearances alone.
>
> (McHugh, 2001, p. 2)

McHugh takes issue with certain DSM diagnoses such as multiple personality disorder and chronic post-traumatic stress disorder. He requests psychiatry give up "appearance driven" diagnosis, as did internal medicine many years ago. McHugh (1999) refers to the "weak-nesses inherent in a system of classification (such as DSM) based on appearances (i.e., symptoms)—and contaminated by self-interest advocacy." He calls for a new method that can "comprehend several interactive sources of a disorder and sustain a complex program of treatment and rehabilitation" (McHugh, 1999, p. 38).

McHugh (2001) illustrates an alternative approach to categorizing and treatment planning for mental disorders. In a structure consisting of interactive perspectives of psychiatry, he attempts to reunite psychosocial components with biology. These interactive sources of disorder include four perspectives for assessment and diagnosis in psychiatric practice:

1. the Disease Perspective, encompassing pathophysiology and pathogenesis;
2. the Dimensional Perspective, including personality, life circumstances, and neurotic symptoms;
3. the Behavioral Perspective including physiologic drive, conditioned learning and choice;
4. the Life Story Perspective, encompassing setting, sequence and outcome (McHugh, 2001).

McHugh (2001) and colleagues at Johns Hopkins hold that these four distinct but interrelated levels of expression constitute the hierarchical organization of human psychological life from the most basic neurological to the most highly developed psychological functioning. Assessment skill demands ascertaining the particular way a person's psychological func-tioning can go awry, as defined by the four perspectives. As Luhrmann's (2000) research reveals, biological theory and psychopharmacology place an inordinate emphasis on the Disease Perspective in contemporary American psychiatry.

The dynamic interactive sources of disorder McHugh proposes for assessing psychological functioning are highly complementary to the assessment factors depicted in the CMHA. In particular, McHugh's four perspectives underscore two key concepts framing the CMHA tool: Basic Life Attachments, and Signals of Distress—concepts from ego psychology, socio-cultural theory, crisis theory, and preventive psychiatry (Caplan, 1964; Hansell, 1976; Hoff, Hallisey, & Hoff, 2009). Together, these two perspectives complement the importance of sensitivity to diversity and spirituality issues, as discussed in Chapter 1 and Kleinman's (1988) "8 questions" for ascertaining the variable meanings of illness and healing across cultures (see also Fadiman, 1997, pp. 251–261).

The complementary perspectives of McHugh and the CMHA will become more apparent in the following case example. Before we proceed with the example, it is important to note that McHugh's work and that of others is consistent with our goal of holistic and collaborative care for patients that present to primary care with emotional/mental health concerns. Primary care providers should be aware of the ongoing thought process and critical analysis in psychiatry that continues with striving to mend the divide between mind and body, e.g. Luhrmann, 2000; Dubovsky, 1997). That said, the realities of a 15–30 minute visit to talk about diabetes, cardiac disease, and the recent loss of a spouse, for example, bring us from academia to the clinical setting.

We have already highlighted the importance of assessing level of safety. The following illustration will take the assessment a step further in addressing psychosocial and mental health needs of a patient in primary care. Although the CMHA 21-item tool was originally designed for use in community mental health settings, it is rooted in the ideal of compre-hensive health (physical and mental) services offered in a smoothly integrated system. Our case illustration demonstrates the importance and value of holistic treatment in all areas of health, convincing the provider it is worth the perceived additional time and effort required.

We note "*perceived*" additional time, because having the information needed to assess life-threatening risk and make an accurate diagnosis as early as possible saves an immense amount of time and expense. The Client Self-assessment form is user friendly (see Figure 2.2.). If intake triage reveals no immediate risk to life, and presuming there is a positive (not dismissive) client–provider relationship, the form could be completed by the patient at home and brought back for discussion during the next visit. Having the patient complete the questions and identify the areas that are problematic sets the stage for planning, action, and holistic treatment. The process also empowers the patient through active involvement, not as a victim, but as part of the solution. Self-mastery and control of one's own destiny is a primary need, and when we capitalize upon that need, it empowers a patient to move forward. Further, with the focus on basic life functions instead of disease, the patient can more easily be engaged in counseling, especially in an era of continued bias against those with mental illness and disparity in insurance coverage for mental health services.

CASE EXAMPLE: ASSESSMENT AND COLLABORATIVE SERVICE CONTRACT

Mr. Brady is a 47-year-old married man who presents for his annual Complete Physical Exam (CPE) 8 months late. He states he is here "to get my wife off my back and get some help to sleep better." His wife has urged him to "see a psychiatrist," which he has resisted.

The review of systems identified that Mr. Brady is experiencing an alteration in his normal sleep cycle for the past six months; he also complains of decreased energy, increased irritability, and decreased sex drive. He is a non-smoker, describes his drinking as sporadic— "sports events," "weddings". Denies illicit drug use. Denies history of substance abuse or legal issues. His CPE is grossly WNL and labs are ordered—including CBC, CMP, TSH, CHOL/Lipid Profile, and a follow-up appointment is set for one month to review lab work. Mr. Brady does have a family history of heart disease; father died of a heart attack at age 55.

As previously discussed, in response to Mr. Brady's presentation, a safety assessment was completed and a recommendation of counseling was made and met with reluctance. Lab work reveals that Mr. Brady has a high cholesterol and triglyceride blood level and this is discussed at his follow-up appointment. He is ambivalent about starting medication, a behavioral plan is recommended and a six month follow up is arranged. His mental health issues remain the same with problems sleeping, lack of energy, and a dejected mood noted. He remains adamant that he does not need to see a "shrink" and "just wants to talk to you about his problems."

At the six month check up, Mr. Brady has gained weight (from 210 to 240 pounds), reports he walked for two days after last appointment and not a day since. His altered sleep cycle has worsened with increased difficulty falling asleep and frequent waking. He has missed 1–2 days of work/month in the past six months, and his previous symptoms of fatigue and irritability have worsened. His sex life was not addressed.

Mr. Brady exhibits slumped posture with intermittent eye contact. When he does look his provider directly in the eye, it is with a look of apathy and unease. He maintains he is not interested in medication for his hypercholesteremia and combats every suggestion for behavior modification with "yeah, but. . ."

How can I help this man? What is really going on? (PCP says to herself: *I have four people waiting for me!*).

Mr. Brady represents the many people who come to the PCP for an annual physical or "sick visit" with physical complaints only to reveal underlying psychosocial needs or concerns. After receiving medical care these clients often continue to return with vague complaints. They are either unable to identify their own psychosocial needs or are looking to be told that they need mental health assistance, which they have thus far rejected seeking.

In providing feedback to Mr. Brady the dialogue may be: "Mr. Brady I am concerned about your physical health as well as your mental health. We've discussed your elevated cholesterol levels and triglycerides, we made a plan and you were unable to follow through with it. I'm concerned that your symptoms of trouble sleeping, lack of energy, irritable mood, and losing interest in sex may represent an underlying emotional issue." This is quickly met with resistance "I'm not crazy if that is what you are implying." "That is not what I said, and I want to talk about your safety. So I need to ask you a few questions. Six months ago when I saw you, you said you were safe from any risk of injury to yourself or others. [see Box 2.1, the five triage questions] You seem to be more down now. Have you been feeling worse lately?" Mr. Brady says, "Yes, but it's not really that bad." PCP: "Is there any chance you've thought about giving up, or hurting yourself?" Mr. Brady: "No, but maybe my wife is right about getting some kind of help."

It is established that Mr. Brady is not at imminent risk of harming himself or another. You assess from his previous comment and his demeanor that if you refer him to a mental health specialist he will not go and this may jeopardize your relationship with him as well. You ask him to take home the Client Self-Assessment Worksheet, complete it and return for a follow-up visit in one week. Figure 2.2 notes Mr. Brady's completion of the worksheet.

Client Self-assessment Worksheet

The following can be used as the initial interview with the client, or as a take-home questionnaire, if an established relationship already exists between the PCP and the client.

1. Physical Health: How do you judge your physical health in general?

1	2	**(3)**	4	5
Excellent	Good	Fair	Poor	Very poor

    Comments: *I have gained some weight and now I have high cholesterol.*

2. Self-acceptance/Self-esteem: How do you feel about yourself as a person?

1	2	**(3)**	4	5
Excellent	Good	Fair	Poor	Very poor

    Comments: *I am a good husband and worker.*

3. Vocational/Occupational (includes student, homemaker, volunteer): How would you judge your work/school situation?

(1)	2	3	4	5
Very good	Good	Fair	Poor	Very poor

    Comments: *I have always stood out in my sales job. Recently some of the younger guys have been getting some of the bonuses I always got. Maybe I'm working too hard, just like my Dad.*

    continued

Figure 2.2 Client Self-assessment Worksheet

4. <u>Immediate Family</u>: How would you describe your relationship with your family?

1	**(2)**	3	4	5
Very good	Good	Fair	Poor	Very poor

Comments: *I don't know what my wife would say but I think we have a good marriage. I sometimes wish we had had kids. Our sex life has diminished a lot over the past two or three years.*

5. <u>Intimacy/Significant Other Relationship(s)</u>: Is there anyone you feel really close to and can rely on if you're very upset or in a life-threatening situation?

(1)	2	3	4	5
Always	Usually	Sometimes	Rarely	Never

Comments: *I can always count on my wife.*

6. <u>Residential/Housing</u>: How do you judge your housing situation?

(1)	2	3	4	5
Excellent	Good	Fair	Poor	Very poor

Comments: *I own a nice home.*

7. <u>Financial</u>: How would you describe your financial situation?

1	**(2)**	3	4	5
Very good	Good	Fair	Poor	Very poor

Comments: *I have always been a good earner but am a little worried about the younger sales force. I don't have the energy I used to and sales are all I know. My wife has an okay job but we couldn't survive on her salary alone.*

8. <u>Decision-making Ability/Cognitive Functioning</u>: How satisfied are you with your ability to make life decisions?

(1)	2	3	4	5
Always very satisfied		Somewhat dissatisfied		Always very dissatisfied

Comments: *I like to make decisions and they usually turn out well.*

9. <u>Problem-solving Ability</u>: How would you judge your ability to solve everyday problems?

(1)	2	3	4	5
Very good	Good	Fair	Poor	Very poor

Comments: *Same as above—fine.*

Figure 2.2 Client Self-assessment Worksheet (continued)

10. <u>Life Goals/Spiritual Values</u>: How satisfied are you with how your life goals (and things you value most) are working for you?

1	2	(3)	4	5

Always very satisfied   Somewhat dissatisfied   Always very dissatisfied

Comments: *Doing this form makes me think about some of the things I wish I had done and I notice I am more worried about my future than I wanted to admit.*

11. <u>Leisure Time/Community Involvement</u>: How satisfied are you with the availability of leisure time and ability to relax and take part in activities beyond everyday duties?

1	2	3	(4)	5

Always very satisfied   Somewhat dissatisfied   Always very dissatisfied

Comments: *I used to exercise 5x a week, golf every chance I could get. I just don't seem to enjoy being active like I used to. I have the time but find it difficult to relax.*

12. <u>Feelings</u>: How comfortable are you with your feelings? (for example, do you often feel anxious or fearful?)

1	2	(3)	4	5

Always comfortable   Sometimes uncomfortable   Always uncomfortable

Comments: *This is new to me, feeling uncomfortable with my own feelings. I was always a friendly confident guy. Now I worry more and am a little paranoid, wondering who wants to "stab me in the back" at work.*

13. <u>Violence/Abuse Experienced</u>: To what extent have you been injured or troubled by physical, sexual, and/or emotional abuse?

1	(2)	3	4	5

Never   Several times recently   Routinely (every day or so)

Comment/describe: *I took my share of beating when I was a kid but that was a long time ago.*

<u>Note</u>: If rating of Item 13 is 2 or above, answer items 19, 20, & 21 below

14. <u>Injury to Self</u>: Do you have any thoughts of suicide or a plan to hurt yourself in any way?

1	(2)	3	4	5

No risk whatsoever   Moderate risk   Very serious risk

Comments/describe: *I don't think I would really ever do it but I have to admit when I have thought of losing my job, the thought of doing myself in has crossed my mind. I have no idea how I would do it.*

Figure 2.2 Client Self-assessment Worksheet (continued)

15. <u>Danger to Other(s)</u>: Do you have any thoughts about violence or a plan to physically harm someone?

(1)	2	3	4	5
No risk whatsoever		Moderate risk		Very serious risk

Comments/describe: *I would never hurt anyone.*

16. <u>Substance Use</u> (alcohol and/or other drugs): Does the use of alcohol and/or other drugs concern you or interfere with your life in any way (work, family)?

1	2	3	**(4)**	5
Never	Rarely	Sometimes	Frequently	Constantly

Comments/describe: *I didn't want to say frequently but since I am being honest, I have been drinking more often and more when I do. My wife has been on my back about drinking and driving. I also got in an argument at a business dinner after I had a few too many.*

17. <u>Legal</u>: What is your tendency to get into trouble with the law?

(1)	2	3	4	5
No	Slightly	Moderately	Greatly	Very much

Comments/describe: *I have gotten a speeding ticket a few times.*

18. <u>Agency Use</u>: How satisfied are you with getting the help you need from doctors or other health providers?

(1)	2	3	4	5
Always very satisfied		Somewhat dissatisfied		Always very dissatisfied

Comments: *When I go, I get great service. I have good health insurance through my job.*

<u>Note</u>: If Item 13, **Violence/Abuse Experienced**, is rated 2 or higher, answer Items 19, 20 & 21.

19. <u>Relationship with Abuser</u>: How would you describe your relationship with the person who has abused you?

(1)	2	3	4	5
No contact or conflict now		Occasional conflict		Great conflict & turmoil

Comments: *My dad died about 7 years ago.*

Figure 2.2 Client Self-assessment Worksheet (continued)

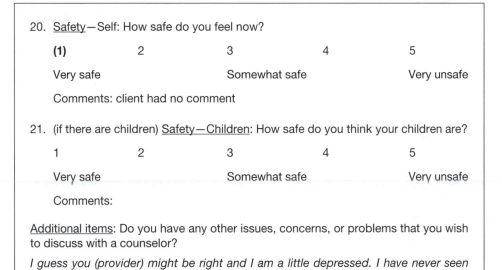

20. Safety—Self: How safe do you feel now?

    (1)   2   3   4   5

    Very safe   Somewhat safe   Very unsafe

    Comments: client had no comment

21. (if there are children) Safety—Children: How safe do you think your children are?

    1   2   3   4   5

    Very safe   Somewhat safe   Very unsafe

    Comments:

Additional items: Do you have any other issues, concerns, or problems that you wish to discuss with a counselor?

I guess you (provider) might be right and I am a little depressed. I have never seen myself as the kind of guy who needs to talk to someone. How about some medication?

Urgency/Importance: Among the items noted, which do you consider the most urgent and/or in need of immediate attention?

I guess I should think about cutting down on my drinking and doing something about my attitude.

Figure 2.2 Client Self-assessment Worksheet (continued)

At Mr. Brady's return visit you review the CMHA with him and discuss his findings. It is evident to the PCP that collateral data from the wife would be helpful, however, not prudent or necessary at this time in order to continue with a plan of action.

The CMHA assessment substantiates your initial assessment of Mr. Brady's need for mental health services. The process of Mr. Brady doing a self-evaluation proved to be thought-provoking and informative, comporting with his ability to identify his displeasure with some areas of his life, and his recent increase in alcohol consumption. He was also able to identify his need for assistance. This may have been different if he had been interviewed by a new provider with whom he did not have an established relationship or the provider seemed in a hurry. Mr. Brady may then have minimized his concerns in order to maintain his dignity. In addition, this self-evaluation makes him feel that he actually has a lot to be thankful for in life and serves as a positive "reality check" for Mr. Brady.

The process of establishing a provider–patient relationship at initial and reoccurring visits illustrates the first step in the problem solving process. Too often the process stops here. The PCP is well aware of the problem, as is the patient. The issue remains: what to do about the problem? The answer lies in the remaining steps of the problem solving process:

- establishing a service/treatment plan;
- implementation of the plan; and
- follow up and evaluation.

The CMHA tool includes a Service Contract to outline the plan of care and consecutive forms for follow up. The follow up forms may be more appropriate for a mental health provider to whom Mr. Brady has been referred. The Service Contract is very appropriate for primary care and is illustrated below. It outlines actions to be taken and serves as a guide for follow-up visits.

The CMHA's quantitative design and client narratives allow for simple prioritization of problems. If a number 3 or higher has been assigned to an item then it needs to be addressed in the Service Contract, illustrated in Figure 2.3, in which the following items were rated 3 or higher (the Crisis rating is from the Initial Contact Form):

Crisis—3
Physical Health—3
Self-acceptance/Self-esteem—3
Life goals—3
Leisure Time/Community Involvement—4
Feelings—3
Substance Abuse—4

We have already established the significant time restraints of the Primary Care Provider. It is recommended that the completed CMHA be sent with referral to a mental health specialist. It is also obvious at this point that the Primary Care Provider is in partnership with other disciplines, that he/she cannot avoid incorporating mental health while providing holistic care. Therefore, the Service Contract of the PCP may look like the following:

Service Contract

Item/Stress Rating	Problem/Issue Specification	Strategies/Techniques
Crisis (3)	Risk of harm to self	Referral to mental health professional
	Cardiac disease	Give number for 24 hotline if available
		Review plan to go to ER if suicidal
		Evaluate safety at every visit
		Education regarding the relationship between physical and mental health
		Recommend abstinence from alcohol
Physical Health (3)	CVD	Referral to nutritionist
	Obesity	Exercise plan
	Alteration sleep cycle	Review medication options
	Decreased libido	Laboratory values/weight
		Recommend abstinence from alcohol
		Consider sleep study in future

Figure 2.3 Service Contract

Substance Abuse (4) Excessive Etoh	Assess family history of substance abuse
	Assess consumption, drinks/ day visit
	Provide education on detrimental effects to both physical and emotional health
	Discuss potential liver damage if treatment for hypercholesterimia is initiated

The following items have been identified and discussed with Mr. Brady with recommendation he seek counseling to address:

Self-acceptance/Self-esteem—3
Life Goals—3
Leisure Time/Community Involvement—4
Feelings—3
Substance Abuse—4

Figure 2.3 Service Contract (continued)

Mr. Brady's ability to identify his need for treatment allows for an easier referral process to a mental health specialist. The fact that Mr. Brady has participated in the procedure also makes it more comfortable to discuss his preliminary diagnosis of: alcohol abuse, dysthymia and R/O major depressive disorder, as well as discussing the direct effects on his physical health. It may be at this time that his libido and sleep disturbances can be discussed and he can be reassured they will be addressed medically if they do not resolve with mental health treatment.

The conversation may be something like this: "Mr. Brady, I very much appreciate how open you have been with me and I think it is invaluable to our ongoing relationship. It is obvious to me that you may benefit from specialized mental health services. I cannot provide you with the counseling I think you need. Of course I could write you a prescription for an anti-depressant medication . . . but I want to emphasize that this might lift your mood for a while but I think it's best to coordinate this with counseling, because we know that the best results from these drugs is in combination with counseling that gets at what's going on in your life and helps you figure out why you came here in the first place. Of course, I'll gladly collaborate with your other providers and continue to see you about your high cholesterol and general medical needs." Mr. Brady responds affirmatively: "I will do it, can you recommend someone?" (See Chapter 3 for further discussion of this case.)

Having an established relationship with a mental health clinic/practice is clearly beneficial in this scenario and will facilitate ongoing collaborative care. It is also paramount to have staff to assist with making the initial appointment. In addition to his initial reluctance to seek additional help, Mr. Brady's symptoms of depression will quite possibly hinder his ability to follow through with the treatment plan (as already witnessed).

Another consideration here is the important issue of detecting impaired cognitive functioning due to brain disease, developmental disabilities (DSM—Axis II, usually requiring legal guardianship) or the aging process which is not the case with Mr. Brady. In the case of developmental disabilities, typical issues include healthcare advocacy, housing and financial support, as well as family "caretaker burden" that can extend to old age of both the disabled person and his or her caretaker. Any symptoms of confusion, inability to coherently answer basic intake questions, or evidence of disorientation as to time, place, and person may signal the PCP's decision to administer the Mini Mental Status Examination (MMSE) in concert with mental health or neuropsychiatric referral. The matter of mental capacity and competency to make healthcare decisions on one's own behalf is discussed more fully in Chapter 12, in the section on cognitive impairments and the role of a designated healthcare proxy for making treatment and end-of-life decisions for persons developmentally disabled in early life with life-long health implications, and those affected by decline of brain function in the usual aging process.

In conclusion, the detrimental effect of untreated emotional/mental health issues on physical health is well documented. Informal mental health assessment in primary care is most likely already part of a complete physical exam. In the setting of multi-system issues and very busy schedules a provider can often feel overwhelmed by patients with emotional issues and either feel frustrated by not having the time to address these issues, and/or feel inadequately trained to assess and address them appropriately and expeditiously.

Utilization of the triage safety assessment and the CMHA provides PCPs with tools to aid in daily interactions with patients, assist with identifying problems, and facilitate planning of appropriate care and/or referrals. The CMHA also serves very nicely as a referral document. It establishes a reason treatment is sought and provides continuity of care, as well as a tool that can be used to re-evaluate progress and provide a common language to facilitate dialogue in collaborative care between providers.

Appendix

Comprehensive Mental Health Assessment Data: Initial, Interim, and Termination Status

Rating Code: 1 = Excellent/Very high functioning/Low stress
   3 = Fair
   5 = Very poor/Very low functioning/High stress

BASIC LIFE FUNCTIONS

1. Physical Health Medical information (chronic/acute illnesses, surgeries, OB/Gyn Hx, accidents, sexual dysfunction, allergies)

   Current primary care provider: Yes _____ No _____

   If yes, name: _____; agency: _____

   Telephone: _____ Date of last visit: _____

   Medications:

	Name	Dosage	Duration	Prescriber
1.				
2.				
3.				
4.				
5.				
6.				

ASSESSMENT RATINGS

Initial   1   2   3   4   5
Comments:
....

Interim   1   2   3   4   5
Comments:
....

Termination 1   2   3   4   5
Comments:
....

2. Self-Acceptance/Self-esteem:

Initial   1   2   3   4   5
Comments:
....

Interim   1   2   3   4   5
Comments:
....

Termination 1   2   3   4   5
Comments:
....

3. Vocational/Occupational:

Employed____ Student____ Homemaker ____ Volunteer ____ Other ____

Initial   1   2   3   4   5
Comments:
....

Interim   1   2   3   4   5
Comments:
....

Termination 1   2   3   4   5
Comments:
....

4. Immediate Family:

Parental status: Children: Yes ____ No ____ How many? _____ Ages ____
(Refer to Child Screening Checklist)

Initial   1   2   3   4   5
Comments:
....

Interim	1	2	3	4	5
Comments:					

. . . .

Termination	1	2	3	4	5
Comments:					

. . . .

5. <u>Intimacy/Significant Others</u>:

   Marital status: Never married ____ Married ____ Widowed ____ Divorced ____
   Separated ____ Living together ____ How long? ____

Initial	1	2	3	4	5
Comments:					

. . . .

Interim	1	2	3	4	5
Comments:					

. . . .

Termination	1	2	3	4	5
Comments:					

. . . .

6. <u>Residential/Housing</u>: Living situation: Lives alone ____ Lives with family ____
   Other ____ (specify) _____

   Significant Other information

   <u>Within household</u>:

   <u>Name</u>   <u>Age</u>   <u>Nature of relationship</u>

   <u>Supportive</u>: <u>Yes No</u>

   <u>Outside household</u>:

   <u>Name</u>   <u>Age</u>   <u>Relationship</u>

   <u>Address</u>   <u>Telephone</u>

Initial	1	2	3	4	5
Comments:					

. . . .

Interim	1	2	3	4	5
Comments:					

. . . .

Termination	1	2	3	4	5
Comments:					

. . . .

7. <u>Financial Security</u>: Source of income _____

Initial	1	2	3	4	5

Comments:

. . . .

Interim	1	2	3	4	5

Comments:

. . . .

Termination	1	2	3	4	5

Comments:

. . . .

8. <u>Decision-making Ability/Cognitive Functioning</u>

Initial	1	2	3	4	5

Comments:

. . . .

Interim	1	2	3	4	5

Comments:

. . . .

Termination	1	2	3	4	5

Comments:

. . . .

9. <u>Problem-solving Ability</u>

Initial	1	2	3	4	5

Comments:

. . . .

Interim	1	2	3	4	5

Comments:

. . . .

Termination	1	2	3	4	5

Comments:

. . . .

10. <u>Life Goals/Spiritual Values</u>

Initial	1	2	3	4	5

Comments:

. . . .

Interim	1	2	3	4	5

Comments:

. . . .

Termination   1   2   3   4   5
Comments:
. . . .

11. Leisure Time/Community Involvement:

Primary leisure & self-care activities_____

Initial   1   2   3   4   5
Comments:
. . . .

Interim   1   2   3   4   5
Comments:
. . . .

Termination   1   2   3   4   5
Comments:
. . . .

12. Feeling Management (coping with anxiety)

Initial   1   2   3   4   5
Comments:
. . . .

Interim   1   2   3   4   5
Comments:
. . . .

Termination   1   2   3   4   5
Comments:
. . . .

SIGNALS OF DISTRESS

13. Violence Experienced: History of physical and/or sexual assault

Date of last assault _____ Description _____

Abuser/assailant (stranger, family) _____ Outcome _____

_____ within last month   _____ medical treatment only
_____ within last 6 months   _____ hospital intensive care
_____ within last year   _____ hospital psychiatric
_____ over 1 year ago   _____ outpatient follow-up
_____ began in childhood   _____ survivor support group
_____ multiple occasions   _____ no treatment or support

Initial   1   2   3   4   5
Comments:
. . . .

| Interim | 1 | 2 | 3 | 4 | 5 |

Comments:

. . . .

| Termination | 1 | 2 | 3 | 4 | 5 |

Comments:

. . . .

14. <u>Injury to Self</u>: History of suicide attempts, ideation, threats, and current risk of suicide

Date of last injury _____ Method _____ Outcome _____

Ideation/threat, no specific plan _____

____ within last month   ____ medical treatment only
____ within last 6 months   ____ hospital intensive care
____ within last year   ____ hospital psychiatric
____ over 1 year ago   ____ outpatient follow-up
                                                         ____ no treatment

| Initial | 1 | 2 | 3 | 4 | 5 |

Comments:

. . . .

| Interim | 1 | 2 | 3 | 4 | 5 |

Comments:

. . . .

| Termination | 1 | 2 | 3 | 4 | 5 |

Comments:

. . . .

15. <u>Danger to Others</u>: History of injury to others, threats, and anti-social behavior

Date of last assault _____ Method/description _____

Outcome (victim injury, arrest, etc.)_____

Ideation/threat, no specific plan _____

Context of assault/aggression (e.g., alcohol abuse) _____

____ within last month   ____ psychotropic drug treatment only
____ within last 6 moths   ____ hospital psychiatric
____ over 1 year ago   ____ outpatient follow-up
____ began in adolescence   ____ batterers treatment group
____ began with intimate partner   ____ no treatment

| Initial | 1 | 2 | 3 | 4 | 5 |

Comments:

. . . .

Interim	1	2	3	4	5

Comments:

. . . .

Termination	1	2	3	4	5

Comments:

. . . .

16. <u>Substance Use</u> (alcohol or other drugs)

<u>Type</u>	<u>Present Use</u>	<u>Past Use</u>	<u>Duration</u>
1.			
2.			
3.			
4.			
5.			

Initial	1	2	3	4	5

Comments:

. . . .

Interim	1	2	3	4	5

Comments:

. . . .

Termination	1	2	3	4	5

Comments:

. . . .

17. <u>Legal</u>

1. Pending court action: Yes _____ No _____ When? _____
2. On probation: Yes _____ No _____ Probation officer _____
3. On parole: Yes _____ No _____ Parole officer _____
4. Conditional discharge: Yes _____ No _____ Requirement _____
5. Other (describe): _____

Initial	1	2	3	4	5

Comments:

. . . .

Interim	1	2	3	4	5

Comments:

. . . .

Termination	1	2	3	4	5

Comments:

. . . .

18. Agency Use
Previous Mental Health Service Contacts

Outpatient: Agency _____ Phone # _____

Contact person _____

Address _____

Inpatient: Agency _____ Phone # _____

Contact person _____

Address _____ Date last Hosp. _____

Reason for admission _____

How often? _____ How long? _____ Avg. length of stay _____

Initial   1   2   3   4   5
Comments:
. . . .

Interim   1   2   3   4   5
Comments:
. . . .

Termination 1   2   3   4   5
Comments:
. . . .

Optional Information

Religious concerns: No ____ Yes ____ What? _____

Ethnic/cultural concerns: No ____ Yes ____ What? _____

Note: Following items to be addressed if rating on Item 13 is 2 or higher

19. Relationship with Abuser

Living with abuser ____
Living in a shelter ____
Living with relative or friend ____
In process of divorce ____
Restraining order in effect ____
In process of seeking counseling ____
No contact with abuser now ____
Other (describe) _____

Initial   1   2   3   4   5
Comments:
. . . .

Interim   1   2   3   4   5
Comments:
. . . .

Termination 1   2   3   4   5
Comments:
. . . .

20. <u>Safety—Self</u>

Safety plan (describe) _____

Initial   1   2   3   4   5
Comments:
. . . .

Interim   1   2   3   4   5
Comments:
. . . .

Termination 1   2   3   4   5
Comments:
. . . .

21. <u>Safety—Children</u>

Children abused: No ___ Yes ___ Date _____ Outcome _____

Children witnessed parental violence: No ____ Yes ____ Date _____

Children in protective custody: No ____ Yes ____ How long? _____

Safety plan for children (describe): _____

Initial   1   2   3   4   5
Comments:
. . . .

Interim   1   2   3   4   5
Comments:
. . . .

Termination 1   2   3   4   5
Comments:
. . . .

A. Do you have any other issues, concerns, or problems that we have not addressed?
    Explain:

B. Major Problems—Client Goals

C. Narrative Summary

D. Composite Stress/Crisis Rating (based on maximum ratings of 21 items)

   Interpretation: Reduction in high stress/crisis scores suggests positive influence of the crisis intervention/counseling process

   Low stress/High functioning   Moderate stress   High stress/Low functioning

1	2	3	4	5
21	42	63	84	105

   Initial:
   Interim:
   Termination:

   Data-based Problem Prioritizing, Goal Setting, and Service Planning: Items with ratings of 5, 4, & 3 are priority areas for intervention/service (see Service Contract form)

References

American Psychiatric Association (APA) (2000). *Diagnostic and statistical manual of mental disorders* (4th ed., rev.). Washington, DC: Author.

Antonovsky, A. (1988). *How people manage stress and stay well*. San Francisco: Jossey-Bass.

Brownlee, S. (2007). *Overtreated: Why too much medicine is making us sicker and poorer*. New York: Bloomsbury, USA.

Caplan, G. (1964). *Principles of preventive psychiatry*. New York: Basic Books.

Caplan, P. (1995). *They say you're crazy*. Reading, MA: Perseus Books.

Cooksey, E.C., & Brown, P. (1998). Spinning on its axes: DSM and the social construction of psychiatric diagnosis. *International Journal of Health Services*, 28(3), 525–554.

Dubovsky, S.L. (1997). *Mind-body deceptions: The psychosomatics of everyday life*. New York: Norton.

Fadiman, A. (1997). *The spirit catches you and you fall down*. New York: The Noonday Press, Farrar, Straus and Giroux.

Hansell, N. (1976). *The person in distress*. New York: Human Sciences Press.

Hoff, L.A. (1990). *Battered women as survivors*. London: Routledge.

Hoff, L. A., & Rosenbaum, L. (1994). A victimization assessment tool: Instrument development and clinical implications. *Journal of Advanced Nursing*, 20 (4), 627–634.

Hoff, L.A., Hallisey, B.J., & Hoff, M. (2009). *People in crisis: Clinical and diversity perspectives* (6th ed.). New York: Routledge.

International Statistical Classification of Diseases and Related Health Disorders, Tenth Revision, (ICD-10). (2004) 2nd Ed. Geneva: World Health Organization.

Kleinman, A. (1988). *The illness narratives: Suffering, healing, and the human condition*. New York: Basic Books.

Luhrmann, T.M. (2000). *Of two minds: The growing disorder in American psychiatry*. New York: Alfred A. Knopf.

McHugh, P.R. (1999). How psychiatry lost its way. *Commentary*, 108(5), 32–39.

McHugh, P.R. (2001). Beyond DSM-IV: From appearances to essences. *Psychiatric Research Report*, 17(2), 1–5.

McHugh, P.R., & Clark, M.R. (2006). Diagnostic and classificatory dilemmas. In M. Blumenfeld & J.J. Strain (Eds.), *Psychosomatic medicine* (pp. 39–45). Philadelphia: Lippincott Williams & Wilkins.

Mezzich, J. (2002). The WPA International Guidelines for Diagnostic Assessment. *World Psychiatry*, 1(1), 36–39.

O'Brien, P.G., Kennedy, W.Z., & Ballard, K.A. (1999). *Psychiatric nursing*. New York: McGraw-Hill.

Peplau, H. (1993). *Interpersonal relations in nursing*. New York: Springer.

Regier, D. (2007). Somatic presentation of mental disorders: Refining the research agenda for DDSM-V, *Psychosomatic Medicine,* 69 (9), 827–828.

Sharma, V.K; Lepping, P.; Cummins, Al, *et al.* (2004). The global mental health assessment tool— Primary care version (GMHAT/PC): Development, reliability and validity. *World Psychiatry*, 3(2), 115–119.

Sugg, N.K., & Inui, T (1992). Primary care physicians' response to domestic violence: Opening Pandora's box. *Journal of the American Medical Association*, 267(23), 3157–3160.

Ustan, T.B. (1999). The global burden of mental disorders. *American Journal of Public Health*, 89(9), 1315–1321.

Watters, E. (2010). *Crazy like us: The globalization of the American psych*e. New York: Free Press.

3 Crisis Care Basics in Primary Care

- Interdisciplinary Theoretical Underpinnings to Crisis Care
- The Crisis Paradigm: A Guide to Understanding and Helping
- Basic Crisis Assessment Skills: Pre-crisis and Acute Crisis States
- Crisis Intervention Strategies in Primary Care: Mental Health Linkage and Follow-up
- Crisis Counseling Strategies: Coordination with Primary Care
- Psychotropic Medication in Crisis Care
- References

This chapter addresses the key features of crisis care with a focus on critical life events, developmental and family issues, prevention, early intervention, and networking, including illustrative case examples. It assumes that such care is an integral facet of comprehensive health and mental health services. Rather than treating people's behavior during crisis as a psychiatric "disorder," it presents the crisis experience arising from stressful life events and socio-cultural factors as a *normal* part of life from birth to death. However, it also recognizes that people with pre-existing psychiatric disabilities are generally more vulnerable to crisis episodes than others—sometimes as a result of misapplied psychiatric diagnoses and/or insufficient support when stressful life events intersect with the burdens of living with mental illness. Also, some horrific events (e.g., war trauma, multiple losses from disasters like Hurricane Katrina, rape, or repeated battering by spouse) fall outside the range of everyday experience for the majority. But people suffering from such physical and emotional traumas should not also be burdened with a psychiatric label such as "personality disorder," especially given the continuing bias and disparity in insurance coverage for those needing mental health services.

We therefore emphasize the smooth integration of crisis assessment and intervention basics into established medical and mental health diagnostic protocols, as illustrated in Chapter 2. Underscoring the chapter's importance is this reality in primary care settings: While a *minority* of clients may present in emotional distress or acute crisis, these patients—especially when risk to life is at stake—can be the *majority*, in terms of stress, anxiety, or

---

* Parts of this chapter are excerpted from Hoff, Hallisey, & Hoff, 2009, *People in crisis: Clinical and diversity perspectives*, 6th Edition, Chapters 2, 3, and 4, and edited for application in primary care practice. Used with permission.

frustration experienced. A primary care practitioner is in a strategic position to identify an impending or acute crisis, offer immediate support and safety, and link an acutely distressed person to crisis specialists and recommended follow-up counseling services.

Crisis theory, assessment, prevention, and intervention strategies are presented around typical scenarios such as serious illness, unexpected death, self-injury, and threats or acts of violence and sexual abuse. Self-destructive behaviors, physical assaults, and sexual abuse are life-threatening and central to crisis assessment and intervention. Key to success in potentially life-threatening situations in primary care is avoiding a mechanical approach or assuming that a "yes or no" question about abuse on intake forms, for example, suffices for crisis assessment. Therefore, we introduce such issues here, but address the topic more comprehensively in Chapters 4 (on suicide) and 5 (on violence), that focus on assessment, early intervention, and networking with crisis and mental health specialists, on behalf of people in life-threatening distress who first present in primary care settings.

Interdisciplinary Theoretical Underpinnings to Crisis Care

The experience of crisis and people helping others in distress is as old as history itself. But as a formal body of knowledge, it is only a few decades old. Not too long ago, when front-line crisis intervention was carried out largely by trained volunteers, some mental health professionals referred to it disparagingly as a mere "band aid," assuming that the real work of helping people in crisis occurred in the offices of psychotherapists, or for those threatening suicide or violence, in the secure and physically constrained premises of psychiatric hospitals.

Today, as a result of major national and international research, health policy decisions, plus teaching and clinical expertise, crisis care comprises a respected body of knowledge in its own right. Thus, most health providers and the general public accept crisis care as an integral part of comprehensive services that should be available to all. The body of knowledge and practices flowing from it are interdisciplinary, representing the following: Public health, emergency medicine and nursing, psychology, social work, psychiatry, sociology, anthropology, and criminal justice.

In no small measure, development of the crisis field as widely known today is traced to work with survivors of disaster and all forms of violence—interpersonal abuse across the life span, and the multiple traumas of war. Primary care providers will be familiar with many of these sources from some of their basic undergraduate and graduate courses in particular practice arenas. Readers are referred to comprehensive crisis texts and online sources for a fuller discussion of crisis theory that space does not allow here (see Hoff, Hallisey & Hoff, 2009). The focus in this chapter is on the intersection of crisis intervention strategies in primary care with the specialized crisis or mental health services needed by some primary care clients. Briefly, we emphasize the importance of distinguishing between stress, predicament, emergency, crisis, and emotional or mental disturbance or breakdown. These definitions clarify distinctions between crisis care and the psychotherapeutic strategies that demand in-depth study of psychopathologies and its treatment by mental health specialists. The distinctions underscore the pivotal position of Primary Care Providers at healthcare entry points, and the necessity of teamwork and community-wide collaboration for effective crisis prevention and resolution.

CASE EXAMPLE: TRIAGE—A CRISIS OR NOT?

The receptionist in a primary care suite receives a telephone call from Fred, a man who is crying and says he wants to talk to someone "right away." Can we assume that this man is in crisis? Not necessarily, without obtaining more information. What we do know from this brief interaction is that he is upset. People experience upsetting incidents in everyday life, but of themselves, most of these incidents do not constitute acute emotional crisis requiring professional help.

On further questioning by the intake nurse, we learn the following about Fred: He is age 40, has chronic kidney disease and a drinking problem, but has managed to keep his stable job as an electrical engineer. He says that today he had a hard time controlling himself from hitting his wife, Angela, as she took off for work. Although he has recently joined Alcoholics Anonymous on Angela's urging, he has gone "off the wagon" twice in the last six weeks. He reports that Angela says she's concerned about their three children and is tired of waiting for him to straighten out his life. On one occasion after a drinking bout and Angela's threat to leave, Fred said he'd kill himself if she left him. From triage questions (see Initial Contact Form, Figure 2.1, and Triage Tool, Box 2.1 Chapter 2) for initial crisis assessment questioning, it turns out that Fred is upset because his wife has just informed him that she wants a divorce. Although he felt an urge to strike Angela, he managed to control himself, denies any history of assaultive behavior, and acknowledges that he needs help to overcome his drinking problem. On further questioning about suicide risk, Fred denies any plan of self-harm and said his previous suicide threat was aimed at keeping Angela from divorcing him. When asked if he could come to the clinic in the next few hours Fred said, "No, I have to go to work, because I can't afford to lose another day's pay."

From this crisis triage information, what do we know about the crisis experience, how it develops, what outcomes we should aim for, and what we should do *immediately*, the *next day*, or *next week*? The case of Fred and his family will be continued in Chapter 9 on substance abuse. Here, we illustrate the basics of crisis development and intervention in primary care, and the intersection between crisis and chronic problems.

Key Definitions

Crisis: An acute emotional upset arising from situational, developmental, or sociocultural sources and resulting in a temporary inability to cope by means of one's usual problem-solving devices. This definition of crisis assumes that emotional upset—for example, when losing one's home in disaster, learning about a life-threatening illness, threat of losing one's spouse (as in Fred's case), or surviving sexual assault or battlefield trauma—following a stressful or life altering event is *normal.* A crisis state should not be equated with a mental "disorder", while acknowledging that diagnosable mental illness leaves one more vulnerable to crisis arising from various life stressors.

Crisis intervention: A short-term helping process focusing on resolution of an immediate, identifiable problem (vs. unconscious conflict or chronic problems), utilizing personal, social, and inter-agency resources.

Psychotherapy: A helping process directed toward changing a person's feelings and patterns of thought and behavior. In contrast to crisis intervention's focus on problem-solving around hazardous events or situations, it involves uncovering unconscious conflict and accompanying symptoms of distress.

Crisis worker (for Natural and Formal Crisis Care): Anyone with the knowledge, skills and attitudes required to assist an individual or family in crisis (e.g., police officer, nurse, social worker, physician, hotline counselor, mental health professional).

Phases of Crisis Development and Preventive Intervention

Psychiatrist Gerald Caplan (1964), sometimes called the father of crisis theory, has shown in his developmental perspective that acute, full-blown crisis can be prevented if its early phases are recognized. Others have built on this early work (e.g., Parad, 1965; Hoff, 1990; Hoff, Hallisey & Hoff, 2009), through work with families and victims of violence and abuse. Thus, for example, it is not only a current hazardous "event" (e.g., threat of divorce) that can trigger emotional crisis, but a hazardous "situation" (e.g., living with an abusive or chronically ill partner, during which one lacked appropriate support and intervention over the years).

There are four phases of development toward an acute, full-blown crisis:

1. A traumatic event causes a rise in one's usual level of anxiety.
2. The person's usual problem-solving ability fails, while the stimulus that caused the initial rise in tension continues.
3. The individual's anxiety level rises further, moving the person to use available resources for problem-solving and to reduce the painful state of anxiety.
4. A state of acute crisis, with the problem remaining unsolved, and anxiety rising to an unbearable degree.

Each phase provides the PCP an opportunity for prevention and early intervention with people presenting in primary care, if the provider knows what questions to ask and how to offer immediate and follow-up service. The cases of Karen and Robert illustrate the progressive phases leading to acute emotional crisis—Phase 4: *Acute crisis* in which internal strength fails, a point at which, without necessary support, a suicide or homicide attempt might be made as a desperate but destructive way to cope.

CASE EXAMPLES AND QUESTIONS TO ASK

Karen: A Battered Woman

Phase 1. The traumatic event of abuse finally erupts, causing a rise in anxiety level. What can Karen and the PCP do to prevent it from happening again, or staying in the hazardous situation?

PCP: "Karen, your eye! It's all swollen. . .What happened?"
Karen: "I just never told you, I think because I kept believing he would change, but this was the worst he's done."
PCP: "I'm so sorry, Karen, but first let's take care of that eye, and go from there."

Phase 2. Karen's usual problem-solving ability fails.

PCP: Explores the situation further, e.g., "How long has this been going on? Who's been there for you when you've been hurt?"
Karen: "I kept trying to talk to him, he refused to talk, I tried to be nice and second-guess his desires, he hit me again"—this time with visible and serious physical injury. She has confided in a friend, but mostly just tried to stick it out on her own.

Phase 3. As a person's anxiety level rises even further, new and unusual coping devices (constructive or unhealthy) are tried: Karen took a tranquilizer, but after "icing" her swollen eye decided she better see her PCP. She deliberately avoided going to the ER, because once before after being battered she had "covered up" what happened when she was treated for a badly bruised arm.

Robert: Facing Divorce Threat after Heart Attack

Phase 1. Robert is a patient being followed for heart problems.

PCP: "Hi, Robert, I thought you'd be coming in a couple weeks from now . . . You seem upset . . . What brings you in today?"

Robert: (choking back tears) "I thought she'd see me through this, but this morning she told me she's leaving and wants a divorce."

PCP: "Oh, Robert . . . What a shock this must be, especially at a time like this since your heart attack . . . I'm so sorry." (In the contrasting example of Fred above—Triage—his wife Angela's threat of divorce came as no surprise, but did serve as a "wake-up call" to get serious about his chronic drinking problem.)

Phase 2. Robert had asked his wife if they couldn't just talk about this when she got home from work, and maybe see a marriage counselor, but she refused.

PCP: Listens patiently, then asks: "Considering your wife's refusal, are you willing to see a counselor on your own?"

Robert replies "yes"—depending on a recommendation he can trust. (In Fred's case, although he has failed twice with his A.A. program, the prospect for a healthy turnaround in solving his drinking problem—and the probability of divorce—is evident from the fact that he called his PCP, thus acknowledging his need for help.) At this phase for Robert, there is promising ground for avoiding further escalation toward an acute crisis.

Phase 3. Robert tried to call his sister, with whom he is very close, but she wasn't home, had a couple of beers, but realized he'd probably be better off if he leveled with his PCP with whom he has a very good relationship, so came in without an appointment.

PCP says: "I'm really glad you came in, Robert . . . Let's figure out what we can do that's best for you. OK?"

Duration of Crisis and Possible Outcomes

In these two scenarios, Karen and Robert are in Phase 3 of crisis development. Considering the importance of strategic intervention and prevention of potentially lethal outcomes, PCPs are in very pivotal positions to foster positive outcomes. This is because one cannot remain in a crisis state indefinitely, as the person must have some relief from the acute emotional pain. Experience with people in crisis reveals that *some* kind of resolution (positive or negative) will occur between *one and six weeks* (Caplan, 1964; Hoff, Hallisey & Hoff, 2009). This clinical reality was the foundation for development of 24/7 crisis services as a norm, just as has been the case historically for medical emergencies. Delays in service for someone in acute crisis could mean the difference between life and death, as discussed in the next section.

There are three possible crisis outcomes, with the first as the ideal goal of providers, and the third to be avoided whenever possible by timely intervention:

1. Return to pre-crisis state, plus growth in resilience and emotional well-being, e.g., learning new and more effective ways to cope with stress and trauma.
2. Return at least to one's pre-crisis state, with little growth, in some cases because of underlying chronic problems requiring psychotherapy which either has been unavailable, or refused by the client.
3. Resolution of crisis by destructive, negative means, e.g., suicide, assault on others, emotional/mental breakdown, substance abuse or addiction.

The Crisis Paradigm: A Guide to Understanding and Helping

These concepts form the basis for *understanding* the person in a pre- or acute crisis state—the foundation for assessment and intervention. The Crisis Paradigm serves two purposes: (1) it depicts the crisis experience from *origin to either positive or negative resolution*; (2) building on such understanding, it provides a *roadmap for the basic steps* of crisis care, whether in primary care or mental health settings:

1. psychosocial assessment of the individual or family, including evaluation of victimization trauma and risk of suicide or assault on others;
2. development of a plan with the person or family in crisis;
3. implementation of the plan, drawing on personal, social and material resources;
4. follow-up, networking, and evaluation of the crisis intervention process and outcomes.

This model depicts the crisis experience and intervention tailored to the origins and subjective responses to stressful life events. It was developed from research with abused women and

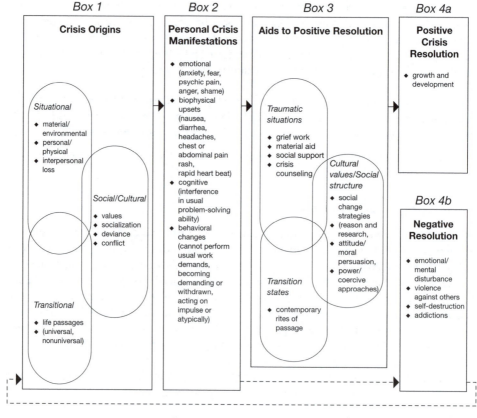

Figure 3.1 Crisis Paradigm. Crisis origins, manifestations, and outcomes and the respective functions of crisis care have interactional relationships. The intertwined ovals represent the distinct yet interrelated origins of crisis and aids to positive resolution, even though personal manifestations are often similar. The arrows pointing from origins to positive resolution illustrate the *opportunity for growth and development* through crisis. The broken line at the bottom depicts the potential *danger of crisis* in the absence of appropriate aids. The loop between Box 4b and Box 1 denotes the *vulnerability* to future crisis episodes following negative resolution.

their children (Hoff, 1990). Earlier theoretical conceptions of crisis focused on crisis originating from unanticipated stressful events and the challenges of life cycle transition states. Typical at the time (mid-twentieth century) was the widely held belief that wife-beating was a "private" family matter, not the business of health providers (see Chapter 5). Since then, a large body of research on psychological trauma from violence and abuse has been incorporated into crisis and mental health texts.

Here we note a significant finding from this research as it pertains to the "origins" of crisis: A key ingredient of emotional healing from traumatic life events is the person's ability to find "meaning" in what happened. The work of Lifton & Olson (1976), for example, underscores the importance of ascertaining how an acutely distressed person answers this question: "Why did this happen to me?" Or as Antonovsky's cross-cultural research reveals (1980, pp. 99–100), one's resistance resources and "sense of coherence" SOC includes the distressed person's *perception* of events as *comprehensible, manageable, and meaningful* in the framework of one's life goals and values.

Diversity of Crisis Meanings

As discussed in Chapters 1 and 2, there is a diversity of meanings that clients attach to stressful or injurious life events that emanate from culture, religion, expected gender-related behavioral norms, etc. Of course, no individual PCP can be expected to know or master details of such extensive cross-cultural differences in multi-cultural healthcare service settings. But for successful crisis care outcomes, it is imperative that providers couch their questions and responses during crisis with sensitivity to these differences, and plan with clients an intervention approach in the context of such diverse meanings and social parameters (some perhaps very restrictive) that influence how clients might respond to PCPs' recommendations in various crisis situations. Some common examples affecting crisis care for diverse immigrant populations include the fear of deportation if an abused person reports interpersonal violence, or the culturally based "shame" that may affect men who seek professional help vs. the expectation of "strength and endurance" in the face of distressing or critical events.

Internationally noted disaster responses in Southeast Asia (the tsunami) and the catastrophic earthquake in Haiti illustrate this point. Accounts of the disaster relief efforts cite the rush to offer much-needed humanitarian assistance—only for the well-intentioned volunteers to depart after a two-week or so stint of relief effort. Also of note is the phenomenon of "psychological ambulance chasing"—in effect, sometimes assuming a "psychiatric disorder" in what is essentially a "normal" response to an extraordinary life event of loss, destruction of home, personal injury, etc. Such pathologizing of disaster responses is counter-productive, especially if done without knowledge of or attention to the traditional healing rites that every community turns to when disaster strikes. Thus, for example, sometimes a blanket, a cup of coffee, information about recovery resources, and simple empathy over tragic loss is what is most appreciated.

Most survivors of such life-altering losses can do without the suggestion that they may need "special psychological services." In the case of Haiti, for instance, the "voodoo" religion (with its African and Christian roots) is a deeply embedded cultural tradition of healing that cannot be easily replaced by Western-trained "crisis responders," who may or may not be attuned to the local culture's healing traditions when confronted with recovery from the devastating losses following an earthquake.

Thus, if the hazardous event is a heart attack, loss of home by fire or natural disaster, or failure in school or work, people typically explain the event as part of life, ("things happen," or for someone religious, "God's will"). If a life-threatening medical diagnosis like lung cancer is related to personal behavior such as smoking, or failure in a college test to one's failure to study, the answer to "Why?" is easier to come by, compared with events of socio-cultural origin for which a typical response was "blaming the victim" for the violence rather than holding perpetrators accountable for their behavior.

In those cases, as the crisis paradigm depicts, the triple origins are intertwined, while crisis care strategies should coincide with the interrelated origins. Thus, for example, a woman who feels trapped in an abusive marriage because of gender-based financial constraints may find limited benefits of individual counseling alone, if the socio-cultural roots of her problem are not also acknowledged, such as with suggestions of resources for personal empowerment around her plight, e.g., referral to a battered women's support group.

When that does not happen, a dangerous downward spiral is set in motion (see Figure 3.2) because the power differential makes the crisis recovery process more challenging—that is, a problem rooted in the *socio-cultural* environment cannot be adequately addressed with *individual* action alone. Therefore, if a person is severely traumatized by abuse rooted in cultural values and social norms permitting it over *centuries*, beyond facilitating individual coping strategies, we must direct explicit attention to the socio-cultural origins of the crisis in order to interrupt the self-blaming that often accompanies these crisis events. The potential for preventing morbidity and mortality underscores the importance of interrupting the downward spiral and addressing the roots of a problem as early as possible (see Chapter 5 for a fuller discussion of this point, and intersection with forensic psychiatry).

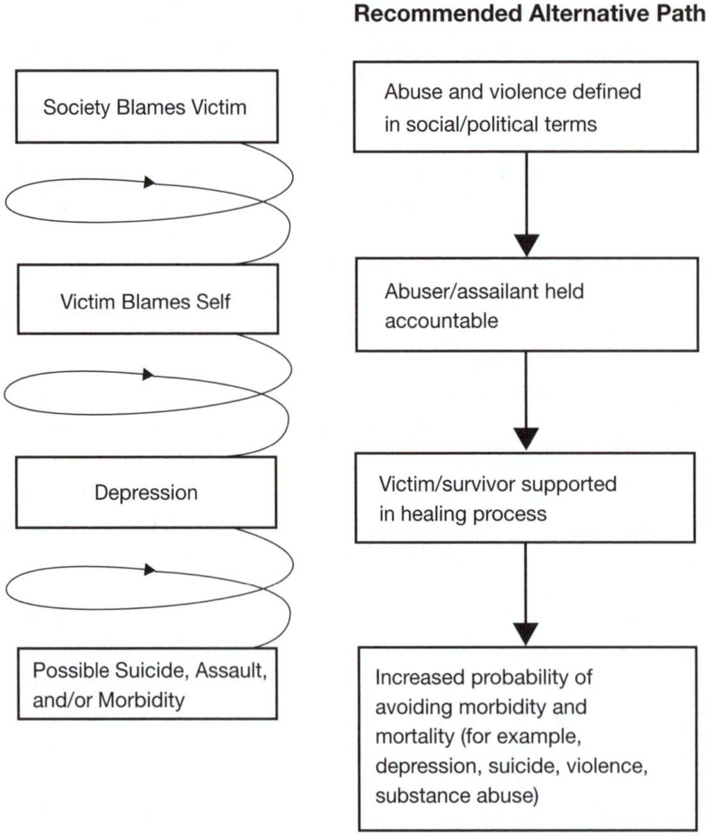

Recommended Alternative Path

Figure 3.2 Abuse, the Downward Spiral, and Alternative Path. *Primary* prevention is ideal, but intervention at *secondary* and *tertiary* levels can also prevent morbidity and save lives.

The crisis paradigm also depicts this important principle: In risk assessment, if medical history reveals serious and persistent mental illness, psychiatric hospitalization, and routine maintenance on psychotropic drugs, such patients are increasingly vulnerable to crisis episodes such as job loss, homelessness, life-threatening upsets with family, etc. (as also revealed in the CMHA Basic Life Attachments and Signals of Distress, Chapter 2). This increased vulnerability to crisis is rooted in (1) the disabling effects of mental illness on self-care, school or employment, and stable social relationships; (2) the lack of sufficient and readily available psychiatric services for many such patients to forestall psychiatric and other life-threatening emergencies; and (3) the global trend toward community-based treatment for all, which often lacks necessary financial support for such service. Box 4b in the paradigm illustrates the propensity for repeat crisis episodes when earlier crisis situations result in negative outcomes—many times for lack of timely crisis intervention.

Together, one result of these factors is psychiatric re-hospitalization and sometimes premature discharge—orchestrated by insurance policies rather than clinical judgment of readiness for discharge—with sometimes tragic outcomes such as violence (Earley, 2006). Predictably, this sad and preventable scenario—traced to the "revolving door" of psychiatric admission and discharge—leaves PCPs in the middle, with major responsibility for psychotropic drug management in an attempt to forestall still another costly psychiatric hospitalization (see Chapters 6, 7, and 8 on anxiety, major depression, and schizophrenia, for detailed discussion of these psychiatric conditions and their treatment in primary care). This is not to say that mentally ill patients should not be treated in primary care settings (see Chapter 1 on interdisciplinary collaboration and Hackley, Sharma, Kedzior & Screenivsan, 2010). Rather, it underscores the need to return to and finally implement nationwide the 1960s ideal of community mental health: i.e., a system in which all people—the usually stable, the disabled, or mentally ill—are entitled to comprehensive services that are smoothly coordinated between medical and mental health facets of the system.

Basic Crisis Assessment Skills: Pre-crisis and Acute Crisis States

Four goals in crisis assessment are paramount for PCPs: (1) to distinguish between healthy and unhealthy responses to whatever has happened; (2) in a related task, ascertain risk to life by suicide or assault on others; (3) acknowledge different levels of assessment in comprehensive crisis care and the particular role of PCPs; (4) to lay the foundation for intervention planning that synchronizes crisis care strategies with the interrelated origins of crisis, as Boxes 1 and 3 of the Crisis Paradigm depict.

Table 3.1 illustrates two levels of assessment and who should do what. The role of PCPs lies squarely in Level 1, based on a vast body of research and clinical practice with this finding: The first contact for most people with *any* problem is not a mental health professional, but rather their physician or clergyperson. This pivotal role of PCPs, however, does not complete the circle of what people in acute crisis need: After initial crisis intervention and safety measures, counseling sessions (up to six or ten) with a crisis specialist or mental health professional are indicated.

But for a variety of reasons (e.g., lack of insurance, resistance to change unhealthy behaviors), this most likely will not occur without commitment to networking and clinical protocols that assure coordination of initial crisis intervention with linkage to follow-up counseling. In other words, PCPs typically are not in a position in terms of either time or professional training to do the whole job of comprehensive crisis care. If they wanted to focus primarily on counseling, they would have chosen a practice arena other than primary care. In most instances, however, without skilled entry-point assessment and safety work in primary care settings, people in crisis can easily "fall through the cracks" of an uncoordinated system, with potentially disastrous results—depending on Level 1 assessment of risk to life.

Table 3.1 Crisis Assessment Levels

	Focus of Assessment	*Assessment Done By*
Level 1	Risk to life • Victimization • Suicide (self) • Assault and/or homicide (against child, partner, parent, health provider, police officer)	Everyone (natural and formal crisis managers) • Family, friends, neighbors • Hotline workers • Frontline workers: clergy, police officers, nurses, physicians, teachers • Crisis and mental health professionals
Level 2	Comprehensive psychological and social aspects of the person's life pertaining to the hazardous event, including assessment of chronic self-harm	Counselors or mental health professionals formally trained in crisis and assessment strategies

As an aid to such assessment, in Chapter 2 we proposed a triage tool (see Box 2.1; Hoff & Rosenbaum, 1994), developed as an adjunct to the original Comprehensive Mental Health Assessment Tool illustrated with the example of Mr. Brady. The intent of this tool is to assure that "risk to life" assessment and immediate safety concerns are integrated with entry point intake protocols, including primary care. This also occurs in emergency settings, with referral to crisis teams.

But beyond emergency care, the basic principle here is to assure that no patient is discharged before such crisis triaging and appropriate linkage to mental health or crisis specialists occurs. Failure to do so is professionally irresponsible and a symptom of the secondary place that mental health often holds in healthcare agencies—a legacy of the historic bias against people needing mental health treatment. There are complex policy implications of holding patients with serious mental illness in emergency settings for hours or even days—usually because psychiatric services are unavailable. Depending on available psychiatric emergency services in particular communities (e.g., large city hospitals may have such *on-site* specialists, while smaller agencies may not), PCPs confronted with an out-of-control patient in primary care may need to call on police if assessment reveals imminent threat to life. Otherwise, it is wise to remember that excessive "power and control" tactics can backfire on the basic human-need principle of personal "self-mastery," and that violence (as in forced constraint) as a response to violence typically begets more violence.

CASE EXAMPLE: MR. BRADY

The interview example of Mr. Brady in Chapter 2 highlights the "signals of distress" noted by psychiatrist Hansell (1976), also referred to as "crisis plumage"—i.e., questions to ask and how to recognize a person in impending or acute crisis and possible risk to life. Information about Mr. Brady from the Triage Tool and Self-Assessment Worksheet revealed the following level of functioning or high stress—ratings number 3 through 5 indicating *Moderate to High Stress and interference with normal functioning*:

Item 11– Leisure Time/Community Involvement: #4 (doesn't enjoy being active anymore)
Item 16—Substance Use: #4 (acknowledges drinking more often and having a few too many)
Item 1—Physical Health: #3 (weight gain, elevated cholesterol, family history of heart disease)

Item 2—Self-acceptance/Self-esteem: #3 (sees himself as good husband and worker . . . does not connect inactivity and drinking with possibility of depression)

Item 10—Life Goals: #3 (more worried about his future than has been willing to admit)

Item 12—Feelings: #3 (worrying more and somewhat distrustful with fellow-workers)

Item 14—Injury to Self: #2. Mr. Brady acknowledges that he has thought about suicide, rating it as low.

Thus, while he is *not* at *immediate risk* of suicide, or otherwise in acute emotional distress, Mr. Brady's ratings on several interrelated factors (self-esteem, feeling expression, laxity with exercise—despite physical and family risk factors for heart disease—plus increased use of alcohol) strongly suggest *underlying emotional issues* about which he could benefit from counseling, and which if not addressed might increase his risk of suicide, as addressed in Chapter 4. Considered together, ratings of 3 or above reveal moderate to high stress levels, and also differentiate between life functions needing *immediate crisis intervention* and underlying problems which, if not addressed, may lead, for example, to suicidal crisis later (see Chapter 2 for Service Plan and Contract with Mr. Brady based on initial assessment).

This case also reveals the PCP's pivotal role in *preventing* crisis through smoothly coordinated referral to a mental health provider, and reassuring Mr. Brady that counseling is important to his overall health. Mr. Brady's case also shows that his acceptance of a referral may not have occurred apart from the good rapport he has with the PCP; that is, when the PCP says explicitly: "I cannot provide you with the counseling that I think you need," he rather grudgingly acknowledges to the PCP that he is a "little depressed," is drinking too much, losing interest in life, and "maybe my wife was right" in suggesting he see a psychiatrist— the very issue presented on admission to primary care!

Crisis Intervention Strategies in Primary Care: Mental Health Linkage and Follow-up

The basics of psychosocial assessment and crisis work in primary care include these essentials:

1. detection of pre-crisis and crisis state through routine inquiry in health assessment protocols, such as the CMHA tool (see Chapter 2);
2. assessment of emotional trauma from victimization and danger of self-injury and/or violence toward others;
3. differentiating between effective and ineffective coping with trauma and crisis;
4. empathic, supportive response to personal emotional pain and the PCP's *public* recognition of trauma from abuse to deflect from self-blame, and place accountability with the perpetrator (see Figure 3.2, the Downward Spiral);
5. safety planning for self, and in cases of violence, any affected children;
6. linkage, referral, and follow-up (with crisis, mental health, and/or trauma specialist);
7. careful monitoring of and coordination with crisis counselors if psychotropic drug prescriptions are indicated.

Let us now consider these elements of crisis care in primary care settings, continuing with the examples of Karen and Robert. Our focus here builds on Box 2 in the Crisis Paradigm: Ascertaining which of the *typical* manifestations of people in crisis—emotional, biophysical, cognitive, and behavioral—apply to a particular individual presenting in primary care, thus laying the foundation for next steps in the crisis care process and *distinguishing between PCP and mental health specialist roles*. Here are examples of questions that can uncover a person's emotional, cognitive, and behavioral responses to distress or trauma: "How do you feel about what happened?" Or, if feelings are already expressed spontaneously: "I can see that you're really upset . . . What did you do when she told you she wanted a divorce? Did you ever consider striking back physically when he abused you?"

CASE EXAMPLES: EARLY INTERVENTION IN PRIMARY CARE

Karen: A Battered Woman (continued)

As noted in the Phases of Crisis Development section, except for rapport with the PCP who asked "What happened?" someone like Karen might have gone to the ER again and offered a cover-up story. While providing support ("I'm so sorry . . .") the PCP should avoid saying "Nobody deserves to be hit or beaten like that." The rationale for avoiding this cliché is this: Some women abused over time come to believe that they *do* "deserve" what they got, because the perpetrator's repeated abuse so erodes her self-esteem that she comes to believe it.

In a busy, time-limited primary care setting, it is inappropriate to attempt to uncover and respond to such underlying dynamics, or to a victim's self-blame for the injury. This is properly the goal of follow-up counseling by violence or trauma specialists. A more appropriate response in primary care is something like this: "What your husband did to you was not right . . . in fact, it's against the law." Or if Karen blames herself for what happened, one might say, "You know, Karen, none of us is perfect, but no matter what you did or said, violence is not acceptable and your husband is responsible for his behavior, not you."

After examining and treating the injured eye, the PCP proceeds with the other triage questions, and also inquires whether her three children (ages seven, five, and two) have ever been witnesses to his violence, and what she has considered doing beyond her belief that he would keep his promises and eventually change. She has never considered suicide "for the sake of the children," says that the abuse has been going on for four years, and occurred only twice in the children's presence.

The PCP says in a non-accusing tone: "Karen, I can see now why you asked me for a tranquilizer last year . . . but I'm really glad you came here today instead of the ER . . . I can see that you've done everything you could to stop his violence, but you know, Karen, you can't really force him to change if he's not motivated to do it on his own." Karen starts to cry. The PCP listens, and says again, "I'm so sorry this has happened to you, Karen, and I know you want to save your marriage. But I'm concerned for your safety and the harmful effects on your children." The PCP then informs Karen about the special services for victim/survivors of domestic violence, and asks her to look over a brochure for same. Karen accepts the PCP's recommendation for an appointment the same day with the trauma/domestic violence counseling service, and also arranges a follow-up visit with the PCP in two weeks. The trauma specialist follows up with immediate safety planning and crisis counseling (see Chapter 5).

Robert: Facing Divorce Threat after Heart Attack (continued)

Robert, age 50, thought he had a reasonably good relationship with his wife, but since their two children completed college and moved out-of-state, had noticed in recent months that she seemed distant and disinterested in doing any of the things they had previously enjoyed—including a satisfying sex life which, however, was cut back temporarily after his heart attack. While Robert had vague suspicions that his wife was cheating on him, he put them aside, refusing to believe that the mother of his children would walk out on him "just like that!" Nor did he want to imagine life without her.

On triage questioning, Robert revealed that he did think about suicide, but had no immediate plan, and that he also never fantasized about hurting his wife despite his suspicions. Robert has basically healthy coping skills; for example, he immediately called on his sister for support after getting the shocking news from his wife. He also refrained from calling his children out of concern for fatherly protection and recognizing their good relationship with their mother. Robert's decision to see his primary care provider, even without an appointment, after a couple of beers was a wise first step in dealing with the shock of his wife's refusal to "talk things out" and maybe see a marriage counselor.

After receiving further emotional support from his PCP, Robert was glad and very relieved for a recommendation of a crisis counselor who could help him through the next few weeks of totally unexpected emotional pain, as well as the opportunity to examine and decide with an empathic person his next steps in re-building his life. Given Robert's history, evidence of healthy coping during acute stress, and ready acceptance of help, his prospects of finding a new and satisfying life look promising.

Crisis Counseling Strategies and Coordination with Primary Care

While the professional counseling indicated for Robert and Karen are properly the realm of mental health and crisis specialists, such services may be under-utilized but for the sound relationship these clients have with a PCP, who facilitates such linkage and continues with the medical care needed. Many call this "holistic" care; i.e., attention to the whole person, not just a physical illness or a serious psychiatric disorder such as schizophrenia, or a crisis of psychosocial origins.

To bolster the PCP's knowledge base and confidence in *facilitating a client's acceptance of referral and linkage for follow-up counseling*, we present a summary of the major facets of crisis counseling beyond what can be provided in primary care and emergency settings:

1. Assist the person through grief work; since loss or threat of loss is a common characteristic of the crisis experience, grieving includes the following:

   - acceptance of the pain of loss; includes dealing with memories of the deceased or other acute loss, e.g., Robert's anticipated loss of his marriage;
   - open expression of pain, sorrow, hostility and feelings of guilt; the person must feel free to mourn loss openly, usually by weeping, and to express feelings of guilt;
   - understanding the intense feelings associated with the loss, e.g., fear of going crazy, as a normal part of the grieving process; ritual expression, as in funerals or a "divorce party," greatly aids in this process;
   - eventual resumption of normal activities and social relationships without the lost person, property, or characteristic such as bodily integrity after surgery, or performance as a worker or student.

2. Be observant for the signs of unresolved grief and depression; e.g., listlessness, prolonged sadness, lack of energy for one's usual functions (school or work), loss of appetite and sexual interest, amenorrhea, sleeplessness and/or early morning waking, suicidal ideation. In such situations, collaboration between the crisis counselor and PCP may result in consideration of anti-depressant medication (see Chapters 4 and 7).
3. Listen actively, with empathy and concern.
4. Encourage the open expression of feelings such as anger, fear, desire for revenge, or misdirected self-blame following abuse.

5. Help the person gain an understanding of the crisis and explore the *meaning* of the hazardous event leading to crisis in relation to one's values and life goals.
6. Help the individual gradually accept reality (e.g., acute loss, abuse, abandonment by parent or spouse, life-threatening danger in the event of an abusive relationship).
7. Explore with the person new ways of coping with problems and avoiding destructive responses such as substance abuse or retaliatory violence.
8. Help the person to link and reengage with supportive resources such as friends, or to find a substitute social network in the event of social isolation following loss or abandonment.
9. Engage the person in decision counseling; for example: What does the person need to go on? What will he or she do, and in what time frame? Who is available for support?
10. Reinforce newly learned coping devices.
11. Agree on a follow-up plan after resolution of the crisis. This should include coordination with the referring PCP, especially when serious medical treatment and psychotropic drug use are part of the overall healthcare plan.

The PCP's knowledge of these basic crisis counseling approaches will also serve to coordinate the medical and mental health facets of treatment. Finally, since there is no such thing as a "perfect counselor or therapist," or the client fails to follow through with counseling, the PCP can encourage continuation or facilitate arrangement for another counselor if the client's dissatisfaction with a counselor appears to be legitimate relative to crisis care standards.

Psychotropic Medication in Crisis Care

Primary care providers are already knowledgeable about the two main drugs that may be indicated for persons in acute crisis—anti-anxiety agents and anti-depressants. Here we offer a brief summary of principles for the responsible use of these drugs in primary care, and cautionary notes about their potential for misuse (or even illegal use) by a person already addicted.

In a culture bombarded with advertisements for drugs as a solution for everyday problems, and a healthcare system in which PCPs are forced into very limited time slots for listening and empathic response to highly distressed persons, the prescription of an anti-anxiety agent can be used as a way out of a crisis situation with potentially life-and-death implications. Combine these cultural and health policy facets with a client in denial about underlying emotional and/or substance abuse problems now presenting in acute crisis, but with a history of little or no motivation to engage in counseling to address these problems, and PCPs are confronted with a potentially dangerous situation. We offer these guidelines and instances for use of an anti-anxiety agent or sleep aid to alleviate acute emotional distress, sleeping problems related to pain, depression, and related problems:

1. when a person is experiencing extreme anxiety, has frequent crying spells, or fears losing control of impulses toward self-harm or hurting others;
2. when a person in acute crisis is so distraught that it is impossible to engage him or her in the problem-solving process;
3. when a person's acute anxiety prevents sleep for a significant period of time.

However, persons unmotivated to deal with underlying problems through counseling may use these psychotropic agents as a way to further avoid counseling or psychotherapy. Or if the person is already chronically dependent on alcohol and other substances as a substitute for healthy problem-solving, a drug prescription offers temporary anxiety relief, but can *increase danger* rather than helping a person in acute crisis to use the occasion as an *opportunity for psychosocial growth.* Primary care providers should therefore use the power of their relationship with clients to persuade them to accept referrals for mental health counseling. This includes limiting a prescription to a short period of time to protect against use for suicide overdose, and with a contingency of evidence that the client has followed through with a referral for counseling. See Chapter 4 for use of anti-depressants for suicidal patients. Early follow-up appointments are critical for these clients presenting in primary care. See also Chapters 6 and 7.

References

Antonovsky, A. (1980). *Health, stress, and coping*. San Francisco. Jossey-Bass.

Caplan, G. (1964). *Principles of preventive psychiatry*. New York: Basic Books.

Earley, P. (2006). *Crazy: A father's search through America's mental health madness*. New York: Berkley Books.

Hackley, B., Sharma, C., Kedzior, A., & Screenivsan, S. (2010). Managing mental health conditions in primary care settings. *Journal of Midwifery & Women's Health*, 55(1), 9–19.

Hansell, N. (1976). *The person in distress*. New York: Human Sciences Press.

Hoff, L.A. (1990). *Battered women as survivors*. London: Routledge.

Hoff, L.A., Hallisey, B.J., & Hoff, M. (2009). *People in crisis: Clinical and diversity perspectives* (6th ed). New York: Routledge.

Hoff, L.A., & Rosenbaum, L.. (1994). A victimization assessment tool: Instrument development and clinical implications. *Journal of Advanced Nursing*, 20(4), 627–634.

Lifton, R.J., & Olson, E. (1976). The human meaning of total disaster: The Buffalo Creek experience. *Psychiatry*, 39, 1–18.

Parad, H. (Ed.). (1965). *Crisis intervention: Selected readings*. New York: Family Service Association of America.

4 Suicidal and Self-destructive Persons

Some people respond to life crises by suicide or other self-destructive acts. Primary care providers are pivotal in helping patients find alternatives to such behavior. Suicide as a response to crisis is used by all classes and kinds of people with social, mental, emotional, and physical problems—possibly including our relatives and neighbors. In short, people of every age, sex, religion, race, sexual identity, and socioeconomic class commit suicide. Perhaps most important of all, in the ethic of most world religions, suicide is generally considered the most stigmatizing sort of death, while suicide prevention is a major public health goal (Wasserman, 2004). In this chapter, suicide and self-destructive behavior are discussed in the contexts of the Judeo-Christian value system and the development of social science, crisis theory, and public health (see Figure 3.1, the Crisis Paradigm, Box 3 and 4b, Chapter 3.)

Incidence and Framework for Understanding Self-destructive Behavior

Suicide is viewed as a major public health problem and leading cause of death in many countries. Suicide among adolescents and young adults continues as a serious problem. The highest rates of suicide in the United States are among older white males (Moscicki, 1999, p. 41). Adolescent suicides constitute about 20% of all suicides nationwide. Among black men, American Indian, and Alaska Natives, however, the highest rates occur between ages

---

* Parts of this chapter are excerpted from Hoff, Hallisey, & Hoff, 2009, *People in crisis: Clinical and diversity perspectives*, 6th Edition, Chapters 9 and 10, and edited for application in primary care practice. Used with permission.

20 and 29 (Moscicki, 1999, p. 41). This suggests racial minority groups' continuing struggle with devastating social and individual circumstances.

There is a strong association between suicide risk and bisexuality in males that is only recently commanding research attention (Remafedi, French, Story, Resnick, & Blum, 1998). Homosexuals are estimated to account for 30 percent of adolescent suicides, despite constituting only 5 to 10 percent of the general population (Remafedi, Farrow, & Deisher, 1991). The rate of suicide for all ages and groups in the United States is about 12 per 100,000 (approximately 30,000 annually) and has remained relatively constant over several decades (National Center for Health Statistics, 2004) (Only those statistical figures reflecting broad trends or changes are cited here. For current official government statistics in the U.S. and internationally, readers are referred to internet sources, e.g., Center for Disease Control [CDC]; and World Health Organization [WHO]).

In the United States, firearms are the suicide method of choice for both men and women, whereas the second most common method used by men is hanging and by women is poisoning. White women's rates peak at around age 50, whereas rates for nonwhite women remain low and fairly constant through old age. Internationally, the wide range of suicide rates reveals further the complexity of the suicide problem. In Canada, the age-adjusted suicide rate is 13.6. In England, France, Italy, Denmark, and Japan, the rates for men are consistently higher than for women. England has the lowest rate for old people, Hungary the highest rates in the world, and Italy the lowest rate for the young.

Suicide attempts occur at least ten times more frequently than suicides, with a total of approximately 300,000 annually in the U.S. Among adolescents, particularly females, the attempt rate may be 20 to 50 times higher. Many of these adolescents have been physically or sexually abused. Stephens' research (1985, 1987) on suicidal women reveals strong links to conflict and abuse in intimate relationships. She suggests that women with histories of exaggerated passivity may be at greater risk of suicide than those who are rebellious. Women have higher rates of depression than men, which are commonly attributed to socioeconomic disparities (Badger, McNiece, & Gagan, 2000). However, research remains to be done on why greater numbers of women who are abused or otherwise disadvantaged do *not* kill themselves.

In the year 2000, approximately one million people died by suicide, a "global" mortality rate of 16 per 100,000. Over the past several decades suicide rates have increased by 60% worldwide, although some of this increase may be attributed to more accurate reporting related to public health attention to the issue. Suicide is among the three leading causes of death for both sexes aged 15–44 (WHO, retrieved 2008). Because reporting systems differ widely, there are probably more suicides than are reported. Cultural taboos, insurance policies, and other factors strongly influence the reporting of suicide. In Japan, there are no religious or state laws banning suicide; hence a significant number of internet-assisted group suicides occur there (Samuels, 2007).

Perspectives, Facts, and Feelings about Self-destructive Persons

A psychosociocultural perspective is most helpful in understanding suicide. Inasmuch as suicide has occurred since the beginning of recorded history, a preventive model contrasts with the tendency to treat suicide primarily as a result of mental illness. Suicide most often occurs during periods of socio-economic, family, and individual crisis situations (WHO, retrieved 2008). Thus, a preventive model should be front and center with treatment of disorders such as subclinical depression or major depressive disorder (MDD) (see Chapter 7).

Nearly everyone has had contact with self-destructive people. Besides suicide and suicide attempts, some people slowly destroy themselves by excessive drinking or abuse of other drugs. Among primary care patients, a certain percentage will have responded to a life crisis by some kind of self-destructive act. Despite public education campaigns to dispel common myths about suicide (Motto, 1999; Shneidman, 1981, pp. 213–214), here are facts that require our attention:

- Although people who commit suicide are usually in emotional turmoil, diagnosable mental illness is not the dominant factor in most suicides.
- Suicide cuts across class, race, age, and sex differences, while comfortable circumstances (e.g., good home and job) do not prevent suicide, as in "Why? He had everything going for him" following the suicide of a talented student.
- Although a significant number of people with sexual identity crisis commit suicide or make suicide attempts, they do so most often because of the prejudice, hatred, and sometimes violence they have endured from mainstream society.
- People who die by suicide almost invariably *talk about suicide or give clues and warnings about their intention* through their behavior, although the clues may not be recognized at the time.
- The majority of people who succeed in killing themselves have a history of previous suicide attempts. Ignoring this history may precipitate another attempt.
- Suicide is much too complex a process to occur as a result of a caring person asking a question about suicidal intent, as in "I'm afraid of putting the idea into his or her head."
- A person's mood or energy level is subjective and difficult to assess. People may kill themselves when depressed or following improvement; *frequent and repeated assessment* is therefore indicated, regardless of the level of depression.

Regardless of these facts, cultural taboos and the strong feelings most people have about suicide, death, and dying may inhibit PCPs from learning more about self-destructive people. After a suicide, several feelings are common among survivors, including PCPs who provided medical services before a patient's death: *anxiety* that something we did or did not do caused the suicide; *relief,* which is not uncommon among family members or therapists who have exhausted themselves trying to help the suicidal person; or *guilt,* which often follows feelings of disgust or relief that the desperate person has died.

Understanding these feelings is crucial if we are to help distressed people find alternatives to suicide. Three perspectives are useful here: social, psychological, and cultural.

Social Perspective

The frustration of PCPs in working with self-destructive people can be traced, in part, to the socialization professionals receive in their role of helping a sick person return to health. Success in this role depends partly on whether patients behave according to expectations of people in the "sick role"—originally defined from the study of people in physically ill conditions (Parsons, 1951, pp. 436–437).

This "sick role" concept is unproblematic if applied to a patient's response to acute pain caused by a fracture or kidney stones. But if so-called "social" illnesses (e.g. STDs) do not fit the traditional sick role–helper model, think of the model's limitations when applied to a person who is self-destructive! Not only do suicidal people defeat the medical role of fostering and maintaining life, but self-injury appears to deliberately flout the natural instinct to live. The self-destructive person is requesting, directly or indirectly, a departure from the usual roles of patient and health service provider. Thus, if helping is limited to medical treatment when the problem is as *philosophical, religious, and social as it is medical*, the trouble that PCPs may encounter when treating suicidal persons is understandable. Attention to these social and sick role concepts is particularly relevant in a time-constrained healthcare system that provides limited insurance coverage for "talk" therapies.

Psychological Perspective

Role conflicts are complicated further if health providers have an unrecognized or excessive need to be needed or to rescue a self-destructive person. Not only is a PCP denied the fulfillment of traditional role expectations, but the suicidal person says, in effect, "I don't need you. How can you save me when I don't even want to save myself?" This is a very good question, considering what we know about the failure of medical treatment or psychotherapy without the client's voluntary collaboration.

The most complex manifestation of the social psychological roots of conflict with suicidal people is in the victim–rescuer–persecutor triangle drawn from transactional analysis (see Hoff, *et al.*, 2009, p. 131). Of all the phases of crisis work, most important here is a provider's sensitivity to a person's basic need for self-mastery, and to control any counter-productive rescue fantasies. Not to do so could result in a vicious cycle of results that is exactly the opposite of our intentions:

- Our misguided rescue attempts are rejected.
- We feel frustrated in our helper role.
- We persecute the suicidal person for failing to cooperate.
- The suicidal person feels rejected.
- The suicidal person repeats the self-injury.
- The helper feels like a victim.

Preventing and interrupting the victim–rescuer–persecutor cycle is one of the most challenging tasks in dealing with self-destructive people.

Cross-cultural Perspective

Suicide universally conveys the value that "death is preferred over life," and has been part of the human condition from the beginning of time. However, particular belief systems will influence how and why suicide occurs and is interpreted in various non-Western societies.

Self-destructive behavior takes on added meaning when placed in a cultural–historical perspective. Views about it—whether it is honorable or shameful—have always varied. In the Judeo-Christian tradition, neither the Hebrew Bible nor the New Testament prohibits suicide. Jews (defenders of Masada) and Christians (martyrs) alike justified suicide in the face of military defeat or personal attack by pagans. Later, however, suicide took on the character of a sinful act. The religious standpoint is complemented now by legal and medical perspectives, with suicide today seen less as a moral offense than as a socially disgraceful act, a response to crisis, or a manifestation of psychiatric illness.

These social, psychological, and cultural facts of life are even more complex when considering the multi-ethnicity of North American and European societies, and an emphasis on preserving one's unique cultural heritage. Dealing with feelings then is a necessary first step towards helping people in suicidal crisis. Team relationships, peer support groups, and readily accessible consultation are also pivotal for PCPs treating self-destructive persons.

Ethical Issues Regarding Suicide

Closely related to coping with feelings about self-destructive behavior is one's position on the right to die and the degree of responsibility for the lives of others. Primary care providers should be familiar with these hotly debated topics (Battin, 1980; Humphrey, 1992; Richman, 1992):

- the right to die by suicide;
- the right to physician-assisted suicide;
- the right and the responsibility to prevent suicide;
- the right to euthanasia and abortion (related topics).

Several ethical and legal questions have implications for PCPs:

- How do we respond to a person's declaration: "I have the right to commit suicide, and you don't have the right to stop me"?
- If our own belief system forbids suicide, how might this belief influence our response to such a person?
- If a person commits suicide, whose responsibility is it?
- If we happen to believe the suicidal person alone is responsible, why do we often feel guilty after a suicide?
- What is the ethical basis for depriving a person of normal, individual rights by commitment to a mental health facility to prevent suicide?
- What do we do if someone close to us requests our assistance in committing suicide?

The intent of these questions is to provide an ethical basis for dealing with these issues without either abandoning our own cherished beliefs or imposing them on others.

Opinions differ regarding the issue of responsibility to save others, the right to determine one's own death, and differentiating between adults and children in regard to rights and responsibilities. The *ethical* and *legal* aspects of certain issues must be distinguished. For example, many people believe that suicide is ethically acceptable in certain circumstances, but regardless of personal beliefs, it is illegal in the United States and in most other countries to assist another in the act of suicide. The passage in Oregon, Washington, and Montana of a ballot measure allowing physician-assisted suicide is an exception to this rule, as is the case in several European countries. Other states are considering similar legislation. Primary care providers must consider the relevance of these debates to their everyday practice with suicidal people. The following case illustrates some of the ethical questions.

CASE EXAMPLE: JOHN—MENTAL HEALTH COMMITMENT

John, age 48, was diagnosed with ALS (Lou Gehrig's disease), and referred to psychiatric services when he became highly suicidal after learning about his wife's death in a car accident. He also had a substance abuse problem, and went on a drinking binge after getting this additional shocking news. He was committed involuntarily to a psychiatric facility with the goal of preventing him from committing suicide. John found the hospital worse than anything he had experienced. John had two very close friends and a small business of his own, but had no contact with his friends while in the hospital. After two weeks, John begged to be discharged. He was no longer highly suicidal but was still depressed. He was discharged with antidepressant medication and instructed to return for a follow-up appointment in one week. John killed himself with sleeping pills (obtained from his primary care provider) and alcohol two days after discharge. The PCP and staff of the mental hospital did not understand how they had failed John.

John's eventual suicide illustrates the care that must be taken in implementing mental health laws on behalf of suicidal people. First of all, the decision to commit a person must be based on a thorough assessment. Second, even if John had been found to be a serious risk for suicide, involuntary hospitalization seemed to contribute to rather than prevent John's suicide. Hospitalization is indicated for suicidal people only when natural social network resources (such as John's friends) are not present.

We offer the following practical guideline to PCPs with respect to rights and responsibilities regarding suicide: each person has the final responsibility for his or her own life, including the right to live as one chooses or to end life. With others, PCPs have a communal responsibility to prevent suicide when it appears to be against a person's own best interests—for example, when suffering from major depression without the benefit of treatment. It also involves examining values and social practices that inadvertently lead people to choose suicide only because they are socially disadvantaged and see no other way out. If ethical arguments do not support legalized physician-assisted suicide, neither does an economic argument. Emanuel and Battin (1998) found that in the wealthy United States, total end-of-life healthcare expenditures would be reduced by only 0.07% if physician-assisted suicide were legalized. The choice of assisted suicide in these instances is not truly free. Our social responsibility does not require that we prevent a suicide at all costs. We need to recognize that misguided savior tactics can result in suicide if overbearing help is interpreted as *control*. However, PCPs have the additional responsibility to learn as much as they can about self-destructive people, and advocate strongly to help a despairing patient find alternatives to suicide.

Characteristics and Major Types of Self-destructive People

To be understood is basic to the feeling that someone cares, that life is worth living. When someone responds to stress with a deliberate suicide attempt, those around the person are usually dismayed and ask *why*. The wide range of self-destructive acts adds to the observer's confusion, especially when considering the many overlapping features of self-destructive behavior. For example, Mary, age 50, has been destroying herself through alcohol abuse for 15 years, but she also takes an overdose of sleeping pills during an acute crisis.

The majority of adolescents who harm themselves have had serious personal, emotional, or behavioral problems. Volumes have been written about suicide—by philosophers, the clergy, psychiatrists and psychologists, nurses, and crisis specialists who have varied opinions regarding the process, meanings, morality, and reasons involved in self-destruction. The focus here is on the *meaning* of self-destructive behavior and the importance of understanding and reaching out to those in emotional pain: the "hurt, anguish, or ache that takes hold of the mind. It is intrinsically psychological; it is the . . . pain of negative emotions, such as guilt, shame, anguish, fear, panic, anger, loneliness, helplessness . . . Suicide occurs when the *psychache* is deemed to be unbearable and when death is actively sought in order to stop the unceasing flow of intolerable consciousness," as described by suicidology founder Edwin Shneidman (1999, pp. 86–87). Our effectiveness in working with suicidal people requires knowledge of these aspects of self-destructive behavior:

- the range and complexity of self-destructive behavior;
- communication and the meaning of self-destructive behavior;
- ambivalence and its relevance to suicide prevention;

- the importance of assessing for suicidal risk;
- sensitivity to ethical and cultural issues as an aid to understanding, assessment, and appropriate intervention.

Self-destructiveness: What Does It Include?

Self-destructive behavior includes any action by which a person emotionally, socially, and physically damages or ends his or her life. The spectrum of self-destructiveness includes biting nails, pulling hair, scratching, cutting one's wrist, swallowing toxic substances or harmful objects, smoking cigarettes, banging one's head, abusing alcohol and other drugs, driving recklessly, neglecting life-preserving measures such as taking insulin, attempting suicide, and committing suicide (Farberow, 1980; Menninger, 1938).

At one end of the spectrum of self-destructiveness is Jane, who smokes but is in essentially good emotional and physical health. She knows the long-range effects of smoking and chooses to live her life in such a way that may in fact shorten it. However, on a lethality assessment scale, Jane would hardly be regarded as suicidal. Smoking by Arthur, who has severe emphysema, is another matter. His behavior could be considered a slow form of deliberate self-destruction. At the other end of the spectrum is James, who plans to hang himself. Unless saved accidentally, James will most certainly die by his own hand.

There are four broad groups of self-destructive people:

1. *Those who commit suicide.* Suicide is defined as a fatal act that is self-inflicted, *consciously intended*, and carried out with the knowledge that death is irreversible. This definition of suicide generally excludes young children because a child's conception of death as final develops around age ten (Pfeffer, 1986). If full information is not available about the person's intentions, it is difficult to determine whether the act is suicidal or accidental. Suicide is not an illness or an inherited disease, as popular opinion and some professional practice seem to imply.

2. *Those who threaten suicide.* This group includes people who talk about suicide and whose suicidal plans may be either *very vague* or *highly specific*; some have made suicide attempts in the past; others have not. All suicide threats should be taken seriously and considered in relation to the person's intention and social circumstances.

3. *Those who make suicide attempts.* A suicide attempt is any nonfatal act of self-inflicted damage with self-destructive intention, however vague or ambiguous. It can also be inferred from behavior. Technically, the term *suicide attempt* should be reserved for those actions in which a person attempts to carry out the *intention* to die but for unanticipated reasons, such as failure of the method or an unplanned rescue, the attempt fails. Other self-destructive behavior can more accurately be defined as *self-injury*—a neutral term we should substitute for the term *suicide gesture* which suggests that the behavior need not be taken seriously or that the person is "just seeking attention."

   Some suicidal persons are in a state of acute crisis—in contrast to some who are chronically self-destructive—and therefore experience a high degree of emotional turmoil. As discussed in Chapter 3, such turmoil makes it difficult for a person to clarify his or her intentions, or it may interfere with making wise decisions about marriage, moving, etc. Certainly, then, it is unwise to make an irrevocable decision such as suicide when in a state of emotional turmoil and crisis.

   The ambiguity arising out of the crisis state should not be confused with a psychotic process, which may or may not be present. Despite issues of impulse control, in the large majority of instances self-destructive behavior is something that people *consciously and deliberately plan and execute.*

4 *Those who are chronically self-destructive.* People in this group may habitually abuse alcohol or other drugs and are often diagnosed with personality disorders. Of special concern to PCPs are people who may destroy themselves by deliberate refusal to follow life-sustaining medical programs for such conditions as heart disease or diabetes. While these behaviors are not explicitly suicidal, individuals who engage in them may become overtly suicidal, thus complicating whatever medical problems already exist.

The concept of *suicidal careers* (Maris, 1981, pp. 62–69) can be seen as "one product of a gradual loss of hope and the will and resources to live, a kind of running down and out of life energies, a bankruptcy of psychic defenses against death and decay" (p. 69). Or as Shneidman (1987) puts it, "People reach 'the point of no return' in response to unendurable psychological pain."

PCPs must distinguish between self-destructive persons and those who engage in *self-mutilating activity* (for example, cutting, scraping, and bruising) that generally has no dire medical consequences, although some may end up killing themselves. Unlike suicidal behavior, self-mutilation typically does not involve an intent to die; rather, it is a way of coping and is usually employed by women. Many of these women are survivors of extreme childhood sexual abuse who have internalized their oppression (see Burstow, 1992, pp. 187–220; Everett & Gallop, 2000).

The Path to Suicide

Suicidal behavior can be viewed on a continuum or as a *highway leading to suicide.* The highway begins with the first suicide threat or attempt and ends in suicide. As in the case of any trip destined for a certain end point, one can always change one's mind, take a different road to another destination, or turn around and come back. The highway to suicide can be conceived either as a short trip—acute crisis—or as a long trip—chronic self-destructiveness extending for years or over a lifetime. But in either case, it suggests that suicide is a process involving:

- one's perception of the meaning of life and death;
- availability of psychological and social resources;
- material and physical circumstances making self-destruction possible (for example, when a gun or pills are available or when a bedridden, helpless person is capable of self-destruction only through starvation).

The continuum concept is also useful in understanding suicides that appear to result from impulsive action, as sometimes happens with adolescents. Even with adolescent suicides, though, examination and hindsight usually reveal a process including, for example, alienation, an acute loss, developmental issues, family conflict, abuse, depression, self-doubt, and cynicism about life.

A destiny of suicide is not inevitable. Whether one continues down the highway to suicide depends on a variety of circumstances. People traveling this highway usually give clues to their distress, so *the suicide continuum can be interrupted at any point*: after a first attempt, a fifth attempt, or as soon as clues are recognized. Much depends on the help available and the ability of the suicidal person to accept and use help. It is never too late to help a despairing person or to change one's mind about suicide.

People who repeatedly injure themselves may be labeled and written off as manipulators or attention seekers. This usually means family members and/or PCPs may conclude that a person who was really serious about suicide would try something that "really did the job."

Individuals thus labeled and ignored will probably continue to injure themselves with progressively more serious medical consequences, signaling increasing desperation for someone to hear and understand their cries for help. They may also engage in the "no-lose game" (Baechler, 1979) which goes something like this: "If they (spouse, friend, family) find me, they care enough and therefore life is worth living. (I win by living.) If they don't find me, life isn't worth living. (I win by dying.)" In the no-lose game, the suicide method chosen is usually lethal but includes the possibility of rescue, such as swallowing pills. No-lose reasoning is ineffective in instances when one cannot reasonably expect rescue (for example, a family member rarely checks a person at two o'clock in the morning). It nevertheless indicates the person's extreme distress and illustrates the logic of the no-lose game.

The Messages of Self-destructive People

Interrupting the continuum or path to suicide depends on understanding and responding appropriately to messages of psychic pain, distress, or despair.

Typically, the communication problems of suicidal people follow two general patterns:

1. In the first pattern, people habitually refrain from expressing feelings and sharing their concerns with significant others, and use the "stiff upper lip" approach to life's problems. Suicide by a person in this group elicits great shock and consternation: "He seemed to have everything. I wonder why. There doesn't seem to be any reason." Yet hindsight usually reveals that there were clues that went unrecognized. Subtle changes in behavior, along with a tendency to repress feelings, there are quiet cries for help, often with no explicit history of suicidal behavior.
2. The second pattern of communication problems is less subtle than the first. Typically, people in this group threaten suicide or have actually injured themselves.

After a person's first suicide attempt, family members and others are usually shocked and more disturbed by a suicide attempt than by anything else the person might have done. Typically, a parent, spouse, friend, or the PCP will say, "I knew she was upset and not exactly happy, but I didn't know she was *that* unhappy." In other words, the first suicide attempt is the most powerful of a series of behavioral messages or clues given over a period of time, such as:

*   "You won't be seeing me around much anymore."
*   "I've about had it with this job. I can't take it anymore."
*   "I'm angry at my mother. She'll really be sorry when I'm dead."
*   "I can't take any more problems without some relief," and may request psychotropic medication from a PCP.
*   "I can't live without my boyfriend. I don't really want to die; I just want him back or somebody in his place."
*   "I can't take the pain and humiliation [from AIDS, for example] anymore."
*   "There's nothing else left since my wife left me. I really want to die."

Behavioral clues may include making out a will, taking out a large life insurance policy, giving away precious belongings, being despondent after a financial setback, or engaging in unusual behavior.

These behavioral, verbal, and affective clues can be interpreted in two general ways: (1) "I want to die," or (2) "I don't want to die, but *I want something to change in order to go on living*," or "If things don't change, life isn't worth living. Help me find something to live for." We can ascertain the *meaning* of suicidal behavior and to identify clues in the distressed person's words and attitudes by *asking*, for example:

• "What do you mean when you say you can't take your problems anymore? Are you thinking of suicide?"
• "What did you hope would happen when you took the pills (or cut your wrists)? Did you intend to die?"

There is no substitute for *simple, direct communication* by a PCP or other person who cares. Besides providing important clinical information, this tells the person we are interested and concerned about her or his motives for the contemplated suicide. Experience reveals that suicidal people are relieved when someone like a PCP is sensitive enough to detect and respond to their despair and help protect them from themselves—including referral for counseling—after initial risk assessment and crisis intervention.

Assessing Suicide Risk and Lethality Levels

While the range of various self-destructive behaviors is very broad, (e.g., substance abuse, failure to take medicine for diabetes or heart disease), the focus here is on ascertaining the immediate and longer-term danger of death by suicide among clients served in primary care.

The Importance of Risk Assessment

The importance of suicide risk assessment can be compared with the importance of diag-nosing a cough before beginning treatment. Failure to assess the degree of suicide risk can result in failure to institute follow-up counseling following emergency medical treatment for self-injury. Another problem arising out of guesswork about suicide risk is unnecessary hospitalization. It is inappropriate to hospitalize a suicidal person when the degree of suicide risk is very low and other sources of protection are available. A person who hopes, by a suicide attempt, to relieve isolation from family may feel even more isolated in a psychiatric hospital, as the case of John, (page 68) illustrates. This is especially true when community and family intervention are indicated instead.

Sometimes health providers hospitalize suicidal people because of their own anxiety about suicide. Unresolved feelings of guilt and responsibility about suicide usually precipitate such action. Conversely, hospitals can be places in which isolation can be relieved and suicide prevented when social supports in the community are lacking. As with personal factors, assumptions about the presence or absence of social supports should not be made without a systematic psychosocial assessment (see Chapter 2).

Ascertaining Client Ambivalence: Weighing Life and Death

Suicidal people usually struggle with two irreconcilable wishes—the desire to live and the desire to die—that is, *ambivalence*. As long as the person is ambivalent about life and death, it is possible to help the individual consider choosing life over death. Suicide is not inevitable. Desperate people can change their minds if they find realistic alternatives to suicide.

The concept of ambivalence is basic to suicide prevention, since those who are no longer ambivalent do not usually come to an emergency service, see their PCP, or call crisis hotlines. An ambivalent person weighing life and death says, in effect, "If no one cares whether I live or die—not even my doctor!—I'd rather die than live." It also affirms the essential interpersonal and social nature of human beings enunciated in Durkheim's classic work

(1951[1897]) published over a century ago, which raises this question: If a person has no more meaningful attachments to a supportive family or community, why not die?

CASE EXAMPLE: SALLY—LISTENING TO CRIES FOR HELP

Sally, age 16, made a suicide attempt by swallowing six sleeping pills. In medical terms, this was not a serious attempt. Although she contemplated death, she also wanted to live. She hoped that the suicide attempt would bring about some change in her miserable family life, so that she could avoid the last resort of suicide itself. Before her suicide attempt, Sally was having trouble in school, ran away from home once, experimented with drugs, and engaged in behavior that often brought disapproval from her parents.

All of these behaviors were Sally's way of saying, "Listen to me! Can't you see that I'm miserable, that I can't control myself, that I can't go on like this anymore?" Sally had been upset for several years by her parents' constant fighting and playing favorites with the children. Her father drank heavily and frequently was away from home. When Sally's school counselor recommended family counseling, the family refused out of shame. Sally's acting out was really a cry for help. After her suicide attempt, her parents accepted counseling. Sally's behavior improved generally, and she made no further suicide attempts.

Had Sally not obtained help, she probably would have continued down the highway to suicide. The usual pattern in such a case is that the attempts become medically more serious, the person becomes more desperate, and finally commits suicide. We can help the ambivalent person move in the direction of life through understanding and response to the *meaning* of the person's behavior.

Risk Assessment Strategies

Listening and responding to emotional and behavioral clues leads to understanding—the foundation for risk assessment, decision, and action. *Suicide risk assessment* is the process of determining the likelihood of suicide for a particular person. *Lethality assessment* refers to the degree of *physical* injury incurred by a particular self-destructive act. *Suicide prediction* is "not very precise or useful" (Maris, 1991, p. 2) and according to psychiatrist Motto (1991, p. 75) should probably be eliminated from scientific terminology. The main focus here is to provide PCPs with risk assessment guidelines based on clinical experience and on empirical and epidemiological findings. Clinical assessment tries to answer this question: What is the risk of death by suicide for *this individual* at *this time*, considering the person's life as a whole?

Lethality Assessment Scales: Research and Clinical Use

Some workers use lethality assessment scales, which are primarily research tools, to assess suicidal risk. Most of these scales are not very effective (Brown & Sheran, 1972), and are too lengthy and time-consuming in a crisis situation. Motto (1985, p. 139) states, "The use of a scale has never been intended to predict suicide, but simply to supplement clinical judgment at the time an evaluation is done." Nor can a rating scale ever substitute for a clinician's sensitive inquiry (Motto, 1991)—for example, "Can you tell me what's happening to cause you so much pain?"

The problem with most scales is that they *do not exclude the non-suicidal population*—a pivotal point revealed in the pioneering research by Brown & Sheran (1972). For example, let us consider depression as a predictive sign. A large number of people who commit suicide (approximately 60%) have been diagnosed as depressed; however, the majority of depressed people do not commit suicide. Of the 20 million or so persons with a depressive disorder, only 0.1% commit suicide; Jacobs (2000, p. 32) notes the striking fact that 99.9% of persons diagnosed annually with depression do not commit suicide. Similarly, the majority of people who commit suicide have made previous suicide attempts, yet eight out of ten people who attempt suicide never go on to commit suicide. These statistics do not invite complacency; they simply indicate the complexity of suicide risk assessment, the limits of psychiatric diagnostic criteria, and the fact that something changed for a particular person at risk—for example, a cry for help was heard.

Signs that Help Assess Suicide Risk

Risk assessment techniques are based on knowledge obtained from the study of *completed* suicides. Such research is among the most difficult of scientific studies, but the study of completed suicides has explained much about the problem of risk assessment. The *most reliable indicators* or signs of suicide risk distinguish people who commit suicide from the population at large and also from those who only attempt suicide (Brown & Sheran, 1972; Maris, 1991). However, since there is not enough research on suicide to warrant general conclusions about suicide for different population groups, one should never be overconfident in applying signs to a suicidal person. It is impossible to predict suicide in any absolute sense; the focus for clinicians should be on assessing *immediate* and *long-term risk*. The chaos of a crisis situation and a PCP's anxiety about suicide can be reduced by thoughtful attention to general evidence-based principles. (See Hoff, *et al.*, 2009, Chapter 9, for in-depth discussion of these signs.)

The classic signs of suicide risk have varied little over the years since Edwin Shneidman's 1960s inauguration of suicidology as a field of scientific clinical study (1985). These principles for assessing suicide risk apply to *any* person in *any* setting contacted through *any* helping situation: telephone, primary care office, hospital, home, work site, jail, nursing home, school, or pastoral care. *Functional* assessment (emotional, cognitive, behavioral—as in the CMHA, Chapter 2) is the focus, although psychiatric *pathology* may be present in some instances. The following discussion is based on research in Western societies; suicide signs and methods vary in other cultural settings (see www.WHO.org). Sensitivity to these differences, however, is important in helping various immigrant and ethnic groups in distress in North America.

Suicide Plan   The majority of persons who die by suicide deliberately planned to do so. Without a high-lethal plan and available means, suicide cannot occur. Regarding the plan, people suspected of being suicidal should be asked several direct questions concerning the following risk assessment criteria:

1. *Suicidal ideas.* "Are you so upset that you're thinking of suicide?" or "Are you thinking about hurting yourself?"
2. *Lethality of method.* "What are you thinking of doing?" or, "What have you considered doing to harm yourself?"
3. *High-lethal methods*

   - gun;
   - hanging;
   - barbiturate and prescribed sleeping pills;
   - jumping;

- drowning;
- carbon monoxide poisoning;
- aspirin (high dose) and acetaminophen (Tylenol);
- car crash;
- exposure to extreme cold;
- antidepressants (tricyclics—most lethal; MAOIs second most lethal; SSRIs less lethal).

4. *Low-lethal methods*

- wrist cutting;
- nonprescription drugs (excluding aspirin and acetaminophen [Tylenol]);
- tranquilizers (anti-anxiety agents).

5. The PCP should also *determine the person's knowledge about the lethality of the chosen method*. For example, a person who takes ten tranquilizers with the mistaken belief that the dose is fatal is alive more by accident than by intent.

6. *Availability of means.* "Do you have a gun? Do you know how to use it? Do you have ammunition? Do you have pills?" Lives have often been saved by removing very lethal methods such as guns and sleeping pills. A highly suicidal person who calls a primary care office or crisis center is often making a final effort to get help, even while sitting next to a loaded gun or a bottle of pills. Such an individual will welcome a direct, protective suggestion by a PCP or counselor, such as, "Why don't you put the gun away?" or "Why don't you throw the pills out, and then let's talk about what's troubling you." When friends and family are involved, they too should be directed to get rid of the weapon or pills. In disposing of lethal weapons, it is important to engage the suicidal person actively in the process, keeping in mind that power ploys can trigger rather than prevent suicide. If trust and rapport have been established with one's PCP, engaging the suicidal person is generally not difficult to do.

7. *Specificity of plan.* "Do you have a plan worked out for killing yourself?" "How do you plan to get the pills?" "How do you plan to get the gun?" A person who has a well thought out plan—including time, place, and circumstances—with an available high-lethal method is an *immediate and very high risk* for suicide. We should also determine whether any rescue possibilities are included in the plan—for example, "What time of day do you plan to do this?" or "Is there anyone else around at that time?" We should also inquire about the person's intent. Some people really do intend to die; others intend to bring about some change that will help them avoid death and make life more livable.

While a specific plan is necessary to cause death, it is a less important sign of risk among people with a history of impulsive behavior, especially among adolescents.

History of Suicide Attempts   In the U.S. and Canadian adult population, suicide attempts occur eight to ten times more often than actual suicide. The rate among adolescents is about 50 attempts to every completed suicide. Among those who attempt suicide but do not go on to commit suicide, usually it is because some change occurs in their psychosocial world that makes life more desirable than death. However, the majority of people who kill themselves have made previous suicide attempts. A history of suicide attempts (65% of those who have completed suicide) is especially prominent among suicidal people who find that self-destructive behavior is the most powerful means they have of communicating their distress to others. Those who have made *previous high-lethal attempts are at greater risk* for suicide than those who have made low-lethal attempts.

Another historical indicator is a *change in method* of suicide attempt. A person who makes a high-lethal attempt after several less lethal attempts that elicited increasingly indifferent responses from significant others is a higher risk for suicide than one with a consistent pattern of low-lethal attempts, especially in the case of suicidal adolescents. Suicide attempts as a risk factor should also be considered in relation to depression. Among the 929 severely depressed patients in the Collaborative Depression Study, suicide attempt was not a predictor of suicide within one year but was a predictor of suicide within two to ten years (Fawcett, 2000, p. 38). This finding underscores a pivotal point in suicide prevention work—the need to *reassess* for suicide risk.

Determining the outcome of previous suicide attempts is also important—for example, "What happened after your last attempt? Did you plan any possibility of rescue, or were you rescued accidentally?" A person living alone who overdoses with sleeping pills and is rescued unexpectedly is alive more by accident than by intent. This person falls into a high-risk category for future suicide if there are other high-risk indicators as well. Suicide risk is also increased if the person has a negative perception of a psychiatric hospital or counseling experience. This finding suggests great caution in employing mental health laws to hospitalize suicidal people against their will, and underscores the pivotal role of a PCP if a patient reports that a mental health counseling referral is "just not working" for whatever reason.

Resources and Communication with Significant Others Internal resources consist of strengths, problem-solving ability, and personality factors that help one cope with stress. External resources include a network of persons on whom one can rely routinely as well as during a crisis. Communication as a suicide sign includes (1) the statement to others of intent to commit suicide and (2) the disruption of bonds between the suicidal person and significant others. People who finally commit suicide typically feel ignored or cut off from significant people around them, as dramatic murder–suicide events in schools and colleges affirm. This is extremely important in the case of adolescents, especially in instances of parent–child communication problems (Evans, Owens, & March, 2005; Goldston, *et al.*, 2008).

Institutionalized racism and the unequal distribution of material resources in the United States appear to contribute to the rapidly increasing rate of suicide among minority groups. This is especially true among young (under 30) people who realize early in life that many doors are closed to them. Their rage and frustration eventually lead to despair, suicide, and other violent behavior.

Others may have apparent supportive resources but serious depression, and the conviction of their worthlessness prevents them from accepting and using such support. Adequate personality resources include the ability to be flexible and to accept mistakes and imperfections in oneself. Some people who kill themselves appear to have happy families, good jobs, and good health, but may also have rigid role expectations imposed by culture, sexual identity, or socioeconomic status. Perceived role failure is usually gender specific—work failure for men (Morrell, Taylor, Quine, & Kerr, 1993) and family or mate failure for women (Stephens, 1985). Such rigidity in personality type is also revealed in a person's *tunnel vision* approach to problem solving: There is only one solution to a problem—suicide (Shneidman, 1987, p. 57). Psychotherapy can help such people to help develop more flexible approaches to problem solving.

Research and clinical experience suggest that providers consider not only the signs of risk but also the complex *patterning* of signs (Brown & Sheran, 1972; Farberow, 1975), in concert with clinical judgment (Motto, 1991). Applying this evidence to the pattern of the signs already noted leads to this risk assessment outcome: If the person (1) has a history of high-lethal attempts, (2) has a specific, high-lethal plan for suicide with available means, and

(3) lacks both personality and social resources, and cannot communicate with available resources, the *immediate and long-range risk for suicide is very high*, regardless of other factors. *Attempts at precise measurement on a scale are of little value if one has inadequate information about these critical signs*. The risk increases, however, if factors summarized in Table 4.1 are also present. See Hoff, *et al.*, 2009, Chapter 9, for a fuller discussion of these factors.

Here, the focus is to differentiate the importance of these signs for three population groups seen by PCPs:

1.   Those at *immediate risk* of suicide, and therefore needing immediate linkage to crisis or mental health specialists.
2.   Those who make non-lethal suicide attempts and, while not at immediate risk, may be at serious risk later if not linked to crisis counseling.
3.   The general population, among whom many experience various degrees of depression but are not at risk of suicide.

Translated to the U.S. population, this means that among 300 million people, approximately 30,000 commit suicide per year. Of course these are tragic and often preventable deaths, but the figures also highlight the role of PCPs in examining the complexity of factors leading to suicide. Two of these factors (physical illness and depression) besides the first four on Table 4.1 are elaborated briefly here and discussed in depth in chapters on depression, anxiety, pain, and substance abuse for their particular relevance to PCPs.

Physical Illness   Studies reveal that many people who kill themselves are physically ill. Some of these victims have been under medical care or have visited their physician within four to six months of their death. The visit to a PCP does not necessarily imply that the person is physically ill. However, it highlights the fact that a large number of people with any problem *seek out either physicians or the clergy*. In the case of suicidal people, the visit may be their last attempt to find relief from distress.

A primary care provider's failure to ascertain the suicide plan or to examine the depression disguised by a complaint with no physical basis often leads to the common practice of prescribing a psychotropic drug without a referral for counseling. An acutely anxious or depressed person may interpret such a response as an invitation to commit suicide. The possibility of suicide is even greater if a diagnosis affects the person's self-image and value system or demands a major switch in lifestyle—for example, AIDS, degenerative neurological conditions, heart disease, breast cancer, amputation of a limb, or cancer of the sex organs (Rodin, 2000).

Depression   Depressed people may experience sleeplessness, early wakening, slowed-down functioning, weight loss, menstrual irregularity, loss of appetite, inability to work normally, disinterest in sex, crying, and restlessness. *Feelings of hopelessness* are an even more important indicator of suicidal danger than depression (Beck, Steer, Beck, & Newman, 1993; Bertolote, *et al.*, 2003). Although not all people who kill themselves show signs of depression, enough suicide victims are depressed to make this an important indicator of risk. This is particularly true for the depressed person who feels worthless and is unable to reach out to others for help. Because most depressed people do not kill themselves (Fawcett, 2000, p. 38) and because a useful predictor must distinguish between the *general population* and those who make *suicide attempts*, we should refrain from declaring depression as a significant predictor of suicide. That said, *depression is a significant avenue for opening direct discussion of possible suicide plans:* "You seem really down. Are you so depressed that perhaps you've considered suicide?" (See Chapter 7.)

Table 4.1 Signs Comparing People who Complete or Attempt Suicide with the General Population

Signs	Suicide	Suicide Attempt	General Population
Suicide plan*	Specific, with available, high-lethal method; does not include rescue	Less lethal method, including plan for rescue; risk increases if lethality of method increases	None, or vague ideas only
History of suicide attempts*	65% have history of high-lethal attempts; if rescued, it was probably accidental	Previous attempts are usually low-lethal; rescue plan included; risk increases if there is a change from many low-lethal attempts to a high-lethal one	None, or low-lethal with definite rescue plan
Resources:* Psychological Social	Very limited or nonexistent; or person *perceives* self with no resources	Moderate, or in psychological and/or social turmoil	Either intact or able to restore them through nonsuicidal means
Communication*	Feels cut off from resources and unable to communicate effectively	Ambiguously attached to resources; may use self-injury as a method of communicating with significant others when other methods fail	Able to communicate directly and nondestructively for need fulfillment
Recent loss	Increases risk	May increase risk	Is widespread but is resolved nonsuicidally through grief work, and so forth
Physical illness	Increases risk	May increase risk	Is common but responded to through effective crisis management (natural and/or formal)
Drinking and other drug abuse	Increases risk	May increase risk	Is widespread but does not in itself lead to suicide
Physical isolation	Increases risk	May increase risk	Many well-adjusted people live alone; they handle physical isolation through satisfactory social contacts
Unexplained change in behavior	A possible clue to suicidal intent, especially in teenagers	A cry for help and possible clue to suicidal ideas	Does not apply in absence of other predictive signs
Depression	60% have a history of depression	A large percentage are depressed	A large percentage are depressed
Social factors or problems	May be present	Often are present	Widespread but do not in themselves lead to suicide
Psychosis	May be present	May be present	May be present

Table 4.1 Signs Comparing People who Complete or Attempt Suicide with the General
Population (continued)

Signs	Suicide	Suicide Attempt	General Population
Age, sex, race, marital status, sexual identity	Statistical predictors that are most useful for identifying whether an individual belongs to a high-lethal risk group, not for clinical assessment of individuals	May be present	May be present

*If all four of these signs exist in a particular person, the risk for suicide is very high regardless of all other factors. If other signs also apply, the risk is increased further.

Assessing Immediate and Long-range Risk

A person might engage in several kinds of self-destructive behavior at the same time. For example, someone who chronically abuses alcohol may threaten, attempt, or commit suicide—all in one day. We should view these behaviors on this continuum: all are serious and important in terms of life and death. The difference is that for some the danger of death is *immediate*, whereas for others it is *long-range*. Still others are at risk because of a high-risk lifestyle, chronic substance abuse, and neglect of medical care.

Distinguishing between immediate and long-range risk for suicide is not only a potential life-saving measure, but also is important for preventing or interrupting a vicious cycle of repeated self-injury. If immediate risk is high, and we do not uncover it in assessment, a suicide can result. Conversely, if immediate risk is low, as in medically non-serious cases of wrist slashing or swallowing a few sleeping pills, but we respond medically as though life were at stake while failing to address the *meaning* of this physical act, we run the risk of *reinforcing* self-destructive behavior. In effect, we say through our behavior, "Do something more serious (medically), and I'll pay attention to you." In reality, *medically non-serious self-injury is a life-and-death issue*—that is, if cries for help are repeatedly ignored, there is high probability that eventually the person will accept the invitation to do something more serious and actually commit suicide. The Collaborative Depression Study (Fawcett, 2000) affirms this decades-long clinical observation.

Table 4.2 Suicide Risk Differentiation

Suicidal Behavior		Ambivalence [fix]Scale	Rescue Plan	Immediate Risk	Long-Range Risk	
Low risk	Life	Desires life more than death	Present	Low	High	
Moderate risk		Life and death seem equally desirable	Ambiguous	Moderate	High	Depending on immediate response, treatment, and follow-up
High risk	Death	Desires death more than life	Absent, or rescue after past attempts was accidental	Very high	High	

The schema in Table 4.2 illustrates suicide risk differentiation at Low, Moderate, and High levels in relation to ambivalence, with all three levels dependent upon immediate response, treatment, and follow-up. It complements the CMHA, (item 14) in Chapter 2, and the Lethality Assessment Tool—Self, Table 4.3. Examples illustrating suicide risk assessment are discussed in the next section along with response according to level of risk.

Comprehensive Service for Self-destructive Persons

The U.S. Department of Health and Human Services, Public Health Service, has published a National Strategy for Suicide Prevention: Goals and Objectives for Action (2001). Internationally, other countries have published similar national strategies. Three kinds of service should be available for all at risk of killing themselves: (1) Emergency medical treatment, (2) crisis intervention, and (3) follow-up counseling or psychotherapy.

Emergency Medical Treatment

Primary care providers are already knowledgeable about emergency medical treatment. Unfortunately, this may be all that is received by some people who attempt suicide. Of course, not everyone who engages in self-injurious acts is in a life-and-death emergency. Therefore, with listening empathically, if the suicide attempt is *medically non-serious*, the PCP's response should not convey a life-and-death urgency. A dramatic and misplaced medical response might reinforce self-destructive behavior while ignoring the problems signaled by the self-destructive act. For example, while suturing a slashed wrist, the physician, nurse, and a PCP should regard the physical injury neutrally, with a certain sense of detachment, an empathic tone, and focus on the *meaning* of self-injury: "You must have been pretty upset to do this to yourself. What did you hope would happen when you cut your wrists?"

Crisis Intervention Strategies

If a person whose suicide attempt is medically serious does not receive follow-up counseling, the risk of suicide within a few months is very high. Emergency and primary care providers should also carefully consider the appropriate use of drugs for suicidal people in crisis (see below), because prescribed drugs are one of the weapons used most frequently for suicide. In agencies where mental health specialists are not available on-site in emergency services, staff should make every effort to link the person to a PCP who can follow through with mental health referral and/or appropriate drug treatment as discussed in Chapter 3.

In addition to the general crisis intervention strategies discussed in Chapter 3, PCPs should be familiar with the several counseling strategies with suicidal persons that may begin in primary care, but usually are enacted by mental health or crisis specialists:

1. *Relieve isolation.* If the suicidal person lives alone and there is no friend or supportive relative with whom the person can stay temporarily, and if the person is highly suicidal, that individual should probably be hospitalized until the active crisis is over.
2. *Remove lethal weapons.* Lethal weapons and pills should be removed either by the counselor, a relative, or a friend, keeping in mind empowerment issues and the active collaboration of the suicidal person in this process. If caring and concern are expressed and the person's sense of self-mastery and control is respected, he or she will usually surrender a weapon voluntarily, so it is safe from easy or impulsive access during the acute crisis. While avoiding power tactics or engaging in the heated debate regarding gun control, all human service providers should calmly inform an acutely distressed

person and the family of this sobering fact: suicide risk increases fivefold and homicide risk increases threefold when there is a gun in the home (Boyd & Moscicki, 1986; Kaplan, 1998).

3. *Encourage alternate expression of anger.* This means actively exploring with the individual other ways of expressing anger short of paying with one's life; e.g., "I can see that you're very angry with her for leaving you. Can you think of a way to express your anger that would not cost you your life?" If anger at the PCP or counselor is connected to the suicide threat, an empathic but not indifferent response is called for: "Of course I'd feel bad, but not guilty. So I'd like to continue working with you around your illness even though you're disappointed right now with our progress."

4. *Avoid a final decision about suicide during crisis.* We should assure the suicidal person that the suicidal crisis—that is, seeing suicide as the only option—is a *temporary* state, and try to persuade the person to avoid a decision about suicide until all other alternatives have been considered during a non-crisis state of mind.

5. *Beware of "no-suicide" contracts.* A cautionary note to PCPs about contracts is in order here. The *no-suicide contract* is a technique employed by some providers in which the client promises to refrain from self-harm between appointments and to contact the provider if contemplating such harm. Since this controversial issue emerged in the suicidology literature, there is growing consensus on this point: Such contracts offer *neither special protection* against suicide *nor legal protection* for the therapist or other provider (Clark & Kerkhof, 1993; Hoff, *et al.*, 2009, pp. 333–334; Reid, 1998). No-suicide contracts may convey a false sense of security to an anxious provider. This is because any value the contract may have flows from the *quality of the therapeutic relationship*—ideally, one in which the provider conveys caring and concern about the client. In no way should a contract serve as a convenient substitute for the time spent in empathetic listening, crisis intervention and counseling, and in careful planning with the client of therapeutic alternatives to self-destruction. Contracts are no more than a mechanistic "quick fix" by time-pressured providers if not incorporated into an overall service plan as discussed here and in Chapters 2 and 3, including such specifics as calling a hotline, or relieving isolation by asking a friend to join in a favorite recreation activity.

6. *Reestablish social ties.* Reestablishing broken social bonds can be done through family crisis counseling sessions or by finding satisfying substitutes for lost relationships. Active links to self-help groups such as Widow to Widow or Parents Without Partners clubs can be lifesaving.

7. *Relieve extreme anxiety and sleep loss.* A suicidal person who is extremely anxious and also has been unable to sleep for several days may become even more suicidal. To such a person, the world looks bleaker and death seems more desirable at four in the morning after endless nights of sleeplessness. A good night's sleep can temporarily reduce suicide risk and put the person in a better frame of mind to consider other ways of solving life's problems.

In such cases, PCPs should consider medication on an emergency basis (Bongar, *et al.*, 1992). This should never be done for a highly suicidal person, however, without daily crisis counseling sessions, since an extremely suicidal person may interpret such an approach as an invitation to commit suicide. An anti-anxiety agent will usually suffice in these instances and thus improve sleep, as anxiety is the major cause of sleeplessness. Antidepressants, in contrast, are more dangerous as a potential suicide weapon. If medication is needed, the person should be given a *one- to three-day supply at most*—always with a return appointment scheduled for crisis counseling.

In general, psychotropic drugs are indicated only if a person is too upset to be engaged in the process of problem solving during crisis (see below and Chapter 3). Nonchemical means of inducing sleep should be encouraged, or alternative therapies, as discussed in Chapter 13. This assumes a thorough assessment and various psychosocial strategies before prescribing drugs. Primary care providers should never forget that many suicide deaths in North America are caused by *prescribed* drugs. Sadly, Rogers' (1971) account of drug abuse ("just what the doctor ordered") is even more applicable today than decades ago (for further discussion, see Chapter 7).

Follow-up Service for Suicidal Persons

Beyond crisis counseling, all self-destructive persons should have the opportunity to receive counseling or psychotherapy as an aid in solving the problems that led them to self-destructive behavior (Bongar, *et al.*, 1992). Primary care providers making referrals should know whether the counselor or psychotherapist is publicly licensed to practice.

Counseling focuses on resolving situational problems, expressing feelings appropriately, and helping the person to change various behaviors causing discomfort, but without deep probing. Psychotherapy involves uncovering feelings that have been denied expression for a long time. It may also involve changing aspects of one's personality and deep-rooted patterns of behavior, such as an inability to communicate feelings or inflexible approaches to problem solving. When hospitalization is also indicated for seriously suicidal persons, health practitioners should observe carefully the standards of care for hospitalized people who are at risk of harming themselves (see Bongar, Maris, Berman, Litman, & Silverman, 1993).

Psychotropic Drug Treatment for Suicidal Persons

Because PCPs are already current on the general topic of psychotropic drugs, readers are referred to other sources (e.g., Dubovsky & Dubovsky, 2007; Garcia & Ghani, 2000). The focus here is limited to the intersection of prescription drugs with suicidal danger, especially for those without specialty training in psychopharmacology.

Antidepressants are not emergency drugs; however, these drugs may be used successfully for some suicidal persons who experience severe, recurring depression. Successful response to antidepressant therapy is highly variable, and debate about the use of psychotropic drugs continues (Brownlee, 2007). Thus, although some people respond favorably to antidepressant treatment, research and controversy continue regarding dosage and the efficacy of such treatment in preventing suicide (Kurdyak, Juurlink & Mamdani, 2007; Salzman, 1999, p. 373). In addition, there is no compelling evidence that antidepressant treatment, even with safer psychotropic agents, has reduced suicidal risk (Baldessarini, 2000, p. 34), whereas the risk of overdosing on antidepressants is well established (Baldessarini & Tondo, 1999, p. 356).

The success of antidepressant agents in persons with bipolar illness is significantly related to the timing of suicidal behavior, which occurs most often during the early course of illness (Baldessarini, 2000, p. 35). It is now well established that the greatest success of drug treatment occurs when used in *combination with psychotherapeutic approaches* (Dubovsky & Dubovsky, 2007; Solomon, Keitner, Miller, Shea, & Keller, 1995). This principle is of the utmost importance when considering the use of psychotropic drugs for anyone, especially adolescents (Elliott, 2006; see Chapters 7 and 11).

Since antidepressant drugs are dangerous, they should be prescribed with extreme caution for suicidal persons—even when explicitly advised of the typical two-week period for symptom relief (Bongar, *et al.*, 1992; Hoff, *et al.*, 2009). When taken with alcohol, an overdose of drugs can easily cause death. People using these drugs can experience side effects, such as feelings of confusion, restlessness, or loss of control. Persons with symptoms of "borderline personality disorder" can have an increase in self-destructive behaviors while treated with antidepressants (Salzman, 1999, p. 379).

Another danger of suicide occurs after the depression lifts during drug treatment. This is especially true for the person who is so depressed and physically slowed down that there is insufficient energy to carry out a suicide plan. Because of all these factors, it is critical to use antidepressant drugs in combination with psychotherapy or psychiatric hospitalization for a depressed person who is highly suicidal, especially if the individual is also socially and physically isolated (see Chapter 7).

CASE EXAMPLE: DRUG TREATMENT

Jack, age 69, a widower living alone, had seen his PCP for bowel problems. He was also quite depressed. Even after complete examination and extensive tests, he was obsessed with the idea of cancer and was afraid that he would die. Jack also had high blood pressure and emphysema. Months earlier, he had had prostate surgery. His family described him as

Table 4.3 Lethality Assessment Tool: Self

Key to Risk Level	Danger to Self	Typical Indicators
1	No predictable risk of suicide now	Has no suicidal ideation or history of attempt, has satisfactory social support system, and is in close contact with significant others
2	Low risk of suicide now	Has suicidal ideation with low-lethal methods, no history of attempts or recent serious loss, has satisfactory support network, no alcohol problems, basically wants to live
3	Moderate risk of suicide now	Has suicidal ideation with high-lethal method but no specific plan or threats, or has plan with low-lethal method, history of low-lethal attempts; for example, employed female, age 35, divorced, with tumultuous family history and reliance on psychotropic drugs for stress relief, is weighing the odds between life and death
4	High risk of suicide now	Has current high-lethal plan, obtainable means, history of previous attempts, is unable to communicate with a significant other; for example, female, age 50, living alone, with drinking history; or black male, age 29, unemployed and has lost his lover, is depressed and wants to die
5	Very high risk of suicide now	Has current high-lethal plan with available means, history of suicide attempts, is cut off from resources; for example, white male, over 40, physically ill and depressed, wife threatening divorce, is unemployed, or has received promotion and fears failure

a chronic complainer. The PCP gave him a prescription for an antidepressant drug and referred him to a local mental health clinic for counseling. Jack admitted to the crisis counselor that he had ideas of suicide, but he had no specific plan or history of attempts. After two counseling sessions, Jack killed himself by carbon monoxide poisoning. This suicide might have been prevented if Jack had been hospitalized. He lived alone, and in the cultural milieu promoting "take pill, feel better," he probably expected to feel better immediately after taking the antidepressant even though the delayed reaction of the drug had been explained. An alternative might have been to prescribe a drug to relieve his anxiety about cancer in combination with a plan to relieve isolation and gain some support by living with relatives for a couple of weeks.

CASE EXAMPLES: ASSESSMENT, CRISIS INTERVENTION, FOLLOW-UP COUNSELING

The following examples illustrate application of risk criteria and comprehensive service for people at moderate risk and high risk of suicide, using the Risk Assessment Tool: Self (Table 4.3)

Moderate Risk: #3, Assessment Tool Application

Susan, an immigrant, age 19, came alone in a taxi to a local hospital emergency department. She had taken an overdose of her antidepressant prescription (three times the usual dose) a half hour earlier. Susan and her three-year-old child, Debbie, live with her parents. She has never gotten along well with her parents, especially her mother. Before the birth of her child, Susan had a couple of short-lived jobs as a waitress. She dropped out of high school at age 16 and has experimented off and on with drugs. Since the age of 15, Susan had made four suicide attempts. She took overdoses of nonprescription drugs three times and cut her wrists once. These attempts were assessed as being of low lethality.

At the emergency department, Susan had her stomach pumped and was kept for observation for a couple of hours. She and the nurses knew one another from emergency service visits after her other suicide attempts. She was discharged with a recommendation that she follow up with her PCP, and seriously consider previous referrals for follow-up counseling. This emergency department did not have on-site crisis or psychiatric consultants. While there, Susan could sense the impatience and disgust of the staff. A man with a heart attack had come in around the same time. Susan felt that no one had the time or interest to talk with her. Twice before, Susan had refused referrals for counseling, so the nurses assumed that she was hopeless and did not really want help.

Suicide risk for Susan

Susan is not in immediate danger of suicide (risk rating: 3). She does not have a high-lethal plan and has no history of high-lethal attempts, although overdosing on a prescription antidepressant signifies a change toward increased risk. Susan's overdose of three times the prescribed dose falls in the moderate-risk category. While Susan's personal coping ability is poor, she is not cut off from her family, despite their disturbed relationship, and has not suffered a serious personal loss. However, because there is no follow-up counseling or evidence of any changes in her troubled social situation, Susan is at risk of making more suicide attempts in the future which, if increasingly medically serious, increases significantly her risk of eventual suicide. On the ambivalence scale, life and death may begin to look the same for Susan if her circumstances do not change.

EMERGENCY MEDICAL INTERVENTION

Treatment for the overdose is stomach lavage.

CRISIS INTERVENTION

Crisis counseling for Susan should include contacts with her parents and focus on the situational problems she faces: unemployment, conflicts with her parents, and dependence on her parents.

FOLLOW-UP SERVICE

Because Susan has had a chaotic life for a number of years, she could benefit from ongoing counseling or psychotherapy, if she so chooses. This might include exploration to continue her education and thereby improve her employment prospects. Family therapy may be indicated if she decides to remain in her parents' household. Group therapy is strongly recommended for Susan.

High-Risk Suicidal Behavior

This includes a threat or a suicide attempt that would probably be fatal without accidental rescue and sophisticated medical or surgical intervention, plus instances when a suicide attempt fails to end in death as intended, as in a deliberate car crash. Ambivalence in high-risk behavior tends more in the direction of death than life. The present and long-range risk of suicide is very high unless immediate help is available and accepted. Chronic self-destructive behavior such as substance abuse increases the risk even further.

Very High Risk: #5, Assessment Tool Application

Edward, age 41 and Caucasian, had just learned that his wife, Jane, had decided to get a divorce. He threatened to kill himself with a gun or carbon monoxide on the day she filed for the divorce. Jane's divorce lawyer proposed that their country home and the 20 adjoining acres be turned over completely to Jane. Edward told his wife, neighbors, and a crisis counselor that his family and home were all he had to live for. Indeed, all Edward could afford after the divorce was the rental of a single shabby room. He and Jane have four children. Edward also has several concerned friends but does not feel he can turn to them, as he always kept his family matters private. Jane's decision to divorce Edward has left him feeling like a complete failure. He has several guns and is a skilled hunter. A major factor in Jane's decision to divorce Edward was his chronic drinking problem. He had threatened to shoot himself eight months earlier after a violent argument with Jane when he was drinking, and Jane kept urging him to get help from A.A.

Applying most significant signs noted above, Edward's case reveals several strong signs of high risk.

1. He has a specific plan with an available high-lethal means—the gun.
2. He threatened suicide with a high-lethal method eight months previously and is currently communicating his suicide plan.
3. He is threatened with a serious interpersonal loss and feels cut off from what he regards as his most important social resources, his family and home.
4. He has a rigid expectation of himself in his role as husband and provider for his family.

He sees himself as a failure and has a deep sense of shame about his perceived role failure.

5. His coping ability is apparently poor, as he resorts to the use of alcohol and is reluctant to use his friends for support during a crisis.

6. He is also a high risk in terms of his age, sex, race, marital status, and history of alcohol abuse.

Suicide risk for Edward

Edward is in immediate danger of committing suicide (highest risk rating, #5). Even if he makes it through his present crisis, he is also a long-range risk for suicide because of his chronic self-destructive behavior—abuse of alcohol and threats of suicide by a readily available, high-lethal means.

EMERGENCY MEDICAL INTERVENTION

None indicated currently. Depending on level of engagement in crisis counseling, an anti-anxiety agent may be indicated for temporary stabilization, as discussed in Chapter 3.

CRISIS INTERVENTION

Remove guns (and alcohol, if possible) or have wife or friend remove them *with* Edward's collaboration. Arrange to have Edward stay with a friend on the day his wife files for divorce. Try to get Edward to attend a self-help group, such as Alcoholics Anonymous, and to rely on an individual A.A. member for support during his crisis. Arrange frequent crisis counseling sessions for Edward, including daily telephone check-in during acute phase.

FOLLOW-UP SERVICE

Edward should have ongoing psychotherapy, both individually and in a group, focusing on his alcohol dependency and his rigid expectations of himself; therapy should help Edward find other satisfying relationships after the loss of his wife by divorce.

Survivors of Suicide

When a suicide occurs, it is almost always the occasion of a crisis for survivors. A "survivor" here refers to all those left behind by someone who commits suicide: family members, primary care provider, psychotherapist, friend, neighbor, the entire community that grieves what might have been a preventable death.

The most immediately affected are usually family, the person's counselor and PCP, and other providers who did all they could to avert the suicide. The anguish, grief, possible guilt or relief felt by survivors is the usual province of mental health professionals. Primary care providers, however, if they have been attuned to family and psychosocial issues in their practice, will probably learn sooner or later about the suicide of a former patient. Given the deeply embedded feelings about death and dying felt by many, some survivors may present to PCPs with physical ailments with no observable or laboratory evidence of pathology. Typically, these ailments may mask unaddressed grief, or perhaps the morbidities and widely noted stress-related physical symptoms of persons caring for a chronically ill spouse or other family member who eventually dies. Such symptoms may be exacerbated if the cause of death was suicide.

Since even a psychotherapist may not be able to plumb the depths of despair that led to suicide, all the more so for a PCP who "after the fact" may recognize clues left unattended. Some survivors may feel enormous guilt and a sense of responsibility for the suicide, or a sense of relief. The latter may occur if relationships were very strained or the person had attempted suicide many times and either could not or would not accept the available help (see Hoff, *et al.*, 2009, for special concerns of child and parent survivors).

To avoid guilt trips or a tendency to "scapegoat" (i.e., find someone to blame), or collude in silence about the suicide, it is important for all professional providers—including PCPs—to convene a team meeting with these three goals: (1) to offer support to the PCP or counselor who treated the person; (2) to ascertain who is best able to contact and offer support to the surviving family members; and (3) to learn, on behalf of others at potential risk, by examining the entire situation for what clues may have been missed, or for possible "system loopholes" that shortchanged the patient.

Some survivors have spent extraordinary energy trying to answer the question: Why? And while critical examination of treatment plans is paramount, we may never know the answer to this question in some cases. It is therefore important to remember that we are not gods, that suicide has been happening for many centuries, and that sometimes people commit suicide despite our best efforts to help them find alternatives.

References

Badger, T. A., McNiece, C., & Gagan, M. J. (2000). Depression, service need, and use in vulnerable populations. *Archives of Psychiatric Nursing*, 14(4), 173–182.

Baechler, J. (1979). *Suicide*. New York: Basic Books.

Baldessarini, R. J. (2000). The complexity of suicide. Grand rounds: Suicide: Clinical/risk management issues for psychiatrists. *CNS Spectrums Academic Supplement: The International Journal of Neuropsychiatric Medicine*, 5 (2, Suppl. 1), 34–38.

Baldessarini, R. J., & Tondo, L. (1999). Antisuicidal effect of lithium treatment in major mood disorders. In D. G. Jacobs (Ed.), *The Harvard Medical School guide to suicide assessment and intervention* (pp. 355–371). San Francisco: Jossey-Bass.

Battin, M. P. (1980). Manipulated suicide. In M. P. Battin and D. J. Mayo (Eds.), *Suicide: The philosophical issues* (pp. 169–182). New York: St. Martin's Press.

Beck, A. T., Steer, R. A., Beck, J. S., & Newman, C. F. (1993). Hopelessness, depression, suicidal ideation, and clinical diagnosis of depression. *Suicide & Life-Threatening Behavior*, 23(2), 120–129.

Bertolote, J. M., Fleischmann, A., De Leo, D., Wasserman, D. (2003). Suicide and mental disorders: Do we know enough? *British Journal of Psychiatry*, 183(5), 382–383.

Bongar, B., Berman, A. L., Maris, R. W., Silverman, M. M., Harris, E. A., & Packman, W. L. (1998). *Risk management of suicidal patients*. New York: Guilford Press.

Bongar, B., Maris, R. W., Berman, A. L., Litman, R. E., & Silverman, M. M. (1993). Inpatient standards of care and the suicidal patient: Part I: General clinical formulations and legal considerations. *Suicide & Life-Threatening Behavior*, 23(3), 245–256.

Boyd, J. H., & Moscicki, E. K. (1986). Firearms and youth suicide. *American Journal of Public Health*, 76, 1240–1242.

Brown, T. R., & Sheran, T. J. (1972). Suicide prediction: A review. *Suicide & Life-Threatening Behavior*, 2, 67–97.

Brownlee, S. (2007). *Overtreated: How too much medicine is making us sicker and poorer*. New York: Bloomsbury.

Burstow, B. (1992). *Radical feminist therapy: Working in the context of violence*. Thousand Oaks, CA: Sage.

Center for Disease Control (CDC) http://www.cdc.gov.

Clark, D. C., & Kerkhof, A. J. F. M. (1993). No-suicide decisions and suicide contracts in therapy. *Crisis*, 14(3), 98–99.

Dubosky, S. L., & Dubovsky, A. N. (2007). *Psychotropic drug prescriber's survival guide*. New York & London: W.W. Norton.

Durkheim, E. (1951[1897]). *Suicide* (2nd ed.). New York: Free Press.

Elliott, G. R. (2006). *Medicating young minds*. New York: Stewart, Tabori, & Chang.

Emanuel, E. J., & Battin, M. P. (1998). What are the potential cost savings from legalizing physician-assisted suicide? *New England Journal of Medicine*, 339(3), 167–172.

Evans, W. P., Owen, P., & Marsh, S. C. (2005). Environmental factors, locus of control, and adolescent suicide risk. *Child and Adolescent Social Work Journal*, 22(3–4), 301–319.

Everett, B., & Gallop, R. (2000). *The link between childhood trauma and mental illness: Effective interventions for mental health professionals*. Thousand Oaks, CA: Sage.

Farberow, N. L. (Ed.). (1975). *Suicide in different cultures*. Baltimore, MD: University Park Press.

Farberow, N. L. (Ed.). (1980). *The many faces of death*. New York: McGraw-Hill.

Fawcett, J. (2000). The complexity of suicide. Grand rounds. Suicide. Clinical/risk management issues for psychiatrists. *CNS Spectrums Academic Supplement: The International Journal of Neuropsychiatric Medicine*, 5(2, Suppl. 1), 38–41.

Garcia, G., & Ghani, S. (2000). Pharmacology update: Newer medications and indications used in psychiatry. *Primary Care Practice*, 4(2), 207–220.

Goldston, D. B., Molock, S. D., Whitbeck, L. B., Murakami, J. L., Zayas, L. H. & Hall, G. C. H. (2008). Cultural considerations in adolescent suicide prevention and psychosocial treatment. *American Psychologist*, 63(1), 14–31.

Hoff, Hallisey, & Hoff, 2009, *People in crisis: Clinical and diversity perspectives*. New York: Routledge.

Humphrey, D. (1992). Rational suicide among the elderly. *Suicide & Life-Threatening Behavior*, 22(1), 125–129.

Jacobs, D. G. (2000). The complexity of suicide. Grand rounds: Suicide: Clinical/risk management issues for psychiatrists. *CNS Spectrums Academic Supplement: The International Journal of Neuropsychiatric Medicine*, 5(2, Suppl. 1), 32–33.

Kaplan, M. S. (1998). Firearm suicides and homicides in the United States: Regional variations and patterns of gun ownership. *Social Science & Medicine*, 46(9) 1227–1233.

Kurdyak, P. A., Juurlink D. N., Mamdani, M. M. (2007). The effect of antidepressant warnings on prescribing trends in Ontario, Canada. *American Journal of Public Health*, 97(4), 750–754.

Maris, R. W. (1981). *Pathways to suicide*. Baltimore, MD: Johns Hopkins University Press.

Maris, R. W. (1991). Assessment and prediction of suicide: Introduction [Special issue]. *Suicide & Life-Threatening Behavior*, 21(1), 1–17.

Menninger, K. (1938). *Man against himself*. Orlando, FL: Harcourt Brace.

Morrell, S., Taylor, R., Quine, S., & Kerr, C. (1993). Suicide and unemployment in Australia. *Social Science & Medicine*, 36(6), 749–756.

Moscicki, E. (1999). Epidemiology of suicide. In D. G. Jacobs (Ed.), *The Harvard Medical School guide to suicide assessment and intervention* (pp. 40–51). San Francisco: Jossey-Bass.

Motto, J. A. (1985). Preliminary field testing of a risk estimation for suicide. *Suicide & Life-Threatening Behavior*, 15(3), 139–150.

Motto, J. A. (1991). An integrated approach to estimating suicide risk. *Suicide & Life-Threatening Behavior*, 21(1), 74–89.

Motto, J. A. (1999). Critical points in the assessment and management of suicide risk. In D. G. Jacobs (Ed.), *The Harvard Medical School guide to suicide assessment and intervention* (pp. 224–238). San Francisco: Jossey-Bass.

National Center for Health Statistics. (2004). *Report of final mortality statistics*. Hyattsville, MD: Author.

Parsons, T. (1951). Social structure and the dynamic process: The case of modern medical practice. In T. Parsons (Ed.) *The social system* (pp. 428–479). New York: Free Press.

Pfeffer, C. R. (1986). *The suicidal child*. New York: Guilford Press.

Reid, W. J. (1998). Promises, promises: Don't rely on patients' no-suicide/no-violence "contracts." *Journal of Practical Psychiatry and Behavioral Health*, 4(5), 316–318.

Remafedi, G., Farrow, J. A., & Deisher, R. W. (1991). Risk factors for attempted suicide in gay and bisexual youth. *Pediatrics*, 87(6), 869–875.

Remafedi, G., French, S., Story, M., Resnick, M. D., & Blum, R. (1998). The relationship between suicide risk and sexual orientation: Results of a population-based study. *American Journal of Public Health*, 88(1), 57–60.

Richman, J. (1992). A rational approach to rational suicide. *Suicide & Life-Threatening Behavior*, 22(1), 130–141.

Rodin, G. M. (2000). Psychiatric care for the chronically ill & dying patient. In H. H. Goldman (Ed.), *Review of general psychiatry* (pp. 505–512). New York; Lange Medical Books/McGraw-Hill.

Rogers, M. J. (1971). Drug abuse: Just what the doctor ordered. *Psychology Today*, 5, 16–24.

Salzman, C. (1999). Treatment of the suicidal patient with psychotropic drugs and ECT. In D. G. Jacobs (Ed.), *The Harvard Medical School guide to suicide assessment and intervention* (pp. 372–382). San Francisco: Jossey-Bass.

Samuels, D. (2007). Let's die together. *The Atlantic*, May, 92–98.

Shneidman. E. S. (1981). Suicide. *Suicide & Life-Threatening Behavior*, 11, pp. 198–220.

Shneidman, E. S. (1985). *Definition of suicide*. New York: Wiley.

Shneidman, E. S. (1987). At the point of no return. *Psychology Today*, 21(3), 54–58.

Shneidman, E. S. (1999). Perturbation and lethality: A psychological approach to assessment and intervention. In D. G. Jacobs (Ed.), *The Harvard Medical School guide to suicide assessment and intervention* (pp. 83–97). San Francisco: Jossey-Bass.

Solomon, D. A., Keitner, G. I., Miller, I. W., Shea, M. T., & Keller, M. B. (1995). Course of illness and maintenance treatments for patients with bipolar disorder. *Journal of Clinical Psychiatry*, 56(1), 5–13.

Stephens, B. J. (1985). Suicidal women and their relationships with husbands, boyfriends, and lovers. *Suicide & Life-Threatening Behavior*, 15(2), 77–90.

Stephens, B. J. (1987). Cheap thrills and humble pie: The adolescence of female suicide attempters. *Suicide & Life-Threatening Behavior*, 17(2), 107–118.

Wasserman, D. (2004). Evaluating suicide prevention: Various approaches needed. *World Psychiatry*, 3(3), 153–154.

World Health Organization (WHO) http://www.who.int/.

5 Violence and Sexual Assault

Prevention, Intervention, and Follow-up

- Overview: Victimization and Violence
- Theories on Violence and Abuse
- Victimization Assessment Strategies
- Crisis Intervention and Follow-up for Survivors of Violence and Abuse
- Assessment of Dangerousness, Assault, and Homicide Risk
- Youth Violence and the Role of Primary Care Providers
- Crisis Intervention with Assailants and those Threatening Violence
- Programs for Violent Men
- Violence and Abuse in the Healthcare Workplace and Forensic Psychiatry
- Primary Prevention of Violence and Anti-social Behavior
- References

Overview: Victimization and Violence

Victimization by violence knows few, if any, national, ethnic, religious, or other boundaries (United Nations, 1996). Despite civil rights legislation, nationally and internationally, violence continues, extending from domestic to community and global arenas, and often originating from bias based on gender, race, disability, and/or sexual identity. Immigrants and refugees usually face triple jeopardy because of social isolation, language barriers, and fear of deportation if they seek help. This chapter addresses violence and abuse from the perspective of victim/survivors (including healthcare workers) as well as their assailants. Its focus is on the pivotal role of primary care providers (PCPs) in prevention, crisis intervention, and on explicit and potentially life-saving linkages with crisis and trauma specialists. The emphasis on early detection in primary care is based on extensive interdisciplinary research and practice with victim/survivors, revealing the risk of serious and often long-term medical and mental health sequelae when support and crisis counseling are lacking at the time of victimization by violence (Campbell, 1998; Dobash & Dobash, 1998; Everett & Gallop, 2000; Figley & Nash, 2005; Herman, 1992; Hoff, 1990; Rynearson, 2006; Stark, Flitcraft, & Frazier, 1979; Wiehe, 1998; and Wilson, 2006).

---

* Parts of this chapter are excerpted from Hoff, Hallisey, & Hoff, 2009, *People in crisis: Clinical and diversity perspectives*, 6th Edition, Chapters 11 and 12, and edited for application in primary care practice. Used with permission.

Incidence and Key Facts: International Perspective

The following brief overview from the above sources and official government statistics (see online resources for current statistics) highlights the urgency of PCPs to address violence issues, not only as guidelines for their practice, but also for their own protection from potentially dangerous persons in the workplace (Hoff, 2010).

BOX 5.1   Violence and Abuse across Cultures

- Around 25% of couples are violent with each other (U.S).
- At least 25% of pregnant women have a current or past history of abuse (U.S. and Canada); about 40% experience the first violent incident when pregnant.
- Battering is the most common cause of injury to women worldwide (PAHO/WHO 2003; UN 1996); in the U.S., the incidence exceeds accidents, muggings, and stranger rape combined.
- Battering and abuse are primary reasons why many women and children are homeless (U.S.).
- Between 60% and 70% of runaways and 98% of child prostitutes have a history of childhood sexual and/or physical abuse.
- Significant numbers of homicides (40% in Canada) are in family relationships; in the U.S. most domestic homicides are by men killing women, with others by women killing men, usually after years of abuse. Killings of women out of jealousy and male ownership or "Honor" occurs across cultures (Husseini, 2009).
- Violence within relationships tends to escalate in severity and frequency over time without early preventive intervention.
- About 50% of boy victims become abusive later, underscoring the fact that later violence is not "inevitable" and early "learned behavior" can be replaced with non-abusive responses to stress.
- Significant numbers of children witness violence.
- Living in a violent home is now considered a form of child abuse.
- Over one million children under age 16 are brought into the international sex trade per year.
- Most violence is committed by heterosexual men against children of both sexes, women, and other men, homophobia notwithstanding.
- Rates of violence by girls and women are increasing, reflecting in part the power of male examples and violence-tinged media influences (U.S. and Canada).
- A majority of rape victims know their attackers.
- Millions of adult and child rape victims have been attacked as the centuries-old "spoils of war" practice and the breakdown of civil order.
- Health professionals were among the last groups to get on board responding to violence as a public health issue after survivors themselves, their advocates, and the legal/criminal justice professions.
- National surveys of nursing schools in the U.S. and Canada reveal that their formal preparation did not adequately prepare them to identify, treat, and care for survivors of sexual abuse and violence (Woodtli & Breslin, 2002; Ross, Hoff, & Coutu-Wakulczyk, 1998).

Such evidence-based "facts" about violence may also be useful in primary care practice as a "reality check" with patients—already injured or vulnerable to abuse—who keep hoping and believing, for example, that "He promised he'd never do it again" . . . "I think he's going to change if I'm patient enough" . . . "I just know it [the violence] will stop if we both stop drinking" or, in the case of sexually abused teens, "I'll just run away as soon as I have a chance."

Violence as a Human Rights Issue

The United Nations has defined violence as a human rights issue, has convened international meetings on the topic, and the United Nations Decade for Women conferences have featured numerous workshops on the worldwide problem of violence against women. The last UN conference was held in Beijing in 1995, with 36,000 women attending, including government representatives from all UN member nations.

In the United States, the U.S. Surgeon General's Workshop on Violence and Public Health (1986) was convened in 1985 to emphasize the fact that victims' needs, treatment of assailants, and prevention of violence should command much greater attention from health and social service professionals than it has until recently. A significant recommendation in the U.S. government's publication of this conference was that all publicly licensed professionals (physicians, nurses, social workers, psychologists) should be trained and *examined* on the topic of violence and victimization as a condition of licensure. Since then, there has been progress on many fronts (for example, the 1999 American Association of Colleges of Nursing position paper noting violence content as *essential* for graduation). However, much is left to be done before curriculum coverage of this topic is addressed beyond the level of particular faculty interest (see Hoff, 2010).

The historical neglect of victimization, and its prevention and treatment in primary care and other health settings, underscores the value placed on family privacy and the myth that the family is a haven of love and security. This pattern of neglect also points to several related issues:

- social values regarding children, how they should be disciplined, and who should care for them;
- social and cultural devaluation of women and their problems;
- a social and economic system in which many elderly citizens often have no worthwhile place;
- a social climate with little tolerance for minority group sexual identity;
- a legal system in which it is difficult to consider the rights of victims without compromising the rights of the accused;
- a knowledge system that historically has interpreted these problems in private, *individual* terms rather than in *public, social* ones.

Many volumes across health, mental health, and criminal justice disciplines have been written on various facets of violence and abuse. The abbreviated coverage in this chapter focuses on the topic's particular relevance to primary care practice. Reflecting a major theme of crisis theory (Hoff, *et al.*, 2009; Hoff, 1990), the term *victim-survivor* is used to acknowledge victimization but to simultaneously convey an abused person's potential for growth, development, and empowerment—a status beyond the dependency implied by *victim* (Burstow, 1992). The terms *violence* and *abuse* are used interchangeably. *Perpetrator* is used to convey the importance of one's accountability for violent or abusive behavior, and the subsequent necessity of collaboration between medical and legal/criminal justice sectors concerned with the rights of both victim/survivors and perpetrators.

Framing violence in a human rights perspective aids in stopping "victim blaming," that occurs even among some victim/survivors who blame themselves for what happened. It also puts a break on "cultural relativism," that is, excusing interpersonal violence as "just a part of *their* culture" and thereby also excusing *us* from action that would defend one's basic human right to safety, while holding abusers of that right accountable. In primary care this means saying something like this to a victim/survivor: "No matter what [your husband] might have said, what happened to you is not right and it's not your fault."

Theories on Violence and Abuse

Earlier theories to explain violence and its prevalence fall into three categories: (1) psycho-biological, (2) social-psychological, and (3) sociocultural (Gelles & Loseke, 1993). Today most violence scholars reject analytical frameworks such as sociobiology, which serve to maintain violence as a private matter. Instead violence is now widely interpreted in psychological, sociological, and feminist terms (Dobash & Dobash, 1998; Segal, 1999). Our position is that violence is predominantly a *social* phenomenon, a means of exerting *power* and *control* that has far-reaching effects on personal, family, and public health worldwide (Hoff, 2010). Accordingly, the term *family violence* is avoided on the grounds that it obscures the fact that most perpetrators in families are men, and most victims are children and women of all ages.

Bio-medical/Psychiatric and Sociocultural Factors Affecting Violence

Many professionals and laypersons have accepted psychological or medical explanations of violence, as revealed in these common sentiments (1) "only a sick man could beat his wife"; (2) child abuse is a syndrome calling for "treatment" of disturbed parents; (3) a "crazed madman" was responsible (and by implication, not accountable) for highly publicized terrorist attacks; (4) "temporary insanity" sometimes excuses murder (even though juries are becoming more skeptical about this plea); and (5) women who kill their abusers are victims of the "battered woman syndrome."

Public debate about biomedical approaches to social problems is increasing (Luhrmann, 2000; Warshaw, 1989). There is growing acceptance of the view that attention to violent persons and their victims in predominantly *individual* terms is at best incomplete and at worst does little to address the *roots* of violence. The view taken here expands on the crisis paradigm (Chapter 3): crises stemming from violence should be treated with a *tandem* approach, taking both individual and sociocultural factors into account. A person in crisis because of violence will experience many of the same responses as those in crisis from other sources. And similar intervention strategies, such as listening, social support, and decision counseling apply as well. However, taking into consideration the sociocultural origins of crises from violence is important in designing prevention and follow-up strategies that do not implicitly blame the victim (Ryan, 1971; Hoff, 1990). For victims of violence, a strictly individual or biopsychiatric approach can compound the problem rather than contribute to the solution (Stark, Flitcraft, & Frazier, 1979).

There is no single cause of interpersonal violence. Rather, there are complex, interrelated *reasons* that some individuals are violent and others are not; psychological, cultural, and socioeconomic factors are often present together, forming the *context* in which violence as a means of control seems to thrive. Children, many seniors, and often wives are economically dependent on their caretakers and in most cases are physically weaker than their abusers. Caretakers of children and older people are often stressed psychologically by difficult behaviors, and socioeconomically by a lack of social and financial resources to ease the burdens of caretaking. In cases of woman battering and sex-role stereotyping, psychological and economic factors intersect at both ends of the social class continuum: poor women are less able to survive on their own, and some women who earn more than their husbands are more vulnerable to attack in a nonegalitarian marriage.

Violence toward others, then, is one way a person can respond to stress and resolve a personal crisis at the same time. For example, a person with low self-esteem who is threatened by the suspected infidelity of a spouse may react with violence. A violent response is not inevitable though; it is *chosen* and may be influenced by such factors as an earlier choice to use alcohol and other drugs. One's use of violent behavior to control another person is influenced by the social, political, legal, and belief and knowledge systems of the violent person's cultural community. The element of choice implies an interpretation of violence as a moral act—that is, violence is *social action* engaged in by human beings who by nature are rational and conscious. Through socialization, humans become responsible for the actions they choose in various situations.

However, consciousness may be clouded and responsibility mitigated by social and cultural factors rooted in the history of human society. Under certain circumstances, a person may be excused from facing the social consequences of his or her behavior, as in cases of self-defense or when a violent act is considered to be irrational. This does not mean that every violent act is a result of mental illness and that the perpetrator should therefore be "treated," as suggested by a popular conception of violence. Nor does it mean that violence can be excused on grounds of racial or economic discrimination; this would suggest that the moral stature of disadvantaged groups is below the standard of responsible behavior. Given the poverty, unemployment, and other tragic results of social inequalities endured by many people—mostly racial minority groups—perhaps in no other instance is the tandem approach to crisis intervention more relevant: violent *individuals* are held accountable for their behavior, while the political and socioeconomic *context* in which much violence occurs is also addressed. Thus, an individual can be held accountable; can be restrained or rehabilitated, while we also address the factors that contribute to a victim's vulnerability and the perpetrator's choice of aggressive behaviors in the first place.

A Contextual vs. Adversarial Approach to Understanding Violence

Attention to perpetrators and why they injure or kill people closest to them forms part of a comprehensive program to reduce violence. Some would argue that programs for perpetrators deflect from the more urgent need of refuge for victims. Violence is a major public health problem as well as a criminal justice issue. At worst, an either-or position damages both victim-survivors and assailants; at best, it constitutes empty polemics. It is therefore not a question of whether we (1) *either* provide refuge and care for battered women *or* provide treatment programs for their batterers, (2) *either* hold parents accountable for the violent and abusive behavior of their children *or* offer parent effectiveness training and socioeconomic support to parents unduly burdened with the task of parenting, or (3) *either* teach inner-city youth anger management skills *or* address the sociocultural and economic roots of their anger. Essentially, either-or debates are adversarial and reflect the *power and control* component of violence itself. These counterproductive arguments have surfaced anew just as progress has appeared in respect to understanding male violence (Adams, 2007). These principles apply regardless of gender, race, ethnicity, religion, or sexual identity.

Violence, then, and PCPs' response to victim-survivors and perpetrators is interpreted here in a multifaceted conceptual framework: moral, social-psychological, legal, and medical. Violence can be defined as an infraction of society's rules regarding people, their relationships, and their property. It is a complex phenomenon in which sociocultural, political, medical, and psychological factors touch both its immediate and chronic aspects. Functioning members of a society normally know a group's cultural rules and the consequences for violating them. Those lacking such knowledge might be publicly excused and receive treatment instead of punishment. Others are excused on the basis of self-defense or the circumstances that alter one's normal liability for rule infractions. A moral society would require restitution to individual victims from those not excused and would design a criminal justice system to prevent rather than promote future crime. A truly moral approach to violence would also avoid or reform practices that discriminate on the basis of race, gender, class, or sexual identity, practices that create a climate in which crime flourishes with the implicit support of society (Brown & Bohn, 1989; Handwerker, 1998).

This theoretical overview assumes a continuum between what happens between family members and intimates and the larger sociocultural factors affecting them. In the following discussion, social-psychological and sociocultural theories will be examined as they apply to crises stemming from violence with respect to:

- prevention;
- intervention during crisis;
- follow-up service (psychosocial care and psychotherapeutic treatment).

Each of these topics is important, but the discussion here focuses on risk assessment, and crisis intervention and follow-up linkage that often may not occur unless initiated by PCPs, with the understanding that specialized follow-up counseling for both victim/survivors and perpetrators is primarily the responsibility of trauma and mental health specialists. Without these important *first steps* in primary care, the *morbidities and mortalities* noted in the Crisis Paradigm, Box 4b in Figure 3.1, and the Downward Spiral, Figure 3.2, may be encountered.

Victimization Assessment Strategies

Providers in various entry points to the health and social service system should incorporate questions about possible victimization trauma into their routine assessments. Bell, Jenkins, Kpo, & Rhodes (1994) state that protocols for such assessments should be mandated by law.

Creating a Climate for Assessment

A first step for PCPs in victim/survivor care is to create a climate that enhances prospects for assessment, since it is legendary that survivors are reluctant to report abuse if for any reason they sense the climate is not receptive to disclosure. Creating such a climate includes the following:

- Beware of a judgmental attitude: Many victim/survivors already feel judged and/or blame themselves for the abuse. Even before learning all the facts of a particular situation, attitudes have a way of speaking louder than words: for example, most people know how it feels to receive a verbal "I'm sorry" or "condolence" wish that does not match the giver's unspoken "cold" attitude.
- Create a space for privacy and time to listen: Survivors recognize the heavy demands and interruptions a PCP faces, and like others will patiently wait their turn in the face of an emergency; but being left in a room alone for 20 minutes or longer with no explanation is anxiety-provoking and unconducive to disclosure.
- Be convinced of the importance of your own role: While not expecting "rescue," for some survivors, a PCP is the first person in the healthcare system to whom they truthfully disclose their plight.

- Examine personal values regarding violence, and deal with a possible history of victimization in one's own life, which has been long buried but which may surface in unexpected ways when confronted with the treatment needs of an abused patient. Such a "wounded healer" may "close down" out of self-protection, or fall into a misdirected "rescue" trap and empowerment issues.
- Be ready to talk *directly* and *empathically* about the violence, using a structured protocol as discussed next.

A Victimization Assessment Tool

In Chapter 2 we introduced a Triage Tool as a foundation for risk-to-life (suicide, victimization, assault/homicide) screening questions to incorporate into all intake questionnaires across healthcare settings. It is replicated here for easy reference by readers focused on victim/survivor care (Figure 5.1), and serves as a baseline for assessing level of trauma from victimization. Table 5.1 presents a Victimization Assessment Tool that builds on data

---

1. Have you been troubled or injured by any kind of abuse or violence? (for example, hit by partner, forced sex)

   Yes____ No____ Not sure____ Refused____ If yes, check one of the following:

   By someone in your family ____ By an acquaintance or stranger____

   Describe:

2. If yes, has something like this ever happened before?

   Yes____ No____ If yes, when?_____

   Describe:

3. Do you have anyone you can turn to or rely on now to protect you from possible further injury?

   Yes____ No____ If yes, who?_____

4. Do you feel so bad now that you have thought of hurting yourself/suicide?

   Yes____ No____ If yes, what have you thought about doing?

   Describe:

5. Are you so angry about what's happened that you have considered hurting someone else?

   Yes____ No____

   Describe:

Figure 5.1 Screening for Victimization and Life-threatening Behaviors: Triage Questions

obtained from the Triage Tool. It complements the tool for suicide risk (Chapter 4), and the Assault/Homicide Tool later in this Chapter, Table 5.2, that form part of the Comprehensive Mental Health Assessment Guide discussed in Chapter 2.

Together, these three tools underscore the interrelationship between violence, victimization, and suicide which, if missed in primary care and other entry points, may shortchange the specialized follow-up counseling indicated for all victim/survivors and perpetrators of violence (Hoff & Rosenbaum, 1994). Questions about suicide and assault potential and resource depletion are often secondary to the *primary* problem of abuse, and may *signal the severity of emotional trauma* from victimization. As the triage questions in Figure 5.1 suggest, such *routine inquiry* could prevent suicide or murder as desperate responses to victimization trauma. For an abuse assessment screen designed specifically for use by health professionals working with women, see Soeken, McFarlane, Parker, & Lominack (1998).

As discussed in Chapter 3, *no crisis assessment is complete without ascertaining the life-threatening risk of suicide, and trauma from victimization and assault.* Research among female suicidal teenagers and adults reveal significant relationships between self-destructive behaviors and histories of childhood sexual abuse and intimate partner violence (Stephens, 1985). Work with battered women, for example, has uncovered the repeated revelation by survivors seeking help: "No one asked." As the study by Sugg and Inui (1992) suggests, physicians, nurses, and others have moved beyond their traditional fear of opening Pandora's Box by inquiring about abuse.

Screening in primary care protocols for intimate partner or other abuse is now common in many U.S. and Canadian healthcare agencies. Yet, such screening is often obscured in a check-off medical history form where it can easily be overlooked in direct interview, especially by PCPs who are unprepared to explore further if the client checked "yes" about abuse or safety in a routine intake questionnaire. On the other hand, lengthy screening tools may be counter-productive in busy emergency and primary care settings (Coker, *et al.*, 2007). Our recommendation to PCPs beyond screening and immediate safety measures is to assure referral and follow-up to crisis counselors based on information obtained from the triage and risk assessment tools discussed here. Trauma counselors may use more in-depth diagnostic tools that are beyond the time boundaries and ordinary expertise of PCPs. An exception to this general pattern might be pediatricians, midwives, and OB/GYN providers who, besides their specialty expertise, function as PCPs and know some of their clients over many years.

Crisis Intervention and Follow-up for Survivors of Violence and Abuse

Once victimization status is identified, it should be followed by in-depth assessment (preferably by mental health professionals with backgrounds in victimology who are also sensitive to gender issues) to ascertain the extent of trauma and the victim-survivor's response (see Hoff, *et al.*, 2009, Chapters 11 and 12, for further discussion of abuse across categories). Also, emergency departments already have established protocols for treatment of various victims, e.g., rape, child witnesses of violence, etc. which should include the follow-up roles of PCPs and trauma specialists (see also Burstow, 1992; Campbell & Humphreys, 1993; Everett & Gallop, 2000; Herman, 1992; van der Kolk, 1987).

The important techniques for PCPs to remember in these and related situations are (1) withhold judgment, (2) offer an empathic, supportive response, (3) assist the victim/survivor with safety planning, and (4) provide information—a card or brochure with the numbers of hotlines, support groups, and counseling services. This seemingly small response is central, for example, to an abused woman's eventual decision to leave a violent relationship because it is empowering to know that others respect her decision, even if it is to stay in the violent relationship for the time being. She also needs explicit recognition from providers that

Table 5.1 Victimization Assessment Tool

Key to Risk	Level of Victimization	Typical Indicators
1	No experience of physical violence or abuse	No memory of violence recently or in the past.
2	Experience of abuse/violence with minor physical and/or emotional trauma	Currently, verbal arguments that occasionally escalate to pushing and shoving or mild slapping. History *may* include past victimization that is no longer problematic or for which a solution is in process.
3	Experience of abuse/violence with moderate physical and/or emotional trauma	Abused several times a month in recent years, resulting in moderate trauma/emotional distress (for example, bruises, no threat to life, no weapons). History *may* include past victimization that is still somewhat problematic (for example, a sexual abuse incident/overture by a parent or stepparent over 2 years ago).
4	Experience of abuse/violence with severe physical and/or emotional trauma	Violently attacked (e.g., rape) or physically abused in recent years, resulting in physical injury requiring medical treatment. Threats to kill, no guns. History *may* include serious victimization (e.g., periodic battering, incest, or other abuse requiring medical and/or psychological treatment).
5	Life-threatening or prolonged violence/abuse with very severe physical and/or emotional trauma	Recent or current life-threatening physical abuse, potentially lethal assault or threats with available deadly weapons. History may include severe abuse requiring medical treatment, frequent or ongoing sexual abuse, recent rape at gunpoint or knifepoint, other physical attack requiring extensive medical treatment.

ultimately it is *her* decision that makes the difference, and that she can take credit for the decision. Because abused women often feel powerless and disrespected, if PCPs convey to them that they are in charge of their lives, such a message may become a premise for their eventual action, even if they currently are not ready for more than medical treatment. Linkage to specialty follow-up services, therefore, cannot be over-emphasized.

General Crisis Intervention Strategies

In addition to the general crisis intervention strategies discussed in Chapter 3, following is a summary of the techniques for victim-survivors whether the injury and abuse is from rape, intimate partner battering, an attack from a stranger, or in the case of frail elders, a family member or caretaker:

- Assure the abused or threatened person of safety and protection through available resources; e.g., police, child and adult protective services.
- In explicit language, assure the victim/survivor that she/he is not to blame for another person's violent behavior.

- Reassure the victim-survivor that one's feelings and reactions to the assault are normal, not a sign of mental illness.
- Inform the person of legal rights and what this realistically means; e.g., a rape victim's right to file charges along with the prospect of what might ensue from an assailant's defense attorney; or, the legal responsibility of health providers to report child and elder abuse.
- Keep in mind the centrality of power dynamics and the person's need to regain a sense of control over one's life.
- While offering empathy and support, refrain from making decisions for the person.
- Provide emergency and other easy-to-understand information, including realistic means of avoiding life-threatening danger. Primary care settings should have this kind of information available to all clients in waiting areas.
- Link the person to specialized self-help groups.

The preventive, crisis, and follow-up aspects of helping victims-survivors should be practiced with a view to their vital connectedness. This triple approach to the problem may not only help end the pain and terror of women who are attacked, but may also remove the negative consequences of violence for children, men, and the entire society.

Mandatory Reporting by Emergency and Primary Care Providers

These principles apply to PCPs, police officers, and others, and raise the controversial question of mandatory reporting of domestic violence (as is required in *all* cases of child and elder abuse or neglect). Such mandatory reporting laws for abused adults exist in four states in the U.S.: California, Colorado, Rhode Island, and Kentucky. Central to this controversy is the issue of empowerment as expressed by female emergency department patients (Rodriques, McLoughlin, Hah, & Campbell, 2001). Nearly half of non-English speaking patients opposed mandatory reporting on grounds of protecting autonomy and socio-political factors like fear of deportation. Mandatory reporting might also be counter-productive in providing a "quick fix" or loophole for emergency department health professionals to avoid linking abused women to crisis and follow-up mental health services.

Also important is assuring abused women that they are not responsible for their victimization, no matter what the person who battered them says to the contrary (see Figure 3.2, Downward Spiral). Even when used in self-defense, a return of violence often escalates rather than decreases the violence. In addition, we should not assume that battered women are routinely in need of psychotherapy, as this could add a psychiatric label to an already heavy burden (Stark, Flitcraft, & Frazier, 1979). If a woman is suicidal, the principles and techniques discussed in Chapter 4 apply.

Once a woman is treated for physical trauma and resolves the dilemma of what to do next, she may be faced with the crises of finding emergency housing, caring for her children, and obtaining money. If a community does not have a safe home network or emergency shelter, if she cannot stay with relatives and has no money, she may have little choice but to return to the violent situation. In such instances, crisis and primary care providers should assist her in developing a survival plan that includes, for example, having a bag packed and getting a key to a friend's house in case of acute danger. We also need to remember that in rural isolated communities worldwide, secure shelters may be non-existent, or that a woman needing protection is expected to rely on kinship or tribal networks.

When a woman decides to leave, up-to-date abuse prevention laws require police to accompany her to her home to get her children, legal documents, and whatever possessions she can bring to an emergency housing situation. Almost invariably, when a woman is battered, her children are affected as well. An important element of helping a mother in crisis, as well as her children, is the availability of child care services, necessary for attention to housing and other problems. The children are often highly anxious and in need of a stable, calming influence as well as appropriate physical outlets and nonviolent discipline (see Humphreys, 1998). Pediatric PCPs caring for children—either physically and/or sexually abused or as witnesses to violence—need firm linkages for referrals to child psychiatric specialists.

Abused women say they do not expect us to rescue them (Hoff, 1990). Rather, they want us to listen to their terror and dilemmas, and offer support as they seek safety, healing, and a life without violence. Because many women call the police and contact emergency medical resources, putting these women in touch with specialized crisis workers is the first and most important thing emergency personnel and PCPs can do after providing medical treatment and safety planning.

Two factors, however, may impede the accomplishment of this task: some women may not acknowledge the cause of their physical injuries, or they provide a cover-up story. There are several reasons for this: (1) the woman may have been threatened by her mate with a more severe beating if she reveals the beating; (2) she may simply not be ready to leave for her own reasons; (3) she may sense the judgmental or unsympathetic attitude of a physician or nurse and therefore not confide the truth. Because of social isolation, prejudice, and fear of deportation, immigrant minority and refugee women who are abused usually face additional impediments to receiving help (Bui & Morash, 1999; Perilla, 1999) (see also Campbell, 1998, "Part VI: Culturally Specific Clinical Interventions").

Sensitivity to these factors will help PCPs to interpret a woman's evasiveness about her injuries and recognize the implausibility of a cover-up story; for example: "When we see women with injuries like this, it's often because somebody hurt them." Besides physical injuries, a battered woman will show other signals of distress and may present with aches and pains or vague symptoms not traceable to specific medical causes (Sugg & Inui, 1992). Primary care providers who use Triage and risk assessment tools can more accurately identify and appropriately respond to a battered woman in crisis. As is true with suicidal persons, *direct questioning* in the context of a trusting relationship usually results in the person's relief to know that someone is caring and sensitive enough to discern one's distress.

While structured counseling sessions are not usually the role of PCPs, the following case illustrates how crisis counseling and follow-up with a battered woman might proceed (excerpted from Hoff, *et al.*, 2009, Chapter 11). It may provide the referring PCP with greater confidence in recommending that their patients pay serious attention to the multiple psychological and social problems often connected to violence and abuse. It also illustrates service planning using the 21-item CMHA tool discussed in Chapter 2, and its use in primary care services specializing in women's health—settings that often include on-site mental health professionals.

CASE EXAMPLE: WOMAN ABUSE BY INTIMATE PARTNER

Sandra Le Claire is a 22-year-old woman who is currently separated from her abusive husband of five years. She came to the U.S. from a country where French was her second language after her native tongue; Sandra is now learning English. She is the mother of two small children, ages two and five. She does volunteer work for pay and is in the process of applying for public assistance. Her husband has been her sole source of financial support, and since their separation nine months ago, his support has been sporadic at best. Sandra presented with cuts and bruises about her face and across her chest and two black eyes, which are swollen shut—all as a result of a beating by her husband. On previous ED visits for minor injuries she was referred to her PCP, but never followed through because of threats by her husband. Sandra says the current beating was the culmination of an argument over her husband's lack of financial support to her and her children. She has never been willing to press charges against her husband out of fear, as he has threatened to kill her; nor has she ever retaliated with violence herself. She has been drinking more frequently and heavily and is becoming increasingly depressed and despondent about her situation. Sandra has suicidal ideation but denies having a specific plan, although in the past she has thought about taking an overdose of Tylenol when upset with her husband. She says her children have not witnessed any of the abusive episodes.

Sandra became pregnant at age sixteen after moving to the U.S. with her parents, and quit high school to get married. She grew up in poverty, the youngest of five children with an alcoholic father and a born-again, church-going mother. Sandra viewed her marriage as a way out.

Although her father worked steadily, he did not earn enough money to support both his family and his drinking. Her mother did not believe in divorce. She raised the children and largely ignored her husband's drinking, sustaining many beatings herself at his hands. Though Sandra feels supported by her mother, who helps her with child care, she does not feel understood. Her mother believes God will provide. She tells Sandra it is just a phase that men go through and that things will improve for Sandra, as they have for her, since Sandra's father has grown less violent over the years. Sandra is not sure she can wait.

Since English is her third language, Sandra has problems with getting financial aid because she cannot complete the forms. Her abusive husband is also a drinker. Sandra had no drinking problem prior to abuse.

Using the Comprehensive Mental Health Assessment (CMHA) and Service Contract forms presented in Chapter 2, the major problems and issues Sandra faces are illustrated and rated for stress levels in Figure 5.2, with safety issues paramount for the PCP's attention.

Date: _____
Code:_____

Stress Rating Code: 1 = low stress/very high functioning   5 = high stress/very low functioning

Item/Stress Rating		Problem/Issue Specification	Strategies/Techniques (planned actions of client and health provider)
20.	Safety—self (5)	Husband threatened to kill her	*Explore* (a) shelter option (b) changing locks (c) restraining order (d) feelings regarding use of these options.
13.	Violence/abuse experienced (4)	Does not seem clear about extent of danger	*Provide information about* (a) shelter number and admission process (brochures/cards) (b) emergency phone number.
14.	Injury to self (3)	Suicidal ideation/no specific or past attempts	*Discuss/listen* to feelings of hopelessness and reluctance to confide in close friend.

Among the issues identified, the PCP's focus should be on items 20, 13, and 14: Victimization, Safety, and Suicidality, and a referral for counseling to address other issues (items 12, 7, 9, and 21 on CMHA). A signed contract includes a one-week follow-up appointment with the PCP, plus Sandra's agreement to call if there are any problems with follow-through on the counseling referral.

Figure 5.2 Service Contract: A Battering Situation

Assessment of Dangerousness, Assault, and Homicide Risk

As in the case of suicide risk assessment, there is no absolute prediction of homicide risk. The topic itself is highly controversial; Monahan (1981, p. 6), for example, cites three criticisms regarding prediction in forensic work:

1. It is empirically impossible to predict violent behavior.
2. If such activity could be forecast and averted, it would, as a matter of policy, violate the civil liberties of those whose activity is predicted.
3. Even if accurate prediction were possible without violating civil liberties, psychiatrists and psychologists should decline to do it, since it is a social control activity at variance with their professional helping role.

Whereas prediction of violence is an issue in forensic work, *assessment of dangerousness and violence potential* can be a matter of life or death in domestic, occupational, and clinical settings. The clinical assessment of risk for dangerousness, assault and homicide is an inherent aspect of police officers' and health and crisis workers' jobs. The average citizen is always calculating safety maneuvers when in known risk areas. This is not the same as making an official prediction of risk as part of the court-requested psychiatric or psychological examination of persons who are detained for crimes and who plead insanity (Halleck, 1987). Although assessment of dangerousness is far from an exact science, health and social service workers do not have to rely *only* on their experience or guesswork. As one hospital trainer put it: "There's nothing out there [but my own experience]." Unfortunately, this person had no exposure to basic risk assessment strategies from either formal or in-service education programs; that is, many may rely on "guesswork" instead of drawing on evidence from crisis, psychiatric, and criminal justice theory and organized data gained through skilled communication with at-risk clients and significant others (see Hoptman, Yates, Patalingug, Wack, & Convit, 1999; Monahan & Steadman, 1994)—assessment based on *principles and data*, not merely on guesswork.

Criteria and Dynamics in Risk Assessment

Based on Monahan's (1981) research, risk assessment criteria include:

1. *Statistics*, for example, men between the ages of 18 and 34 commit a much higher percentage of violent crimes than older men or women of any age. Statistical indicators, however, should be viewed with the same caution as in suicide risk assessment.
2. *Personality factors*, including motivation, aggression, inhibition, and habit. For example, once a habit of response to upsets by verbal threats and physical force is established, it lays a foundation for further, potentially lethal violence.
3. *Situational factors*, such as availability of a weapon or behavior of an unwitting potential victim.
4. *The interaction* between these variables.

Toch (1969) claims that the *interaction* factor (in several stages) is crucial to influencing violence. First, the potential victim is classified as an object or a potential threat—essentially, a dehumanization process. Based on this classification, some action follows, after which the potential victim may make a self-protective move. Whether or not violence occurs depends on the interaction of such variables as the effectiveness of the victim's self-protection or the would-be attacker's interpretation of resistance as an "ego" threat demanding retaliation.

Establishing a bond, therefore, between a victim and assailant or terrorist can counteract dehumanization and thus serve to prevent an attack, although that strategy should not be relied on in all cases. This is the basis for a widely held principle in crisis intervention and hostage negotiation: *time* and keeping *communication* channels open—rather than precipitous action, taunts, or threats—are to the benefit of the negotiator and can save the lives of victims, terrorists, suicidal persons, and healthcare providers threatened at work by their patients or disgruntled family members.

Clearly, assessing danger is no simple matter, but lives can be saved by taking seriously the fact that only potentially dangerous people make threats of assault or homicide. A careful read of newspaper accounts of murders reveals almost invariably the assailant's verbal and other cues that were either ignored or misinterpreted as not being serious. Thorough training in crisis assessment and intervention is therefore paramount for health providers and others who work with disturbed or potentially violent people. This includes alertness to cues such as an angry outburst and agitation, and *always* inquiring about the *meaning* of verbal threats that too many times are dismissed by family, friends, and sometimes even professional colleagues. Health and social service providers should educate their clients and the general public about this safety issue.

When the indicators of dangerousness described in Table 5.2 (developed and tested in the 1970s—see Chapter 2) were introduced for routine use in community mental health clinics, staff were astounded at how many clients were entertaining violent fantasies. But crisis workers also noted the clients' openness to receiving help in dealing with their anger and violent impulses. These findings apply with respect to three major categories of abusive and violent assailants: (1) the international increase in violence and antisocial behavior among young people; (2) violence and abuse in the workplace; and (3) programs for men who batter and emotionally abuse their women partners.

Besides their usefulness in standard criminal justice and police work, the criteria for assessing the degree of danger and risk of assault apply in a number of situations:

1. in crisis, emergency, mental health, and forensic services;
2. in primary care settings;
3. in the event that a healthcare worker is threatened with violence or is being taken hostage, or stalked at home;
4. in all domestic disputes.

While acknowledging that violent people can learn to resolve conflict non-violently, *past violent behavior* is still a powerful indicator of future behavior. As the triage questions in Figure 5.1 indicate, routine screening for assault and homicide potential is gender neutral; therefore, an abused woman's own potential for assaulting or killing her assailant following abuse must also be ascertained.

Translated into everyday practice, the following criteria are helpful as guidelines to assess for risk of assault or homicide:

- history of homicidal threats;
- history of assault;
- current homicidal threats and plan, including on the internet;
- possession or easy availability of lethal weapons;
- use or abuse of alcohol or other drugs;
- conflict in significant social or clinical relationships—for example, infidelity, threat of divorce, labor-management disputes, authoritarian approaches to mentally ill patients;
- threats of suicide following homicide.

Application of Criteria: An Assessment Tool

Assessing for dangerousness, assault, and homicide risk is aided by use of an assessment tool, Table 5.2, excerpted from the Comprehensive Mental Health Assessment form presented in Chapter 2.

Table 5.2 Assault and Homicidal Danger Assessment Tool

Key to Danger	Immediate Dangerousness to Others	Typical Indicators
1	No predictable risk of assault or homicide	Has no assaultive or homicidal ideation, urges, or history of same; basically satisfactory support system; social drinker only
2	Low risk of assault or homicide	Has occasional assault or homicidal ideation (including paranoid ideas) with some urges to kill; no history of impulsive acts or homicidal attempts; occasional drinking bouts and angry verbal outbursts; basically satisfactory support system
3	Moderate risk of assault or homicide	Has frequent homicidal ideation and urges to kill but no specific plan; history of impulsive acting out and verbal outbursts while drinking, on other drugs, or otherwise; stormy relationship with significant others with periodic high-tension arguments
4	High risk of homicide	Has homicidal plan; obtainable means; history of substance abuse; frequent acting out against others, but no homicide attempts; stormy relationships and much verbal fighting with significant others, with occasional assaults
5	Very high risk of homicide	Has current high-lethal plan; available means; history of homicide attempts or impulsive acting out, plus feels a strong urge to control and "get even" with a significant other; history of serious substance abuse; also with possible high-lethal suicide risk

Youth Violence and the Role of Primary Care Providers

Aggressive, antisocial, and violent behavior among children and adolescents is gaining international attention. Overall crime rates in the United States and western Europe have declined sharply for several years, while dramatic shootings by school children have captured international attention. Bullying, cyber harassment, and mobbing—usually child-on-child aggression—continue to create terror in schools and have even been associated with suicide (Hoover & Juul, 1993). Youth violence has moved parents, social scientists, journalists, legislators, and others to debate and soul-search about the cultural climate and other factors that have spawned these tragedies. Research on bullying in Europe traces such behavior to a combination of factors in the home (e.g., inconsistent discipline, abuse, alcohol); the school (more antisocial behavior in the worst schools); and the characteristics of individual victims and perpetrators. Together, these factors underscore the *interactional* character of aggression and its sequelae. Paralleling adult patterns, the majority of bullying and antisocial behavior is perpetrated by males against both males and females (Ellickson, Saner, & McGuigan, 1997). Pediatric primary care providers are in strategic positions for early detection and prevention of youth aggression and violence (see Chapter 11 for further discussion of this topic).

Crisis Intervention with Assailants and those Threatening Violence

All of the principles of crisis intervention apply to the violent or potentially violent person at home, in school, or prison, and the workplace to help ensure safety of self and others. The application of these principles to aggressive, antisocial, or violent people are summarized as follows:

1. Keep communication lines open. As long as a person is communicating, violence usually does not occur.
2. Facilitate communication between a disgruntled employee or patient, for example, and the person against whom he or she is threatening violence. While hospital security personnel have designated crisis intervention roles, health workers' premature engagement of a security officer may backfire if excessive physical force is used to gain control of a potentially dangerous situation. Remembering the principle that "violence begets more violence," when physical containment is indicated, humane and respectful behavior is fundamental to safety.
3. Develop specific plans—*with* the dangerous person—for nonviolent expression of anger, such as time-out, jogging, punching a pillow, or calling a hotline, whether at home or in a psychiatric or substance abuse treatment unit.
4. Communicate by telephone or behind closed doors whenever possible when dealing with an armed person, especially until rapport is established and the person's anxiety subsides. This includes applying the risk assessment criteria as in Table 5.2.
5. If dangerous weapons are involved, collaborate with police for their removal whenever possible; implement emergency policies and procedures for appropriate application of force by a security officer or police, and by mobilizing a team effort to warn fellow workers. Failure to work in teams can be life threatening.
6. Insist on administrative support and emergency backup help; refuse any assignment that requires working alone in high-risk settings—for example, psychiatric wards or crisis outreach visits. If home visits are indicated, obtain information about potential danger whenever possible via telephone and team consultation *before* arriving at home premises.
7. Make hotline numbers and emergency call buttons readily available.
8. Examine social and institutional factors influencing violent behavior—for example, harsh authoritarian approaches to employee relations, which may trigger revenge and violence by an upset patient or a disgruntled worker; failure to help disturbed persons seek professional help as an alternative to violence; and rigid structures and rules for geriatric and psychiatric patients.
9. Warn potential victims of homicide, based on risk assessment and the principles of the Tarasoff case (Van de Creek & Knapp, 1993). A general guideline for warning potential victims is a rating of "moderate—#3," or "high—#4 or #5" on the Risk Assessment Tool (Table 5.2).
10. Remember that a violent person who is also threatening suicide is a greater risk for homicide.
11. Conduct follow-up. Engage in social and political activity to prevent violence.

Several factors, however, may become obstacles to providing aid to these people in crisis: (1) the sense of contempt or loathing one may feel toward a criminal or patient who has threatened a health or social service worker, (2) the fear of the prisoner or other person threatening violence, and (3) the need to work within the physical and social constraints of a detention setting or workplace where one does not anticipate interaction with disturbed or violent persons. People working in these settings, therefore, must assess and deal with crises according to the circumstances of their particular situations. The works of Adams (2007); Meloy (1992); and Tavris (1983) are particularly recommended.

Programs for Violent Men

Newspaper accounts reveal that restraining orders have not prevented the murders of women by their intimate partners. In fact, clinical work with abused women reveals that they are perhaps in greatest danger after filing for a restraining order, particularly in cases in which the woman's partner feels that he owns her and is now confronted with an external force threatening his need to control her. This underscores the need for caution among PCPs and others in persuading a woman to seek court protection; for trusting the woman's own judgment of the man's potential for violence; and attention to the contextual factors that may infuriate him to the point of violence.

Moving beyond the debate about whether perpetrators should receive treatment or serve time in jail, the both-and approach discussed earlier should generally be the norm, even when the women who have been battered—especially those intent on salvaging their relationship and marriage—just want the violence to stop, by whatever means. To carry out that approach, the health and criminal justice aspects of domestic violence must be synchronized, culturally sensitive, and include systematic follow-up through probationary and court systems. In a public health and crisis prevention framework, any program for abusive men must include three facets:

1. the need to assess and reassess their potential for further assault or homicide, as suggested in Table 5.2;
2. the importance of holding the perpetrator accountable for his violent behavior, regardless of mental pathology and any excuses, such as that the woman's behavior provoked him to violence;
3. a focus on the *roots* of the problem, *power and control* over one's partner, not just "anger management," since anger is a "trigger" not typically used except against the intimate partner.

These program elements imply regular supportive contact by a PCP or crisis counselor with the woman who was abused and is possibly still at risk, particularly if she has filed a restraining order and in instances when men present themes of jealousy, desperation, and ownership of their partner (Meloy, 1992).

Court-mandated counseling has led to a proliferation of batterer programs illustrating a variety of intervention systems (Gondolf, 1999). Despite progress in evaluating the effects of these programs, results are still mixed (Adams, 2007; Babcock & Steiner, 1999). However, those who have developed standards for and researched batterer programs assert that accountability and victim safety are central, regardless of competing perspectives (Bennett & Piet, 1999). Outcome measures of effectiveness reveal that the longest, most comprehensive program demonstrated the lowest re-assault rate; this nine-month program of weekly group counseling also includes an extensive clinical evaluation, in-house substance abuse treatment, individual psychotherapy for emotional and mental problems, and casework with women partners (Gondolf, 1999, pp. 44–45). Since effective programs are designed to confront and diffuse power and control dynamics, short "anger management" can be dangerous—especially to the abused spouse—if led by someone without knowledge and expertise about this core feature of violence (Dempsey, 2003). These findings can be used effectively by any PCP working with abused women who may simply rely on "hope and trust" that a violent partner will change.

In most programs for men who batter, group counseling is the preferred mode (Adams, 2007), usually including other men who have been violent in the past but are no longer violent. This approach underscores the premise that violence is not inevitable but is learned and reinforced through parenting practices and its pervasiveness in the sociocultural milieu. For abused women who believe "couples counseling" is the answer to stopping violence, PCPs should note that this highly controversial approach tends to obscure violence as the primary problem (Bograd & Mederos, 1999) and implies a counselor's "neutrality" in regard to criminal behavior. If couples counseling is used, safety, ownership of responsibility for violence, and a *prior* intention of reconciliation must first be established (Edleson & Tolman, 1992, pp. 88–107).

Although programs for batterers and refuges for victims must be supported, these secondary and tertiary measures would be much less costly in financial and human terms if primary prevention and "restorative justice" were more valued and promoted (see Earley, 2006). Primary care providers serving the families and children of prisoners also need to pay special attention to the medical sequelae of chronic social and economic stress traceable to imprisonment of a spouse or parent.

Violence and Abuse in the Healthcare Workplace and Forensic Psychiatry

One of the first principles in crisis work is safety—for ourselves, our clients, significant others, and the general public. Moving from the global to everyday work life, violence as an occupational health hazard has gained public attention (Levin, Hewitt, & Misner, 1992; Lipscomb & Love, 1992; Merchant & Lundell, 2001). Police officers, health, mental health, crisis, and other workers make up a special category of victims. The potential danger to PCPs from clients and/or abuse by one's colleagues (lateral violence) embroils us in the controversial relationship between crime and mental illness (forensic psychiatry). Despite numerous debates on this topic, the distinctions between crime and mental illness overlap with relevance to life crises and the safety of PCPs, police, security personnel, and other workers often caught in the middle. With greater skills in applying risk assessment knowledge in the workplace, many injuries from violence might be avoided, since mentally ill people are probably no more violent than they were in the past, and their rates of violence are comparable to those of the general public (Friedman, 2006).

While some people who commit crimes are mentally ill, therefore entitling them to leniency before the law, many insanity pleas leave much room for doubt. Insanity is a *legal*, not a mental health, concept. Difficulties with this issue in the United States are complicated by a criminal justice system that often denies a decent standard of treatment to criminals. The humanitarian impulse of most people is to spare even a violent person an experience that seems beyond the deserts of the crime. It is paradoxical, then, that the tendency to only *treat* a person rather than also holding him or her responsible for violent behavior, exists in concert with the movement to assert the rights of mentally ill patients (Earley, 2006). We cannot have it both ways. One cannot, on the one hand, exercise the freedom to reject treatment and hospitalization for behavioral disorders and, on the other hand, plead temporary insanity when one then fails to control violent impulses and commits a crime (or in psychiatric and primary care settings, assaults a staff member who may or may not press criminal charges). The following case illustrates this point, as well as the need for mental health and health professionals to examine their misplaced guilt feelings when they hold clients accountable for their violent behavior.

CASE EXAMPLE: MENTAL STATUS AND ACCOUNTABILITY

Connie, age 51, was being treated in a private psychiatric facility for a drinking problem and depression following a divorce. A mental status examination revealed that Connie was mentally competent and not suffering from delusions or other thought disorders, though she was very angry about her husband's decision to divorce her because of her drinking problem. When Connie, therefore, decided to check out of the residential treatment facility against medical advice, there was no basis for confining her involuntarily, according to any interpretation of the state's mental health laws. A discharge planning conference was held, at which follow-up therapy sessions were arranged through a special program for alcoholic women. Connie failed to keep her counseling appointments. One week after leaving the psychiatric unit, Connie attempted to demolish her former husband's car by crashing her own car into it. She endangered the lives of other people by driving on sidewalks, where pedestrians successfully managed to escape her fury. Connie was arrested and taken to jail. While the judge preferred committing Connie to the psychiatric unit where she had been treated, testimony by a mental health professional supported this decision: Mental status examination and Connie's intact physical capacity provided no basis on which to keep her from being a further menace to society by psychiatric vs. criminal justice containment. Connie was furious with her counselor for not offering psychiatric grounds for avoiding a jail term.

This case suggests spillovers of violence from home to workplace, as well as using alcohol as an excuse from accountability for violent behavior. A biomedical versus public health response to workplace violence may help perpetuate the problem if the larger social ramifications of the issue remain unaddressed. Obviously, this takes us well beyond an injured healthcare worker's responsibility. Yet, safety in one's workplace and our common humanity in a violent society demand such a two-pronged approach to this serious issue (see Arnetz & Arnetz, 2001).

Too often the signs of impending assault or homicide are either not recognized or are ignored until it is too late, as documented in widely publicized massacres at schools and worksites. It is important to note that murder does not occur in a cultural or social vacuum; it does not "just happen." Typically, it is planned, although impulse may play a part.

Fortunately, the days of assaulted health workers having to absorb their injury and emotional trauma as "part of the job" appear to be coming to an end (O'Sullivan, *et al.*, 2008). Research has uncovered the relationship of workplace injury to gender, race, and class factors, as well as to the work environment itself—for example, inadequate staffing and lack of structured supervisor support. Guidelines from the Occupational Safety & Health Administration and labor union action portend the prospect of redressing the neglect of many victimized workers who have been largely on their own in the process of recovering from the trauma of such mostly preventable violence (Rosen, 2001; Runyan, 2001). Post-trauma support programs for injured workers are also gaining attention. For further discussion, see Hoff (2010), Chapters 11 and 12, including vicarious traumatization of staff.

Primary Prevention of Violence and Anti-social Behavior

So long as loopholes exist in the criminal justice system's response to interpersonal violence such as battering, refuges are no less than lifesaving for many women at risk. Similarly, residential treatment programs for out-of-control youth are necessary. But the very fact that an entire system of residential programs for battered women has been established speaks to the tendency, especially in the United States, toward *reactive* rather than *preventive* approaches. History reveals that all societies establish rules for how to treat deviant members.

The fruits of such reactive policy recommendations (Hoff, 1990) are underscored by a study in 29 cities documenting that the lives saved by the shelter system are mostly those of men—that is, murders are prevented because women receive help through hotline, shelter, and legal services before reaching the point of using deadly force against their abusers. However, if the male partners do not receive help, they are more likely to kill the women (Dugan, Nagin, & Rosenfeld, 2001). In other words, refuges for abused women are just that—an emergency resource, not primary prevention. But moving beyond emergency measures will yield limited results without the community-wide endeavors, generally intrinsic to primary approach to healthcare in the following arenas.

Personal and Socio-psychological Strategies

When sincerely addressing the issue, individuals may become overwhelmed by the pervasiveness of violence and withdraw out of a sense of helplessness, self-protection, burnout, or what is sometimes referred to as *vicarious traumatization*—that is, internalizing the psychic pain that victimized patients share with empathic providers. It is important therefore that PCPs and clients at risk focus on selected actions and obtainable goals including, for example:

1. adopting nonviolent language in everyday social interaction;
2. using nonviolent ways of disciplining children; attending parent effectiveness training groups to assist with difficult child-rearing challenges;
3. providing all workers with violence prevention information and emergency protocols, including how to recognize and respond humanely to an upset or disgruntled client or co-worker with antisocial tendencies;
4. remembering that since violence and victimization are deeply rooted in sociocultural, economic, and political contexts, individual efforts *alone*—while necessary—are not sufficient to address the problem.

Socio-political Strategies

These strategies are most successful when combined with personal and social-psychological approaches on the premise that people need grounding in information and self-confidence in order to stand firm against obstacles in the political arena.

1. *Educating the public through schools, community organizations, and churches.* For example: How many people who have attended church, synagogue, or mosque, for example, have heard a sermon condemning violence against women and children, or have sponsored programs to explicitly address such issues?
2. *Contacting legislators and organizing for a change in laws that may be outdated or otherwise do not address the issues local people face.* In the United States, for example, addressing the powerful gun lobby, or the high rate of incarceration among African-American youth as opposed to Caucasian youth for comparable offenses.

3. *Using advocacy and systematic organizing around racial and economic justice.* This includes seeking equality in educational opportunities and addressing the media influence on violence (see Sorenson, Peterson, & Berk, 1998).

Professional Strategies

In the United States, the Surgeon General's report (U.S. Department of Health and Human Services, 1986) recommended that all licensed professionals be required to study and pass examination questions in violence prevention and the treatment of various victims of violence. As a complement to this public policy statement, PCPs and their teachers can exert leadership and advocacy within their own groups for curriculum and in-service program development to systematically address this topic. At present, such educational endeavors are incidental at best (Hoff, 2010). The American Association of Colleges of Nursing (1999) has produced a position paper underscoring the need for inclusion of violence content in all nursing education programs. Similar programs have been developed for criminal justice professionals in North America and other countries.

The vast knowledge already available to professionals must be combined with personal strategies in order to:

- widely disseminate new knowledge about this poignant topic to the public;
- change the values and attitudes that have served as fertile soil for nurturing and normalizing violent and antisocial behavior;
- effect broad policy and functioning of social institutions through the political process necessary to bring about needed change.

References

Adams, D. (2007). *Why do they kill? Men who murder their intimate partners.* Nashville, TN: Vanderbilt University Press.

American Association of Colleges of Nursing. (1999). *Position paper: Violence as a public health problem.* Washington, DC: Author.

Arnetz, J. E., & Arnetz, B. B. (2001). Violence towards health care staff and possible effects on the quality of patient care. *Social Science and Medicine, 52,* 417–427.

Babcock, J., & Steiner, R. (1999). The relationship between treatment, incarceration, and recidivism of battering: A program evaluation of Seattle's coordinated community response to domestic violence. *Journal of Family Psychology, 13*(1), 46–59.

Bell, C. C., Jenkins, E. J., Kpo, W., & Rhodes, H. (1994). Response of emergency rooms to victims of interpersonal violence. *Hospital and Community Psychiatry, 45*(2), 142–146.

Bennett, L., & Piet, M. (1999). Standards for batterer intervention programs: In whose interests? *Violence Against Women, 5*(1), 6–24.

Bograd, M., & Mederos, F. (1999). Battering and couples therapy: Universal screening and selection of treatment modality. *Journal of Marital and Family Therapy, 25*(3), 291–312.

Brown, J. C., & Bohn, C. R. (1989). *Christianity, patriarchy, and abuse: A feminist critique.* New York: Pilgrim Press.

Bui, H. N., & Morash, M. (1999). Domestic violence in the Vietnamese immigrant community: An exploratory study. *Violence Against Women, 5*(7), 769–795.

Burstow, B. (1992). Radical feminist theory: Working in the context of violence. Thousand Oaks, CA: Sage.

Campbell, J. C. (Ed.) (1998). *Empowering survivors of abuse: Health care for battered women and their children.* Thousand Oaks, CA: Sage.

Campbell, J. C., & Humphreys, J. H. (1993). *Nursing care of survivors of family violence.* St. Louis: Mosby-Year Book.

Coker, A. L., Flerx, V. C., Smith, P. H., Whitaker, D. J., Fadden, M. K., Williams, M. (2007). Partner violence screening in rural health care clinics. *American Journal of Public Health*, 97(7), 1319–1325.

Dempsey, K. (2003). Do batterer programs "work"? *Victim Impact*, 4(1), 6—7,11.

Dobash, R. E., & Dobash, R. P. (Eds.) (1998). *Rethinking violence against women*. Thousand Oaks, CA: Sage.

Dugan, L., Nagin, D., & Rosenfeld, R. (2001). Explaining the decline in intimate partner homicide: The effects of changing domesticity, women's status, and domestic violence resources. Paper presented at the 1997 meeting of the American Society of Criminology.

Earley, P. (2006). *Crazy: A father's search through America's mental health madness*. New York: Berkley Books.

Edleson, J. L., & Tolman, R. M. (1992). *Intervention for men who batter: An ecological approach*. Thousand Oaks, CA: Sage.

Ellickson, P., Saner, H., & McGuigan, K. A. (1997). Profiles of violent youth: Substance use and other concurrent problems. *American Journal of Public Health*, 57(6), 985–991.

Everett, B., & Gallop, R. (2000). *Linking childhood trauma and mental illness: Theory and practice for direct service practitioners*. Thousand Oaks, CA: Sage.

Figley C. R. & Nash, W. P. (Eds.). (2005). *Combat stress injury*. New York: Routledge.

Friedman, R. A. (2006). Violence and mental illness: How strong is the link? *New England Journal of Medicine*, 355(20), 2064–2066.

Gelles, R. J., & Loseke, D. R. (Eds.) (1993). Current controversies on family violence. Thousand Oaks, CA: Sage.

Gondolf, E. (1999). A comparison of four batterer intervention systems: Do court referral, program length, and services matter? *Journal of Interpersonal Violence*, 14(1), 41–61.

Halleck, S. L. (1987). The mentally disordered offender. Washington, DC: American Psychiatric Press.

Handwerker, W. P. (1998). Why violence? A test of hypotheses representing three discourses on the roots of domestic violence. *Human Organization*, 57(2), 200–208.

Herman, J. (1992). *Trauma and recovery: The aftermath of violence*. New York: Basic Books.

Hoff, L. A. (1990). *Battered women as survivors*. London: Routledge.

Hoff, L.A. (2010). *Violence and abuse issues: Cross-cultural perspectives for health and social services*. London: Routledge.

Hoff, Hallisey, & Hoff (2009). *People in crisis: Clinical and diversity perspectives*. 6th Ed., London: Routledge.

Hoff, L. A., & Rosenbaum, L. (1994). A victimization assessment tool: Instrument development and clinical implications. *Journal of Advanced Nursing*, 20(4), 627–634.

Hoover, J. H., & Juul, K. (1993). Bullying in Europe and the United States. *Journal of Emotional and Behavioral Problems*, 2(1), 25–29.

Hoptman, M. J., Yates, K. F., Patalingug, M. B., Wack, R. C., Convit, A. (1999). Clinical prediction of assaultive behavior among male psychiatric patients at a maximum-security forensic facility. *Psychiatric Services*, 50(11), 1461–1466.

Humphreys, J. (1998). Helping battered women take care of their children. In J. C. Campbell (Ed.), *Empowering survivors of abuse: Health care for battered women and their children* (pp. 121–137). Thousand Oaks, CA: Sage.

Husseini, R. (2009). *Murder in the name of honor*. Oxford: One World Oxford.

Levin, P. E., Hewitt, J. B., & Misner, S. T. (1992). Female workplace homicides: An integrative research review. *American Association of Occupational Health Nursing Journal*, 40(5), 229–236.

Lipscomb, J. A., & Love, C. C. (1992). Violence toward health care workers: An emerging occupational hazard. *American Association of Occupational Health Nursing Journal*, 40(5), 219–228.

Luhrmann, T. M. (2000). *Of two minds: The growing disorder in American psychiatry*. New York: Knopf.

Meloy, R. (1992). *Violent attachments*. Northvale, NJ: Aronson.

Merchant, J. A., & Lundell, J. A. (2001). Workshop violence intervention research workshop, April 5–7, 2000, Washington, DC: Background, rationale, and summary. *American Journal of Preventive Medicine*, 20(2), 135–140.

Monahan, J. (1981). *Predicting violent behavior: An assessment of clinical techniques*. Thousand Oaks, CA: Sage.

Monahan, J., & Steadman, H. J. (Eds.). (1994). *Violence and mental disorder: Developments in risk assessment*. Chicago: University of Chicago Press.

O'Sullivan, M., Siqueira, C. E., Sperrazza, K., Koren, A., Melillo, K. D., Hoff, L. A., White-O'Sullivan, E. M., & Slatin, C. (2008). It's part of the job: Healthcare restructuring and the healthy and safety of nursing aides. In L. McKee, E. Ferlie and P. Hyde (Eds.), *Organizing and reorganizing: Power and change in health care organizations* (pp. 99–111). Basingstoke: Palgrave Macmillan.

PAHO/WHO (2003). *Violence against women: The health sector responds*. Washington: Author.

Perilla, J. L. (1999). Domestic violence as a human rights issues. The case of immigrant Latinos. *Hispanic Journal of Behavioral Sciences*, 21(2), 107–133.

Rodriguez, M. A., McLoughlin, E., Hah, G., Campbell, J. C. (2001). Mandatory reporting of domestic violence injuries to the police: What do emergency department patients think? *Journal of the American Medical Association*, 286(5), 580–583.

Rosen, J. (2001). A labor perspective of workplace violence prevention: Identifying research needs. *American Journal of Preventive Medicine*, 20(2), 161–168.

Ross, M., Hoff, L. A., & Coutu-Wakulczyk, G. (1998). Nursing curricula and violence issues: A study of Canadian schools of nursing. *Journal of Nursing Education*, 37(2), 53–60.

Runyan, C. W. (2001). Moving forward with research on the prevention of violence against workers. *American Journal of Preventive Medicine*, 20(2), 169–172.

Ryan, W. (1971). *Blaming the victim*. New York: Vintage Books.

Rynearson, E. K. (Ed.). (2006). *Violent death: Resilience and intervention beyond the crisis*. New York: Routledge.

Segal, L. (1999). *Why feminism? Gender, psychology, politics*. New York: Columbia University Press.

Soeken, K. L., McFarlane,J., Parker, B., & Lominack, M. C. (1998). The abuse assessment screen: A clinical instrument to measure frequency, severity, and perpetrator of abuse against women. In J. C. Campbell (Ed.) *Empowering survivors of abuse: Health care for battered women and their children* (pp. 195–203). Thousand Oaks, CA: Sage.

Sorenson, S. B., Peterson, J. G., & Berk, R. A. (1998). New media coverage and the epidemiology of homicide. *American Journal of Public Health*, 88(10), 1510–1514.

Stark, E., Flitcraft, A., & Frazier, W. (1979). Medicine and patriarchal violence: The social construction of a "private" event. *International Journal of Health Services*, 9, 461–493.

Stephens, B. J. (1985). Suicidal women and their relationships with husbands, boyfriends, and lovers. *Suicide & Life-Threatening Behavior*, 15(2), 77–90.

Sugg, N. K., & Inui, T (1992). Primary care physicians' response to domestic violence: Opening Pandora's Box. *Journal of the American Medical Association*, 267(23), 3157–3160.

Tavris, C. (1983). *Anatomy of anger*. New York: Simon & Shuster.

Toch, H. (1969). *Violent men*. Hawthorne, NY: Aldine de Gruyter.

United Nations (1996). *The Beijing declaration and the platform for action*. New York: Author.

U.S. Department of Health and Human Services (1986). *Surgeon General's workshop on violence and public health: Report*. Washington, DC: Author.

U.S. Surgeon General (1986). *Surgeon General's workshop on violence and public health: Report*. Washington, DC: U.S. Department of Health and Human Services.

Van de Creek, L., & Knapp, S. (1993). *Tarasoff and beyond: Legal and clinical considerations in the treatment of life-endangering patients* (Rev. ed.). Sarasota, FL: Professional Resource Press.

Van der Kolk, B. A. (1987). *Psychological trauma*. Washington, DC: American Psychiatric Press.

Warshaw, C. (1989). Limitations of the medical model in the care of battered women. *Gender and Society*, 3(4), 506–517.

Wiehe, V. R. (1998). *Understanding family violence: Treating and preventing partner, child, sibling, and elder abuse*. Thousand Oaks, CA: Sage.

Wilson, J. P. (Ed.) (2006). *The posttraumatic self: Restoring meaning and wholeness to personality*. New York: Routledge.

Woodtli, A., & Breslin, E. (2002). Violence-related content in the nursing curriculum: A follow-up national survey. *Journal of Nursing Education*, 41(8), 340–348.

6 The Anxious Patient

Anxiety is a common, normal and useful response to life's challenges and dangers, and is therefore part of the human experience. It is usually experienced as a vague sense of uneasiness. When we are confronted with a danger, anxiety causes us to get out of the way of the danger. When we are faced with a test, either in an educational setting, or a test of our skills in the workplace, anxiety may be the driving force behind our preparation to meet this challenge; without the anxiety we might not prepare and therefore might fail the test! Anxiety can become overwhelming and cause problems with our ability to function. When this happens in a transient situation, we are often able to deal with the situation and then move on to other issues in our lives. When the feeling of being overwhelmed continues for more than a brief period of time, it can become problematic. Fear is different than anxiety. Fear is generally thought of as a response to a known, external, definite threat, while anxiety is a response to an unknown or internal threat.

Anxiety in a Complex World

Most adults have experienced anxiety. Things such as intense worry or fear, difficulty concentrating, a "keyed up" feeling, accompanied by physical symptoms such as sweating, palpitations, dry mouth, hot flashes or chills, dizziness, trembling, restlessness, shaking and muscle tension are common when one is anxious. Anxiety has an effect on the general health of an individual. Anxiety can also affect thinking, perception and learning. It can result in confusion and distortion of perceptions, which can affect learning.

Many people talk about stress rather than using the term anxiety. There are physiological responses that occur when the body is under stress detailed by Hans Selye (1956) in the General Adaptation Syndrome (GAS) including the alarm stage (fight or flight), the resistance/recovery stage, and the exhaustion stage. Psychological defense mechanisms such as denial, projection, rationalization, and intellectualization are the psychological system's response to anxiety that threatens our physical, mental, and social selves. An individual's perception of an event as well as the person's coping mechanisms is what determines how stressful an event is to that person and how much anxiety the person may experience.

Anxiety in American society was dramatically changed on September 11, 2001. As people worldwide witnessed the attacks in New York, Pennsylvania, and Washington, D.C. and sat glued to their television sets, we entered a new age of anxiety. Prior to these events, anxiety was primarily a personal issue related to the stressors of everyday living. Current difficulties related to the financial state of one's country bring anxiety to the forefront as people become anxious about their ability to provide for food and shelter for their families. Anxiety about diverse issues is common across cultures.

It is important for primary care providers to differentiate between anxiety about a common life situation, and anxiety as a symptom of a psychiatric illness. Additional information about the person, one's family, and life circumstances will assist the primary care provider to develop an understanding of the problems and appropriate questions to pursue in assessment of the individual (see Chapter 3, Crisis Care Basics). Severity of the anxiety, as well as duration of the symptoms and effect on how the person functions in daily activities, can help determine the need for treatment and follow-up care.

Prevalence and Description of the Problem

Anxiety disorders are the most common mental health problem in the U.S., affecting an estimated 40 million adults. Anxiety problems are highly treatable, yet only one-third of those suffering with anxiety receive any treatment (ADAA, 2008). The National Co-morbidity Study (National Institute of Mental Health, 2009) reported that one in four people in the U.S. met the diagnostic criteria for at least one anxiety disorder, and that the prevalence rate for anxiety disorders was 18 % in a six-month period. Women have a higher level of anxiety than men and the prevalence of anxiety decreases with higher socioeconomic status.

Anxiety problems cost the U.S. more than $42 billion a year, accounting for almost one-third of the country's mental health bill of $148 million (ADAA, 2008). Over half of this amount is associated with the use of healthcare services. People with anxiety problems most often seek care from primary care providers first for symptoms that mimic physical illnesses. People with anxiety are three to five times more likely to go to the doctor and six times more likely to be hospitalized for psychiatric disorders than those without anxiety (ADAA, 2008). Common somatic signs of anxiety are listed in Box 6.1.

Anxiety in Primary Care Settings and Differential Diagnosis

Anxiety is common in any primary care practice. Who among us has not gone to a medical appointment as the result of some symptoms and feared for the worst outcome? When people feel that their physical well-being is in a state of change, perhaps putting them at risk for some unknown disease, it can strike fear in their hearts and cause great anxiety. In primary care settings more than half of the medical visits are for somatic complaints, which are most often associated with anxiety or depression.

There is some evidence that chronic anxiety can lead to long-term health problems. The Framingham Heart Study found connections between anxiety and hypertension in men aged 45–59 (Kubzansky, 2009). Other studies have examined the association of anxiety to heart attacks. In a 2005 study, women aged 65 and older with anxiety were found to have more difficulty with activities of daily living (Sareen, Cox, Clara, & Asmundson, 2005).

BOX 6.1 Somatic Signs and Symptoms of Anxiety

- Anorexia
- Backache
- Butterflies in the stomach
- Chest discomfort
- Diaphoresis
- Diarrhea
- Dizziness
- Dyspnea
- Palpitations
- Vomiting
- Faintness
- Pallor
- Dry Mouth
- Tachycardia
- Fatigue
- Flushing
- Headache
- Hyperventilation
- Light-headedness
- Muscle tension
- Nausea
- Urinary frequency
- Paresthesia
- Sexual dysfunction
- Shortness of breath
- Sweating
- Tremulousness

Box 6.1 lists the most common somatic signs and symptoms of anxiety. Many people come into a primary care setting presenting with these symptoms and never endorse problems with anxiety or worry unless asked about these problems. Questions related to life events and changes in everyday functioning may assist in determining anxiety as a problem. Often, laboratory tests will be needed to rule out any medical cause of the anxiety.

Additionally, several medical conditions (Box 6.2), intoxication or withdrawal from certain drugs and/or alcohol, as well as side effects of several medications (Box 6.3) may cause symptoms related to anxiety. Complete physical work-up of these conditions should take place, based on presenting symptoms, physical examination, and thorough history before arriving at a diagnosis of anxiety (see Assessment and Screening Tools).

BOX 6.2   Medical Illnesses that Mimic Symptoms of Anxiety

- Respiratory Illnesses
  - Asthma
  - COPD
  - Hypoxia from any cause
  - Pulmonary embolism

- Endocrine Disorders
  - Acute intermittent porphyria
  - Carcinoid syndrome
  - Cushing's syndrome
  - Hyperthryroidism
  - Hypoglycemia
  - Insulinoma
  - Hypothyroidism
  - Pheochromocytoma
  - Menopause

- Cardiovascular Disorders
  - Angina
  - Arrhythmias
  - Atrial tachycardia
  - Mitral valve prolapse
  - Myocardial infarction

- Orthostatic hypotension
  - Congestive heart failure
  - Coronary artery disease

- Neurological Disorders
  - Aura of migraine
  - Cerebral neoplasia
  - Delirium
  - Demyelinating disease
  - Early dementia

- Metabolic Disorders
  - Acidosis
  - Electrolyte abnormalities
  - Substance Abuse/Dependence
  - Hyperthermia
  - Pernicious anemia
  - Wilson's disease

- Partial complex seizures
- Vestibular disturbance
  - Brain tumor
  - Cerebral syphillis
  - CVA
  - Huntington's chorea
  - Multiple Sclerosis
  - Pain

Source: Adapted from Pollock, Otto, Bernstein & Rosenbaum, 2004; Saddock & Saddock, 2003

BOX 6.3 Medication Side Effects that Mimic Symptoms of Anxiety

- Analgesics
- Antibiotics
- Digitalis
- Anabolic steroids
- Anticholinergic agents
- Antidepressants
- Antihypertensives
- Antiparkinson agents
- Anticonvulsants
- Antihistamines
- Anti-inflammatory agents
- Aspirin
- Caffeine
- Coritcosteroids
- Neuroleptics
- Indomethacin
- Ephedra
- Theophyllin
- Chemotherapy agents
- Sympathomimetics
- Thyroid supplements
- Bronchodilators and decongestants
- Cocaine
- Epinephrine
- Cannabis
- Oral contraceptives
- Anesthetics
- Toxins

- Intoxication and/or withdrawal from:
  - Analgesics/narcotics
  - Alcohol
  - Sedative/hypnotics
  - Benzodiazepines
  - Nicotine
  - Opiates
  - Methamphetamine
  - Phencyclidine (PCP)
  - Ecstacy (MDMA)

CASE EXAMPLE: ANXIETY IN THE FAMILY

Maria Rodriguez is a 23-year-old single woman from Puerto Rico. She comes to see her primary care provider (PCP) only to find out that the provider, a nurse practitioner (NP) who cared for her for the last year and a half, has moved out of state, and she has been assigned to a new NP. She is very quiet in her presentation, has no eye contact and is looking suspiciously around the room as if thinking about running out of the room. She is very hesitant in her responses to medical questions; when asked about her mood, substance abuse, or any family history of mental illness she gets up and starts pacing in the room. The main reason for the visit is that she has been experiencing abdominal pain for about a week and a half. The nurse practitioner is beginning to think that there may be a mental health problem and is not sure at all how to proceed since Maria is not being very cooperative with the history.

The nurse practitioner finally says to Maria that she seems very nervous and that she wonders if there is something she is worried about. At this point, Maria bursts into tears and says that her beloved aunt Tina had bad abdominal pain just like she is experiencing and that when she went to the doctors to find out about the pain she was diagnosed with liver cancer and died within three months of that visit. Maria is terrified that she also has liver cancer.

This scenario is more common than most professionals would predict and is rarely the kind of information that patients offer freely. The necessity of paying attention to the mood of each individual patient and asking clearly about the mood can often elicit information that would not be revealed otherwise. The intervention may be very brief, as it was in this case, allowing the PCP to move on to other parts of the assessment. Reassurance that the similar symptoms would make anyone frightened and the fact that making the appointment quickly after the appearance of symptoms was the right thing to do, may be all that is necessary to do at this point. Following a physical exam and other tests, the nurse practitioner was able to rule out the liver cancer.

Presentation of Anxiety Disorders

Anxiety Disorders are classified in the DSM-IV-TR (APA, 2000) as: Acute Stress Disorder, Generalized Anxiety Disorder, Panic Disorder, Social Phobia, Specific Phobia, Obsessive-Compulsive Disorder, and Post-traumatic Stress Disorder. There are also anxiety problems associated with medical conditions and their treatments and anxiety problems associated with medications and substance use and withdrawal (Boxes 6.2 and 6.3).

Acute Stress Disorder   Acute stress disorder is characterized by the development of anxiety and other symptoms, within one month of exposure to a traumatic stressor. This includes personal experience of an event involving a threat (actual or perceived) of death or personal injury, witnessing such an event, or learning about an unexpected or violent death, serious harm or threat of death experienced by someone close to you such as a family member or close associate. The response to the stressor must include intense fear, helplessness, or horror. The individual will also show signs of re-experiencing the event, such as recurrent images, thoughts, dreams, illusions, or flashbacks. The person will also avoid any stimuli associated with the event and experience numbing and symptoms of arousal such as difficulty sleeping, irritability, poor concentration, hypervigilance, motor restlessness or exaggerated startle response (APA, 2000). The DSM-IV-TR criteria requires that there must be significant distress or impairment of functioning over at least two days and less than four weeks, occurring within four weeks of the event to be classified as an acute stress disorder (APA, 2000).

Generalized Anxiety Disorder (GAD)   Generalized anxiety disorder presents with excessive uncontrollable worry and anxiety over everyday issues. People with this problem can agonize over job responsibilities, finances, health issues, personal appearance, and family well-being and relationships. This excessive worry can affect daily functioning and can cause multiple physical symptoms. The focus of the worry and anxiety may shift from day to day. The intensity, duration, and frequency of the worry is disproportionate to the real situation; the person is often aware that the fears are out of proportion to the situation; yet is not able to control the anxiety. People who have this problem may be very irritable, restless, and complain that they feel on edge, are easily tired and have trouble sleeping. Normal daily activities may become impossible to maintain. GAD affects 2–3% of the U.S. population (Swartz, 2006). GAD commonly occurs with other anxiety disorders, depression, and substance abuse. It can be difficult to diagnose since it lacks the dramatic presentation seen with a panic attack.

Panic Disorder   Panic disorder is twice as common in women as in men. It affects approximately 2.7% of the U.S. population or six million people. Attacks usually begin in the late teens or early twenties and often are not diagnosed. Only about one in four people with panic attacks receive adequate treatment.

Many otherwise healthy people may experience an isolated panic attack and never experience one again; this does not signify a diagnosis of panic disorder. A panic attack is an abrupt onset of an episode of intense fear or discomfort that peaks in about ten minutes and lasts only about 20–30 minutes. People experience a feeling of imminent danger and the need to escape, as well as physical symptoms such as: palpitations, sweating, trembling, shortness of breath, a choking feeling, chest pain or discomfort, dizziness, lightheadedness, a sense of things being unreal or feeling detached, a fear of losing control or "going crazy," a fear of dying, tingling sensations, and/or chills or hot flashes. The intensity of these physical symptoms frequently brings patients to an emergency setting. In the popular movie *Something's Gotta Give* Jack Nicholson portrays a man who presents to the ER with chest pain that is a panic attack.

Panic disorder is diagnosed when the person has recurrent and unexpected panic attacks accompanied by persistent concerns about having more attacks, continued worry about the meaning or implications of the attack, and a change in the person's behavior due to the attack. A complication of panic is agoraphobia—the fear of being in public places. This fear may have developed as a result of trying to avoid situations and places that have triggered panic attacks. Panic disorder with agoraphobia can severely restrict a person's life. Panic disorder occurs co-morbidly with depression, substance abuse, and suicidal thinking.

Social Phobia   Social phobia is also called social anxiety disorder and describes people who have extreme and persistent anxiety in social situations. This can include performance anxiety and fear of public speaking. The main problem is the fear of embarrassment or ridicule that accompanies the anxiety. The person is able to recognize that the fear is not reasonable or is out of proportion to the situation, but the anxiety persists and the person will either avoid or tolerate the situation with great discomfort. Anticipatory anxiety is often a problem with the person experiencing significant anxiety for days or weeks prior to the event.

Social phobia is more common in women, typically beginning in childhood or adolescence and associated with shyness and social inhibition. Approximately 15 million people (in the U.S., or 6.8% of the population) are affected by social phobia (ADAA, 2008). A stressful public experience may intensify the problem (Swartz, 2006).

Specific Phobia   Up to 8% of the adult U.S. population may suffer from one or more specific phobias. Usually phobias develop during childhood and may persist for years or decades.

Specific phobias do not generally develop as the result of a single traumatic event. Instead there is often evidence of a phobia in another family member and/or social or vicarious learning of phobias (Swartz, 2006). Panic attacks may also be involved in the development of specific phobias.

The DSM-IV-TR describes specific phobia as a marked and persistent fear of the presence or anticipation of a specific object or situation; the fear is excessive or unreasonable and is often recognized as unreasonable by the person (APA, 2000). The avoidance of the specific object or situation causes significant distress and interferes with the person's functioning.

Obsessive-Compulsive Disorder (OCD)   Obsessive-compulsive disorder is characterized by recurrent, repetitive thoughts (obsessions), or behaviors (compulsions), or both. The person recognizes these thoughts or behaviors as unreasonable and intrusive, and that they interfere with ability to function in job, school, and/or relationships. The obsessions and compulsions must take at least up to an hour a day, every day, and interfere with normal social and occupational functioning to meet DSM criteria for diagnosis (APA, 2000).

"Obsessions are defined as recurring and persistent thoughts, ideas, images, or impulses, sometimes of an aggressive nature, that seem to invade a person's consciousness" (Swartz, 2006, p. 51). The thoughts are experienced as intrusive and inappropriate and cause anxiety or distress. Some of the more common examples of obsessions include fear of contamination from germs, thoughts of aggressive or violent behavior or fear of harming oneself, and a fear of making a mistake.

Compulsions are repetitive and ritualistic behaviors that are performed following a specific set of rules or patterns. The behaviors are aimed at reducing distress or preventing some dreaded event or situation. The behavior temporarily relieves whatever tension is brought about by obsessive thoughts. Some of the more common types of compulsive behavior include checking and rechecking to make sure that doors are locked, windows closed, appliances are turned off, repetitive hand washing accompanied by an obsession with germs and dirt and excessive neatness, cleanliness and organization, and hoarding behavior.

OCD occurs in about 1–2 % of the population, up to 2.2 million adults in the U.S. One-third of people with OCD first experience symptoms as children. OCD occurs equally among men and women, and accounts for 6 % of the $148 billion yearly mental health bill (ADAA, 2008). Mild OCD may allow people to function with only minimal interference with their daily activities, while severe OCD may be incapacitating. Common comorbid psychiatric problems that occur with OCD include depression and substance abuse.

Post-Traumatic Stress Disorder (PTSD)   Post-traumatic stress disorder is a chronic problem that follows an exposure to a traumatic event such as a natural disaster, rape or another violent crime, an accident, war, or terrorism. The event must have involved actual or threatened death or serious injury, and the response of the person was intense fear, helplessness, or horror. Witnessing such events is known to be as stressful as being personally affected by the event. The symptoms associated with PTSD include:

- recurrent, intrusive, distressing dreams and memories of the event;
- flashbacks and a sense that the event is recurring;
- extreme distress when stimuli that symbolize or elicit memories of the event are encountered;
- avoidance of thoughts, feelings, and activities associated with the event;
- inability to remember parts of the event;
- markedly diminished interest in normal activities;
- feeling of detachment or unreality; dissociation;

- hyperarousal, hypervigilance, exaggerated startle response;
- low expectations of the future;
- insomnia, nightmares, and excessive fatigue;
- extreme irritability;
- inability to concentrate;
- significant distress and impairment in functioning (APA, 2000; Swartz, 2006).

If these symptoms persist for over a month after the event and are associated with severe distress or functional impairment, a diagnosis of PTSD is made. Symptoms usually occur within three months of the event but there may be a delayed onset of symptoms that occurs six months after the event. The chronic nature of this problem adds to the difficulties that a person faces such as low self-esteem, a sense of hopelessness and being permanently damaged, difficulties in relationships, difficulties with work and abuse of substances, including alcohol and illicit or legal drugs.

In the general population the prevalence of PTSD in one year is 3.6% with women being twice as likely as men to have this problem. Among those exposed to extreme trauma, about 9% develop PTSD (Satcher, 2008). Hoge and colleagues (2004) studied members of the armed services deployed in Iraq and Afghanistan either before combat or three to four months after their tour of duty. They found major depression, generalized anxiety, and post-traumatic stress disorder (PTSD) among these troups, based on standardized screening, with the highest rates in the group following duty in Iraq. The largest difference was in the screening for PTSD. It is anticipated that as the war goes on, more veterans will be diagnosed with PTSD. Hoge also found that only 23–40% of the participants sought mental healthcare.

Co-morbid Psychiatric Problems and Anxiety

Nearly one half of people diagnosed with a depressive disorder are also diagnosed with an anxiety disorder (ADAA, 2008). These illnesses can occur at the same time or one may precede the other. One diagnosis may be the primary diagnosis and the other secondary. For example, someone with social anxiety disorder may become anxious about not being able to attend family gatherings and therefore may become depressed. The combination of the two problems may result in greater disability and decreased functioning than either alone.

Additionally, anxiety and substance misuse or abuse are also common co-morbid problems. The desire to self-medicate anxiety may lead to a long-term problem with substances, and the effect of the substances and/or detoxification from the substances may contribute to ongoing symptoms of anxiety. In a study of primary care patients 58% of the patients with a substance use disorder met the criteria for another mental disorder. The most common co-morbid disorders with alcohol misuse were depression and agoraphobia, and with other drug use disorders the most common disorders were specific phobia and agoraphobia (Olfson, *et al.*, 1997). Other research has indicated that social anxiety disorder and PTSD are common co-morbid problems with alcoholism (ADAA, 2008). Having both an anxiety disorder and substance abuse problem may result in a vicious circle effect causing the person to use a substance to deal with the anxiety, and then experiencing more anxiety as a side effect of the substance use, leading to further use of the substance. The implications for treatment are that both problems must be addressed simultaneously for treatment to be effective, and to break the vicious circle.

The National Epidemiological Survey on Alcohol and Related Conditions conducted by the National Institute on Alcohol Abuse and Alcoholism (NIAAA, 2006) reported that about 20% of those with an anxiety or mood disorder have a current alcohol or substance abuse problem. Additionally, this study found that the vast majority of people with both alcohol and other substance abuse and anxiety experience the problems independently, with only some or none of the anxiety being induced by the alcohol or drugs. People with an anxiety disorder are two to three times more likely to have a problem with alcohol or other substances than the general population (ADAA, 2008).

People with alcohol and anxiety problems are at risk for many complications including:

- additional problems such as hospitalization, financial problems, and medical illnesses;
- lower treatment adherence;
- increased risk of relapse;
- increased risk of dangerous interactions between drugs and prescribed medications;
- more pronounced withdrawal symptoms.

Assessment Issues

Failure to recognize the problem of anxiety in primary care settings contributes to inadequate adherence to medical treatment recommendations and can result in increased medical visits and hospitalizations, and the overuse of medical resources. During the course of routine medical visits, questions about anxiety and preoccupation with concerns or fears should be included in the history. A question such as "Do you tend to be anxious or nervous?" is a general screening question and a positive response indicates the need for further questioning. Further questions can include:

- "Have you ever had to limit your activities because of anxiety?"
- "Have you ever had a panic attack?"
- "Do you have any problems with excessive hand-washing or checking things over and over?"
- "Do any of these problems significantly interfere with your life?"

Careful questioning about recent or remote life events related to the anxiety is important, as well as any family history of anxiety problems (as noted in Chapter 2).

Ruling out any medical or substance related problems that can cause symptoms of anxiety is the first step in assessing for a problem with anxiety (Boxes 6.2 and 6.3). Review of use of caffeine and over-the-counter medications and remedies, as well as any herbal supplements should be part of the assessment process (see Chapter 13). Additionally, review of developmental issues given the patient's age, and the sociocultural context of the patient and family, is essential in the assessment of symptoms related to anxiety. Discussion of the hazards of labeling and inadequate assessment is included in Chapters 2 and 3, and is of great importance in the discussion of anxiety.

In the fast-paced primary care setting, the focus is on a diagnosis and treatment within a short period of time. The need to move people in and out of a practice setting can result in an over-reliance on medication, when what anxious clients really needs is someone to talk to about their life situation and their feelings. In the case of Maria as described above, it is easy to imagine that the PCP did not take the time to address her behavior and consequently would have missed a vital component of the problem, and perhaps recommended medication inappropriately.

Psychiatric Evaluation

Anxiety clearly is a part of life, so the psychiatric assessment of anxiety must focus on the magnitude of the symptoms of anxiety, the distress the anxiety causes for the individual, and the impact on the person's ability to function. Questions about when the anxiety occurs, what happens when the person becomes anxious, any warning of impending anxiety, the duration of episodes, and what helps resolve the episodes are all important, brief questions that can be included in an examination.

The Primary Care Anxiety Project, a longitudinal study of 539 individuals in primary care in New England who had anxiety disorders, revealed that 52% of the patients were receiving treatment. Of that group 24% were receiving both psychopharmacological treatment and psychotherapy, 21% were receiving only medication and 7.2% were receiving only psychotherapy (Weisberg, Dyck, Clupepper, & Keller, 2007). Patients receiving pharmacological treatment received similar treatment whether or not the prescriber was a primary care physician or a psychiatrist, with the exception that *primary care physicians were less likely to prescribe benzodiazepines*. Those receiving medications from a primary care prescriber were less likely to be receiving psychotherapy. Given the evidence that providing both pharmacologic and psychotherapy treatment provides the best results, this study highlights the need for *more collaborative care approaches in primary care settings*.

Screening Tools and the Context for Assessment

There are several screening tools designed for rating anxiety levels. These tools were developed primarily with a focus on research and may not have been utilized widely in clinical situations. Screening tools also may use valuable clinical time in a primary care setting and therefore are not often utilized in this setting. A screening tool provides a snapshot of what is occurring at a given point in time, and therefore a discussion of symptoms as they have developed over time may provide a greater window into the presence of a problem with anxiety. The most widely used anxiety-related screening tools include the following:

- Hamilton Anxiety Rating Scale (HAM-A)
- Yale-Brown Obsessive-Compulsive Scale (Y-BOCS)
- Brief Psychiatric Rating Scale (BPRS).

Perhaps one of the most important factors in the assessment of anxiety is for the provider to remain calm and use a matter-of-fact approach. Severe anxiety can become contagious and may result in the provider hurrying through the assessment process, to end his or her own discomfort. A therapeutic approach is another key factor in the assessment process. It enhances a patient's comfort in talking about feelings.

For screening in primary care, the Comprehensive Mental Health Assessment tool (CMHA) (see Chapter 2) addresses anxiety specifically in question #12: *Feelings: How comfortable are you with your feelings?* (or, *Do you often feel anxious or fearful?*). Additionally, questions about decision-making ability (#8) and problem-solving ability (#9) examine how the person feels about ability to manage problems. This is of great importance in assessing the level of anxiety since the person's *perception* of the situation is of primary importance in understanding one's ability to cope with the feelings.

Laboratory Tests

While there are no specific laboratory tests related to anxiety, there are several general tests that may be useful in ruling out medical problems, which may present with symptoms of anxiety. In general a CBC with a differential, electrolytes, and thyroid function tests is useful and included as a part of many general medical examinations. Ruling out exposure to any anxiety-inducing substance such as caffeine is an important first step in determining a lifestyle related problem. Serum bicarbonate levels may be decreased, while chloride levels may be increased in panic disorders. Use of a urine toxicology screening test may assist in ruling out an addictive disorder. An EKG may be indicated in ruling out a cardiac problem when a person has panic symptoms. Many people (up to 40%) of people with a panic disorder may have mitral valve prolapse (Saddock & Saddock, 2003). See Boxes 6.2 and 6.3 for other medical illnesses and medications that may indicate the need for further laboratory or other screenings, when ruling out a medical condition related to the symptoms of anxiety.

CASE EXAMPLE: COLLABORATIVE CARE

Jean was a 28-year-old Caucasian woman with a two-year-old daughter. She had a diagnosis of HIV disease (high CD4 count and low viral load), depression, and poly-substance abuse (in remission for three years) and was being followed by a primary care provider and a psychiatric clinical nurse specialist (CNS) associated with the practice. Jean was being treated with Zoloft for her depression and was seen in weekly psychotherapy sessions; her depression was stabilized after four months but she elected to continue therapy for support and to explore some issues in more depth. The therapist suspected an abuse history, but Jean answered the screening questions related to abuse as not applicable. One day she walked into the primary care providers' office demanding to be seen, and once seen, she told the PCP that her anxiety was keeping her awake at night, and that she needed medication immediately. The PCP arranged for an emergency appointment with her CNS since he did not feel comfortable prescribing any medication without further assessment.

Jean followed up with the appointment and began talking and demanding medication as soon as she sat down with the CNS. She became resistant to questions about when the anxiety began and focused only on the medication. She began shouting at the CNS that "You won't give me anything for anxiety because I am an addict! It's not fair!" The CNS said, "I see that you are very upset about something, but any time I try to ask a question so I can understand what is going on, you yell at me. I am not sure what to do, since I do not understand what is upsetting you so much."

At that point Jean began to sob and said that her former boyfriend, the father of her daughter, was stalking her, and that she was really frightened about what might happen to her. The CNS and Jean developed a safety plan including where she might go to be safe and people to call to help her get there. They decided together that frequent contact with the CNS and continuation of the Zoloft was the best support, and that use of other medication might keep her less alert than she needed to be of any signs of impending danger. They discussed the fact that this stress did put her at increased risk of relapse and she increased her attendance at N.A. (Narcotics Anonymous) meetings and talked more frequently to her sponsor. Jean did not want to consider a shelter; she was living at the time in supported HIV housing, and did share this information with the housing staff of the shelter.

Jean did not ever stop contact with her former boyfriend, but did end the intimate relationship at one point. She dropped out of treatment many months later, despite several attempts to contact her, to at least have a meeting to discuss termination of the therapy. About two years later the CNS was informed that she had relapsed, did get additional substance abuse treatment, and was killed by her former boyfriend, the day that she was discharged from inpatient treatment.

This situation, while not common, does address the need to always try to determine the *cause of anxiety*, particularly if it is a new symptom as was the case in this example.

This example also demonstrates the usefulness of a collaborative practice model in handling complex patient problems. If the primary care provider had simply responded to the initial request for medications it would have eliminated the possibility of determining the serious underlying cause of the anxiety that emerged in the work with the CNS. On the other hand, sometimes—aside from our best efforts—circumstances beyond our control determine tragic outcomes such as Jean's.

Treatment: Psychotherapeutic and Pharmacologic

Anxiety is best thought of as a continuum from mild to moderate anxiety, to severe and then panic. Use of self-management techniques and other interventions are most helpful when introduced early on, when the anxiety is at a mild to moderate level. Minarik (1996) and Leavitt and Minarik (1989) introduced a Hierarchy of Anxiety Interventions with mild to moderate levels of anxiety, focusing on prevention strategies, and moderate to severe anxiety including panic, focusing on treatment strategies. Examples of prevention strategies include providing concrete information, increased opportunities for self-control, increased patient and family involvement in care, and encouraging hope. Examples of treatment strategies include use of a support person, provision of accurate information for restructuring fearful ideas, teaching of anxiety reduction techniques, and repetition of realistic reassurances.

Treatment recommendations suggest that a combination of psychotherapy and pharmacological interventions are the most successful treatments for anxiety. However, treatment does not always require medication. Use of anti-anxiety drugs often depends on the patients' ability to tolerate the anxiety, while learning to manage the symptoms of anxiety. The effect of the anxiety on an individual's ability to function in daily living is also a key determinant in the use of medication. Despite the recommendations, combined treatment is not always presented to patients as the optimal treatment regimen. Additionally, stigma about mental healthcare, lack of access to mental health providers and inadequate insurance reimbursement may contribute to the over-reliance on medication treatment without psychotherapy.

Awareness of treatment guidelines and community and professional standards of care for treatment of anxiety is essential for primary care providers. Treatment guidelines for anxiety are widely available on the internet including the commonly used American Psychiatric Association guidelines (www.psych.org) and U.S. government guidelines (www.guidelines. gov).

Treatments recommended for anxiety include: elimination of anxiety-causing stimulants such as overuse of caffeinated beverages or stimulating over-the-counter medications, participation in psychotherapy, especially cognitive-behavioral therapy, pharmacological treatments including antidepressants, anxiolytic and antipsychotic agents, and patient self-management techniques including herbal remedies. Brief descriptions of the therapeutic modalities, pharmacological therapies, and self-management strategies will follow.

Psychotherapeutic Modalities

Psychotherapy offers people the opportunity to identify the various factors that may contribute to, or exacerbate their anxiety, and learn new techniques and strategies to manage the anxiety. Over the past few decades there has been an increased focus on time-limited therapies for anxiety problems that focus on coping abilities, rather than exploring unconscious conflicts, as is done with psychodynamic therapies (Surgeon General's Report on Mental Health). Both individual and group therapy are effective treatment modalities for anxiety disorders.

Cognitive-behavioral therapy, behavioral therapy, and supportive psychotherapy will be discussed briefly.

Cognitive-behavioral therapy helps people evaluate the apparent cause and effect relationships between thoughts, feelings, and behaviors, and also helps them develop strategies to decrease symptoms. Exposure to situations that increase anxiety may be included as a part of the therapy, and enhancement of mastery over the anxiety is a goal of treatment.

Behavioral therapy is an important treatment modality for some of the anxiety problems. Systematic desensitization is among the most effective treatments for some anxiety disorders such as panic disorder with agoraphobia. The therapist and patient define the phobic stimulus and then work together to expose the patient to events that stimulate the anxiety and progressively move to increasing levels of anxiety, while assisting the patient in the mastery of the anxiety. Behavioral treatment is most often provided in a specialized therapy practice, although elements of behavioral treatment may be utilized by a number of therapists.

Supportive psychotherapy is a part of most therapeutic relationships and is important in treating anxiety problems. The development of a trusting relationship with the therapist is important if the patient is going to be able to confront the anxiety that has resulted in discomfort and disability. Additionally, the ability to investigate new coping strategies, rehearse and utilize them in an appropriate manner at the right time (usually at an early stage when the anxiety-provoking stimulus is identified) are all activities that come under the rubric of supportive therapy.

Anti-anxiety Medications

Antidepressant medications have become the first line of treatment for anxiety disorders. Box 6.4 lists the medications used in the treatment of specific anxiety disorders. Selective Serotonin Reuptake Inhibitors (SSRIs) and Selective Norephinephrine Reuptake Inhibitors (SNRIs) are considered the first line of treatment for anxiety disorders. More detailed discussion of antidepressant medications is included in Chapter 8. Initiation of treatment for anxiety with an antidepressant medication occurs commonly in primary care settings. Careful explanation that the medication may take up to four weeks to relieve anxiety is essential; this long delay may contribute to lack of adherence, or premature discontinuation of treatment if not carefully discussed, with the option of a return visit to the primary care setting if anxiety remains acute. Often practitioners may also prescribe benzodiazepines if rapid control of symptoms is necessary, and then taper the benzodiazepine as the antidepressant takes effect in control of the anxiety. Many patients who may be used to the immediate effect of a benzodiazepine may be resistant to treatment with an antidepressant or Buspirone since these medications have a longer time of onset.

Benzodiazepines are thought to relieve anxiety by enhancing the effects of the neurotransmitter GABA. Most often a longer acting benzodiazepine is utilized for ongoing treatment of an anxiety disorder. Generally the side effects of benzodiazepines are considered to be mild including minor disturbances of cognition, decreased coordination, and drowsiness. Patients should be advised to avoid operating machinery or driving when adjusting to a dose of a benzodiazepine (either when starting a new medication or following an increase in dosage).

The most troublesome side effects of benzodiazepines are the development of tolerance to the drug, both physical and psychological, and withdrawal symptoms if the medication is suddenly discontinued. Withdrawal symptoms generally occur within one to two days of the last dose with short acting benzodiazepines, and within five to ten days of the last dose for long acting benzodiazepines. The withdrawal syndrome includes symptoms such as irritability, agitation, restlessness, insomnia, tremor, muscle aches, confusion, and seizures. Therefore tapering of dosages following treatment is necessary to avoid a withdrawal syndrome; usually anyone who has been on regular benzodiazepine doses for a period of about a month should be tapered from the medication. Patients can also become addicted to benzodiazepines and therefore these drugs should be used with caution with patients with an addictive disorder (see Box 6.4).

BOX 6.4 Types of Medications Used in Treating Anxiety

Medication	Indication for use	Daily average doses
Antidepressants		
SSRIs Paroxetine (Paxil)	OCD, panic, social phobia, PTSD, GAD	20–60 mg.
Sertraline (Zoloft)	OCD, panic, social phobia, PTSD	50–200 mg.
Fluoxetine (Prozac)	OCD, panic, social phobia	40–60 mg.
Escitalopram oxalate (Lexapro)	social anxiety disorder	10–20 mg.
Citalopram (Celexa)	anxiety in elders	20–40 mg.
SNRIs Venlafaxine (Effexor)	GAD	150–375 mg.
NRIs Bupropion (Wellbutrin)	GAD	10–30 mg.
TCAs Amitriptyline (Elavil)	panic, GAD	
Imipramine (Tofranil)	GAD, phobias	75–200 mg.
Trazadone (Desyrel)	GAD	150–400 mg.
Clomipramine (Anafranil)	OCD	50–125 mg.
MAOIs Phenelzine (Nardil)	panic, social phobia	30–90 mg.
Tranylcypromine (Parnate)	panic, social phobia	20–60 mg.
Isocarboxazid (Marplan)	panic, social phobia	10–30 mg.
Beta-Blockers Propanolol (Inderal)	social phobia	30–140 mg.
Atenolol (Tenormin)	social phobia	50–100 mg.
Alpha-Blocker Prazosin (Minipress)	PTSD (nightmares)	low doses
Anxiolytics		
BNZ Alprazolam (Xanax)	panic disorder, GAD, phobias	1–4 mg.
Lorazepam (Ativan)	panic disorder, GAD, phobias	2–10 mg.
Clonazepam (Klonopin)	social phobia, GAD, phobias	1–4 mg.
Diazepam (Valium)	GAD, panic, phobias	4–40 mg.
Non-BNZ Buspirone	GAD, OCD	10–30 mg.
Atypical Anti-psychotics Olanzapine (Zyprexa)	augmentation	low doses
Quetiapine fumurate (Seroquel)	augmentation	
Risperidone (Risperidal)	augmentation	
Ziprasidone (Geodon)	augmentation	
Arupiprazole (Abilify)	augmentation	

Source: Adapted from Anxiety Disorders Association of America; Swartz, 2006

Buspirone has been utilized to treat anxiety disorders, specifically GAD. It is a 5-HT 1A receptor partial agonist and requires two to three times a day dosing. It has a longer onset (up to two to four weeks) and patients may need treatment with a benzodiazepine during this period of time. Unlike the benzodiazepines it does not have the sedative, hypnotic, muscle-relaxant or anti-convulsant effects, is not associated with a withdrawal phenomenon, or cognitive impairment and has a low potential for abuse. The most common side effects are headache, nausea, dizziness, and insomnia. Occasionally patients may report a feeling of restlessness from Buspirone (see Box 6.4).

The *beta blockers* are utilized primarily with social phobia and fear of public speaking. The side-effects are minimal with these drugs that for the most part are used only occasionally. The *alpha-blocker,* pazosin has been used effectively to treat nightmares with PTSD. More recently second generation anti-psychotic medication (see Box 6.4) has been utilized to augment therapy when symptoms of anxiety have shown only partial response to treatment.

CASE EXAMPLE: NEED FOR FURTHER TREATMENT

Doug is a 45-year-old African-American man who comes into the primary care practice with vague complaints of abdominal discomfort, headaches, fatigue, and occasional palpitations. He is healthy otherwise and has been followed in the primary care practice for many years. He denies any alcohol use other than a couple of beers a week with friends and denies any other substance use. As the primary care provider reviews the past year since the last physical exam she learns that he and his wife have separated and that he has not been doing well at work for the last six months.

He is fearful that he will lose his job. He does not present as depressed but says that he worries constantly that he will not have enough money to pay child support and maintain his apartment (he moved out of the home he and his family lived in). He has difficulty concentrating at work (he is a machinist) and is worried that he might actually hurt himself at work since he has had a few minor accidents already. He has not been able to see much of his kids (ages five and eight) and has taken on a second job to cover expenses. As the primary care provider asks more questions he reveals that he has been much more irritable and has gotten into a recent argument with his boss and later was furious with himself for doing this. He says that his sleep has been even worse since this happened and that he is becoming more and more concerned about his job. He says that he has never experienced this much worry in his life.

The primary care NP decides that he meets the criteria for Generalized Anxiety Disorder and attempts to discuss some self-management strategies with Doug, but quickly realizes that he is too anxious to be able to use these strategies effectively at this point. She prescribes Paroxetine for the anxiety and sets up a phone appointment in a week and a regular appointment in two weeks. At the time of the phone appointment, Doug is continuing to have acute anxiety and not sleeping well. At this point the NP adds Clonazepam 0.25 mg twice a day for one week and reaffirms the appointment for the following week. When Doug comes in the following week he is continuing to have difficulty at work, difficulty sleeping and is very worried most of the time about work, his ability to straighten things out with his wife, his lack of contact with his children, and a number of other issues. The NP is clear with Doug that she thinks that psychotherapy would be extremely important to add to the medication treatment and Doug clearly does not want to do this. The NP spends a great deal of time talking to him about how combined treatment (psychotherapy and psychopharmacology) yields the best results, but he is still resistant.

Doug leaves the office with another prescription for a week of Clonazepam and Paroxetine and a return appointment in one week. When he returns he says that he had used up all the Clonazepam a day early and that he needs more. At this point, the NP tells Doug that she insists that he connect with a therapist for the most effective treatment and that she will only continue prescribing the medication if he also sees a therapist; she then is able to walk him down the hall to set up an appointment with the therapist (who is in the same building) for a week and a half later. The NP increases the Clonazepam to 0.25mg three times a day, gives Doug a prescription to carry him through the time of his appointment with the therapist, and sets up an additional appointment with herself (the NP) on the same day (following the appointment with the therapist). She leaves a phone message for the therapist (while Doug is present) describing all of this and asking for the therapists' recommendations after the initial meeting with Doug.

The example of Doug presents a reasonable approach by the primary care NP to deal with anxiety in the primary care setting. It also acknowledges that the time involved and the minimal response to treatment of this patient would indicate the need for a referral to a specialist. This kind of collaborative care is not always so readily available. Development of contacts with psychiatric providers is essential for being able to provide collaborative care to patients with combined medical and psychiatric problems.

Self-management Strategies

There are a wide variety of appropriate self-management strategies for use in dealing with anxiety and other chronic mental health issues. Basic self-care such as getting adequate sleep, exercising, and avoiding caffeine and alcohol are important measures that may decrease anxiety. Family and self-management support is achieved through collaborating with patients and families to help them acquire the skills, confidence, and motivation to manage the problem of anxiety. Providing the tools for management, enhancing the patient's own coping mechanisms, and providing close follow-up to address the challenges, successes and failures of self-management strategies are examples of the collaborative model of care necessary in chronic illness management. Support groups for both patients and families are additional supports and ways to identify other means for managing the anxiety. The National Alliance of Mentally Ill (NAMI) provides patients and families with education and advocacy services.

Providers should assume that each patient has tried a variety of self-management techniques even before seeking medical help, so questioning about what has been tried, what works and what does not work should be part of the initial assessment. Regular exercise has been demonstrated as an effective way to relieve anxiety. Use of massage, touch, distraction, relaxation techniques, breathing techniques, focusing techniques, music therapy, and guided imagery and visualization are all self-management techniques that can be introduced by the primary care provider. Learning to use these techniques in the early stages of an episode of anxiety requires some practice and encouragement. Use of support groups or group sessions to teach and review these techniques is a good way to provide care to several people at one time and also build supportive networks for patients.

Use of complementary alternative therapies is detailed in Chapter 13. Valerian, L-theanine, passion flower, fennel, hops, motherwort, heather, and kava are all herbal remedies that have been associated with reducing anxiety. Patients should be told that report of use of any of these herbal remedies is important since they are not necessarily benign substances and may interact with other medications that are being prescribed for the patient.

In summary, utilization of a wide variety of approaches when managing anxiety can be the most beneficial approach to treatment. The collaborative relationship between patient and provider, and primary care provider and mental health provider works best when all the approaches are geared towards improving the function of the individual patient. Communication among all members of the healthcare team is essential in providing the optimum treatment and management of the problem.

References

American Psychiatric Association (APA). (2000). *Diagnostic and statistical manual of mental disorders* (4th Ed.) DSM-IV-TR. Washington, D.C.: American Psychiatric Association.

Hoge, C. W., Castro, C. A., Messer, S. C., McGurk, D., Cotting, D. I., & Koffman, R. L. (2004). Combat duty in Iraq and Afghanistan, mental health problems, and barriers to care. *New England Journal of Medicine*, 351(1), 13–22.

Kubzansky, L. (2009). Going to the heart of the matter: Do negative emotions cause coronary artery disease? *Journal of Psychosomatic Research*, 48(4), 323–337.

Leavitt, M., & Minarik, P. (1989). The agitated, hypervigilant response. In Rigel, B., & Ehrenreich, D. (Eds.) *Psychological Aspects of Critical Care Nursing*. Rockville, MD: Aspen, pp. 49–65.

Mental Health: A Report of the Surgeon General-Chapter 4. www.surgeongeneral.gov/library/mentalhealth/chapter4/sec2_1.html (accessed on October 11, 2008).

Minarik, P. (1996). Psychosocial intervention with ineffective coping responses to physical illness: depression-related. In Barry, P. D. (Ed.). *Psychosocial Nursing Care of Physically Ill Patients and their Families*. New York: Lippincott Raven, pp. 323–339.

National Institute of Mental Health (2009). *www.nimh.nih.gov/* (accessed on July 12, 2010).

National Institute on Alcohol Abuse and Alcoholism (NIAAA) (2006). National epidemiological survey on alcohol and related conditions. http://pub.niaaa.nih.gov/publications/AA70/AA70.pdf (accessed on July 1, 2010).

Olfson, M., Fireman, B., Weissman, M. M., Leon, A. C., Sheehan, D. V., Kathol, R. G., Hoven, C., & Farber, L. (1997). Mental disorders among patients in a primary care group practice. *American Journal of Psychiatry*, 154 (12), 1734–1740.

Pollack, M. H., Otto, M. W., Bernstein, J. G. & Rosenbaum, J. F. (2004). Anxious patients. In Satcher, D. (1999). Mental health: A report of the Surgeon General. http://www.surgeongeneral.gov/library/mentalhealth/resources.html (accessed on 1 July 2010).

Saddock, B. J., & Saddock, V. A. (2003). Kaplan & Saddock's *Synopsis of psychiatry: Behavioral sciences/clinical psychiatry* (9th Ed.). Philadelphia, PA: Lippincott Williams & Wilkins.

Sareen, J., Cox, B. J., Clara, I., & Asmundson, G. J. (2005). The relationship between anxiety disorders and physical disorders in U.S. National Comorbidity Survey. *Depression and Anxiety*, 21, 193–2020.

Selye, H. (1956). *The stress of life*. New York: McGraw Hill.

Stern, T. A., Fricchione, G. L., Cassem, N. H., Jellinek, M. S., & Rosenbaum, J. F. (Eds.). *Handbook of general hospital psychiatry* (5th Ed.). Philadelphia, PA: Mosby.

Swartz, K. L. (2006). *The Johns Hopkins White Papers: Depression and anxiety*. Baltimore, MD: Johns Hopkins Medicine.

Weisberg, R. B., Dyck, I., Clupepper, L., & Keller, M. B. (2007). Psychiatric treatment in primary care patients with anxiety disorders: A comparison of care received from primary care providers and psychiatrists. *The American Journal of Psychiatry*, 164(2), 276–282.

7 Problems of Depression and Mood Disorders

- Prevalence and Description of Mood Problems
- Depression as a Co-morbid Condition with Medical Disorders
- Illnesses and Medication Effects Commonly Mistaken for Depression
- Assessment Issues and Screening Tools
- Treatment of Depressed Persons: Psychotherapeutic and Pharmacologic
- Patient Self-management, Family, and Alternative Therapy Approaches
- References

Almost all humans have some understanding of and experience with the alteration in mood patterns. The experience of "the blues" is a common part of the human condition, but bears little resemblance to the profound feelings experienced by those with major depressive disorder. This common experience can both enhance the understanding of the experience and lead to lack of assessment for the more serious consequences of mood or affective problems. William Styron in describing his own depression discussed the "basic inability of healthy people to imagine a form of torment so alien to everyday experience. For myself the pain is most closely connected to drowning or suffocation—but even those images are off the mark" (1990, p.17).

The mood problems as described by the DSM-IV-TR (APA, 2000) include major depressive disorder, dysthymic disorder, and bipolar disorder. This chapter will define these problems, the prevalence of the problems, and costs to society. Descriptions of the diagnostic criteria for each of these disorders are included; however, the chapter's major focus is on depression, since depression is commonly seen in primary care settings. Information about assessment, diagnosis and treatment, both pharmacologic and non-pharmacologic, is provided. Collaborative care with psychiatric mental health professionals is discussed and suggestions for appropriate referrals are included throughout the chapter.

Prevalence and Description of Mood Problems

Problems of depression and mood are common in the U.S. with approximately 20.9 million American adults, or 9.5 % of the population having what has been labeled a mood disorder in a given year (National Institute of Mental Health [NIMH]). The median age for onset for mood disorders is 30 years. Depression often co-occurs with anxiety and substance abuse problems.

Major Depressive and Other Mood Disorders

Major Depressive Disorder (MDD)   This mood disorder is the leading cause of disability in the U.S. for those in the age group 15–44 and the fourth leading cause of disability in the world (WHO, 2001). Over the next 20 years depression is projected to become the second leading cause of disability in the world and the leading cause of disability in high income nations such as the United States (Mathers & Loncar, 2006). It affects about 6.7 % of the adult population in the U.S. or approximately 14.8 million citizens in a given year. Major depressive disorder is more common among women than men and the median age of onset is 32 years of age (NIMH). This condition ranks first for psychiatric hospitalizations, and accounts for 23.3% of all hospitalizations. It has been estimated that 80% of people with depression are either treated by primary care providers or not treated at all (Reiger, Goldberg, & Taube, 1978; Young, Klap, Sherbourne, & Wells, 2001). The fact that mental health professionals are not sought out as the providers may be due to several factors, including stigma and the fact that many people with depression report more physical symptoms than emotional states (Stewart, Ricci, Chee, Hahn, & Morganstein, 2003).

Major depressive disorder can affect up to 10% of males and 25% of females. It affects people's ability to work and can result in an estimated 5.6 hours of lost work per week with a cost of $24 billion in annual wages (Stewart, Ricci, Chee, Hahn, & Morganstein, 2003). Approximately 80% of people with depression report some problems with functional impairment related to their depression and, of that group, 27% report serious problems at work or home (CDC). There is a relationship between MDD and increased use of health services, including medical appointments, laboratory tests, inpatient and outpatient services, and other diagnostic and treatment services. The cost in quality of life includes the effect of MDD on school or career performance, functional ability, family relationships, and an increased risk of alcohol and substance abuse, as well as injuries and accidents that may be the result of decreased concentration and attention.

When one or more chronic medical problems are present the prevalence of depression is even greater. The more severe the chronic medical problem, the more likely it is that depression will complicate the illness. Failure to treat depression that accompanies a medical illness can result in prolonged hospitalization, incomplete treatment of the illness, and increased risk of complications and death. For example, depression in the presence of cardiac disease has been associated with an increased risk of cardiac arrest, and early death (Lesperance & Frasure-Smith, 2000). Depression is often co-morbid with anxiety and anxiety may also be a common symptom of depression.

Dysthymic Disorder   This disorder is viewed as chronic milder depression than major depressive disorder. The course of dysthymia is usually two years or longer and people with dysthymia may have one or more episodes of MDD. Although dysthymia may not disable a person, it does affect function and feelings of well-being. It affects approximately 1.5% of the adult population or about 3.3 million Americans in a given year. The median age of onset is 31 years of age (NIMH). Dysthymic disorder has an insidious onset, often has a chronic course of illness, but is not as disabling to the person as MDD.

Bipolar Disorder   Bipolar disorder affects approximately 5.7 million American adults or about 2.6% of the U.S. population in a given year. The median age of onset for Bipolar disorder is 25 years of age (NIMH). The lifetime prevalence of bipolar disorder for men and women is about equal; the average age of onset for bipolar disease is mid-to late twenties.

Presentation of the Problem

Major Depressive Disorder   Major depressive disorder includes a period of at least two consecutive weeks where a person experiences a change from previous functioning that includes either a depressed mood or a loss of interest or pleasure in nearly all activities (APA, 2000). A person with these symptoms must also present at least five or more of the following symptoms for a diagnosis of MDD:

1.   depressed mood most of the day, nearly every day;
2.   diminished interest or pleasure in any or all activities;
3.   significant weight loss or weight gain;
4.   insomnia or hypersomnia;
5.   psychomotor agitation or retardation;
6.   fatigue or loss of energy nearly every day;
7.   feelings of worthlessness or inappropriate guilt nearly every day;
8.   diminished ability to concentrate, or indecisiveness, nearly every day;
9.   recurrent thoughts of death, suicidal ideation or a suicide attempt or plan (APA, 2000).

These symptoms are not related to a medical condition, are not the result of effects of a substance or a general medical condition, and are not the results of bereavement following a loss. Together, these symptoms cause significant impairment in social and occupational functioning (APA, 2000).

Most often the person's appetite is decreased, resulting in weight loss. Some individuals will have an increase in appetite and crave certain kinds of food, often sweets or other carbohydrates. The sleep changes that occur often involve insomnia with early morning awakening, or nighttime wakening with difficulty returning to sleep as the most common sleep difficulties seen in depression. People may also present with hypersomnia or increased sleep during the day and night. Psychomotor changes can either be in the form of agitation, which can include an inability to sit still, or retardation, which is a slowing down of movement and speech; these changes in the psychomotor presentation should be observable by outsiders. A change in energy level often takes the form of fatigue that is so profound that even the smallest task seems to require a major effort by the person. These changes are referred to as the vegetative signs of depression.

Depression is often co-morbid with anxiety and this co-morbid condition is two to three times more common in women than in men. Co-morbid depression and anxiety results in greater severity of illness, increased chronicity, higher relapse rates, poorer response to treatment, and an increased risk of suicide (Kessler, *et al.*, 2003, 1994). Routine screening of depression should include assessment of anxiety as well (see Chapter 6).

People with depression often may have negative evaluations of their worth as human beings and be preoccupied with feeling guilty over minor past failings. This sense of worthlessness may reach delusional proportions in some depressed people. Many people with depression report impaired ability to concentrate or attend to normal pursuits. Recurrent thoughts of death may range from a feeling that others would be better off without the person, to specific plans to commit suicide (see Chapter 4 for assessment of suicide risk).

There is a recurrent nature to depression and a 50–80% chance that a second depressive episode will follow the first (Greden, 2001). Additionally, there is an 80–90 % chance that a third episode will follow a second episode. Approximately 15% of people who have MDD will eventually commit suicide (Hirschfeld, 1997). Questions about previous episodes of depression (diagnosed or not) are very important in the initial interview.

Dysthymic Disorder   This disorder is described as "a chronically depressed mood that occurs for most of the day more days than not for at least two years" (APA, 2000, p. 376). When depressed, diagnosis of the person requires two additional symptoms present such as: poor or excessive appetite, insomnia/hypersomnia, decreased energy or fatigue, low self-esteem, difficulty with concentration and/or decision-making, and feelings of hopelessness. These symptoms may have persisted for so long that people often feel that they have been this way for a long time and may consider the feelings part of their personality.

Bipolar Disorder   Formerly known as manic/depressive disorder, bipolar disorder is characterized by one or more manic episodes or mixed episodes with both manic and depressive symptoms. A manic episode is a distinct period of time during which an individual has an elevated, expansive, or irritable mood for at least one week. For diagnosis the mood change must be accompanied by at least three of the following symptoms: inflated self-esteem or grandiosity, decreased need for sleep, pressured speech, flight of ideas, distractability, psychomotor agitation, and an excessive pursuit of pleasurable activities that have a high potential for painful consequences such as sexual activity, spending, or gambling (APA, 2000).

The elevated mood may initially seem charming and pleasant, but the expansiveness and unending enthusiasm can pervade all areas of life. An irritable mood and lability of the mood is also frequently seen and may be overlooked as part of the symptom presentation. Frequently the decreased need for sleep may be the first symptom identified. The person may go for days without sleep, yet not be the least bit tired and feel full of energy. Speech is also commonly affected and people present with loud, rapid, pressured speech and providers may not be able to interrupt the person. Racing thoughts moving faster than the person may be able to speak can result in a flight of ideas. Poor judgment can lead to financial, legal, and family problems. Often a report of family and/or friends may be necessary to obtain an understanding of the impairment, since grandiosity may prevent the patient from even acknowledging the situation as problematic.

Hypomania is described as similar to a manic episode with the same changes in mood and behavior as described for mania, but the symptoms are not significant enough to cause impairment in social or occupational functioning, or to require hospitalization. The disturbances in hypomania must represent a change in the person's usual mood and behavior and persist for at least four days. Many people may like this experience, find that it may increase their ability to work and/or be creative, and not report it as a problem.

Bipolar disease encompasses a range of mood disturbances and has been delineated as either bipolar I or bipolar II by DSM-IV-TR. Bipolar I includes simple mania, mixed episodes of mania and depression, and hypomania with the history of a previous episode of mania. Bipolar II presents with no previous episode of mania and at least one past episode of major depression and past or current hypomania (APA, 2000).

Bipolar disease often is compounded by a problem with substance use/misuse. The lethal mix of grandiosity or severe depression with mind-altering substances can decrease a person's impulse control and increase the risk of suicidal ideation and actual suicide attempts (see Chapter 4 for further discussion of risk assessment for suicide).

Depression as a Co-morbid Condition with Medical Disorders

Depression is recognized as a cause of increased morbidity and mortality in chronic medical illness. A bi-directional relationship between depression and some medical illnesses suggests that depression may be either an antecedent and/or a consequence of some illnesses such as cardiac disease, HIV/AIDS, cancer, epilepsy, diabetes, arthritis, and stroke (Benton, Staab, &

Evans, 2007). Many chronic illnesses also include symptoms that overlap with symptoms of depression, therefore making the diagnosis of depression difficult. Sleep and appetite disturbances, fatigue, lack of energy or interest in activities may all be symptoms related to the medical condition and not symptoms indicating depression.

Depression is cited as a risk factor as well as a common co-morbid condition of cardiac diseases including coronary artery disease, unstable angina, acute myocardial infarction, congestive heart failure, and following coronary artery bypass surgery (Benton, Staab, & Evans, 2007). Depression is more common among patients with cancer than the general population and is associated with a poorer prognosis and increased morbidity in this population. Many of the chemotherapeutic drugs associated with cancer can cause mood-related symptoms. Pain and depression are often co-morbid conditions in chronic and life-limiting illnesses, and inadequate treatment of each of these issues can impact the treatment of the other. Depression is common with HIV/AIDS. Depression, symptoms of depression, and stress have been associated with poor adherence to retroviral treatment, decreased psychosocial functioning, more rapid progression of the disease and mortality in HIV/AIDS (Robins, *et al.*, 1984).

Depression has been noted in increased numbers in many neurological diseases such as cerebrovascular disease, Parkinson's disease, multiple sclerosis, Huntington's disease, Alzheimer's disease, and epilepsy. A significant increase in the suicide rate has been identified in people with epilepsy. Depression is common with people who have had a stroke, particularly a stroke in the left frontal area of the brain (Swartz, 2006). Post-stroke depression treatment has been associated with improvements in cognitive functioning. Depression in people with Alzheimer's disease has been associated with increased nursing home placements, rapid decline, and increased mortality (Benton, Staab, & Evans, 2007).

Patients with depression and arthritis who received collaborative care had reduced depression, pain intensity and interference in daily activities due to pain, and had improved overall health and quality of life after 12 months of treatment of depression (Lin, Katon, Von Korff *et al.*, 2003). Depression increases the risk for diabetes and also worsens the course of diabetes if untreated (Lin, *et al.*, 2005).

Endocrine disorders, specifically hypothyroidism and Cushing's disease, can present with symptoms similar to depression and can also lead to depression. Vitamin deficiency such as insufficient folic acid, vitamin B6, or vitamin B12 have also been linked to depression (Swartz, 2006).

Diseases such as chronic fatigue syndrome and fibromyalgia have been associated with depression. Often diagnosis of these diseases occurs after many years of seeking treatment and after patients have seen a number of providers including psychiatric providers.

The research related to co-morbid medical conditions and depression has exploded over the past two decades and will continue to increase in the coming years, resulting in the need for increased focus and education about depression for all practitioners. Polsky, *et al.* (2005) found that people with serious diseases such as cancer, heart disease, chronic lung disease or arthritis were at risk for developing significant depression following their diagnosis with the medical problem. Increased assessment skills and development of collaborative practices between psychiatric and primary care providers will be essential in treating the whole person.

CASE EXAMPLE: DIFFERENTIAL DIAGNOSIS

Mrs. T is a 61-year-old African-American woman who has been widowed for five years. Her husband's death was very sudden; he developed pneumonia and died after a three day hospitalization. She was brought into her primary care provider (PCP) accompanied by her daughter who has been increasingly worried about her mother's behavior change. Mrs. T has been an active member of her church for decades and over the last three months has not gone to church, or engaged in any of her other regular activities. She has gradually become more secluded at home; when the daughter has gone to check up on her mother she has observed that Mrs. T has not been cleaning her home, or taking care of herself as she always had in the past. She has lost about 12 pounds since her last visit a year ago, and the PCP notes that she has a flat affect, slowed verbal responses, and seems to have psychomotor retardation.

The PCP begins to suspect depression and/or dementia and asks Mrs. T about her mood; Mrs. T says her mood is "fine." She has no previous episodes of depression and no family history of depression. She is able to complete all of the mental status questions appropriately, although in a slow manner. Mrs. T's daughter does not feel that her mother is depressed, but thinks that something is definitely wrong. She agrees to have her mother see a counselor in the clinic and she also meets with the counselor.

The counselor completes an evaluation and is concerned about the fact that Mrs. T is so guarded about discussing the details of her husband's death and suspects a complicated grief reaction or unresolved grief. Further questioning about her husband's death reveals that he died of AIDS and the family does not ever talk about this. Mrs. T consents to an HIV test, which is positive and she has a CD4 count of 150 meaning that she also has the diagnosis AIDS. A diagnosis of HIV dementia or encephalopathy is made and treatment with anti-retroviral medications is initiated; after four to five months of treatment Mrs. T has returned to church, has a much greater range of affect, an improved appetite, and started cleaning her house again. During this period of time she was also seen weekly in counseling at the clinic and benefited from having someone to talk to about her diagnosis and how she could manage her fears and the stigma associated with a diagnosis of HIV disease.

In this situation the immediate concerns about depression or dementia were appropriate for a differential diagnosis. The involvement of the counselor helped fill in the missing data that was not obtained on an initial visit with the PCP, but essential to the treatment. This is an example of how integrated mental healthcare in primary care settings can make a major difference in assessment, diagnosis, and treatment of patients.

Illnesses and Medication Effects Commonly Mistaken for Depression

There are several medical illnesses and/or treatments characterized by a significant change in mood that is the direct result of a physiological change related to that illness or agent. Patients may present with a delirium related to the medical condition that includes symptoms commonly associated with depression such as sleep and appetite disturbance, difficulty with concentration, or psychomotor retardation. These illnesses are displayed in Box 7.1.

Additionally, many medications have been associated with symptoms of depression. These medications are displayed in Box 7.2. Thorough assessment is discussed in the next section and is of utmost importance in differentiating between depressive symptoms as part of a medical problem or treatment, and the diagnosis of depression. Psychiatric consultation liaison programs in the hospital or other healthcare settings specialize in providing differential diagnosis and treatment of such problems, and focus additionally on staff education and support for management of such problems.

BOX 7.1 Medical Conditions with Symptoms of Depression

- Tumors
  - Primary cerebral
- Trauma
  - Cerebral contusion
  - Subdural hematoma
- Infections
  - Cerebral (meningitis, encephalitis, HIV, syphilis)
  - Systemic (sepsis, urinary tract infection, pneumonia)
- Cardiac and vascular
  - Cerebrovascular (infacts, hemorrhage, vasculitis)
  - Cardiovascular (congestive heart failure, shock)
- Physiologic or metabolic
  - Hypoxemia, electrolyte disturbance, renal or hepatic failure, hypo or hyper glycemic
  - Postictal states
- Endocrine
  - Thyroid or glucocorticoid disturbances
  - Cushing's disease
- Nutritional
  - Vitamin B12 deficiency, folate deficiency
- Demyelinating
  - Multiple sclerosis
- Neurodegenerative
  - Parkinson's disease, Huntington's disease
- Pain, especially chronic pain conditions
- Mononucleosis
- Diabetes mellitus
- Pernicious anemia
- Pancreatitis
- Hepatitis
- Human Immunodeficiency Virus (HIV)

Source: Adapted from Saddock & Saddock, 2003; Fortinash & Holoday Warrett, 2008

BOX 7.2 Medications and Agents Causing Symptoms of Depression

- Drug intoxication from alcohol or sedative-hypnotics
- Anti-psychotics
- Metoclopramide, H2-receptor blockers
- Antihypertensives (especially agents such as methyldopa, clonidine, reserpine guanethidine, hydralazine, hydrochlorthiazide, propanolol)
- Sex steroids (oral contraceptives, anabolic steroids)
- Coticosteroids (prednisone)

- Antidyskinetics (levodopa, carbidopa, amantadine)
- Bromocriptine
- Chemotherapeutic agents
- Digitalis
- Thiazide diuretics
- Benzodiazepines (such as alprazolam, chlordiazepoxide, diazepam, clonazepam, lorazeapam, oxazepam)
- Disulfarim
- Sulfonamides
- Opiates
- Antiretrovirals (such as abacavir, atazanavir, efavirenze, enfuviritide, lamivudine-Zidovudine, lopinavir-ritonavir, ritonavir, saquinavir)
- Drug Withdrawal
  - Nicotine
  - Caffeine
  - Alcohol or sedative hypnotics
  - Cocaine
  - Amphetamines
  - Marijuana

Source: Adapted from Saddock & Saddock, 2003; Fortinash & Holoday Warrett, 2008

Issues Commonly Associated with Depression: SAD, Grief, Suicide, and Stigma

Despondency in the face of a medical illness is common and prevalent in primary care settings. Recognition of this reaction to severe medical problems is certainly important in providing additional supports for patients. Peer support groups and internet resources have expanded the possibilities for support, yet many people suffer alone. Medicalization of the despondency and associated reactions can occur if providers are unaware of the support options available to patients and only offer medication or referrals for psychiatric care. Many people have received excellent support and maintain life-long connections with other members of peer support groups.

Some people will develop depressive symptoms, may meet criteria for major depressive disorder (MDD), and may require psychopharmacological intervention, yet will still benefit over the long-term from the support obtained from peer support groups. When patients utilize the services provided by psychiatric mental health counselors, the psychiatric diagnosis of adjustment disorder often is utilized in this kind of situation. Adjustment disorder with depressed mood or anxious mood are typical examples of diagnoses but are usually of shorter duration than the criteria for MDD or anxiety disorder. Use of such diagnoses may assist patients in gaining insurance coverage for psychiatric care; however, some patients may resist referrals to psychiatric providers due to the stigma and labeling associated with such care (see Chapter 3).

Seasonal Affective Disorder (SAD)   SAD usually presents with symptoms of depression that develop during October or November and decrease in March or April. Changes in circadian rhythm, or internal biological clocks, are affected by changes in the amount of daily sunlight. In some people less sunlight can cause depression probably due to changes in melatonin.

People with SAD will frequently have excessive eating and sleeping patterns, crave sugar or starchy foods and have no symptoms during the spring and summer months when more sunlight is available.

Grief Both grief and depression involve symptoms of sadness and feeling lost or blue; however, they are different. Grief is considered a normal part of life in that it is a response to loss—loss of a loved one, a move to an unfamiliar place, loss of opportunity, or developing a life-threatening or chronic illness. Chronic progressive illnesses can be viewed as a series of losses that a person must master in order to adjust to, and live with, the illness.

The grieving process produces a wide range of feelings. Societal expectations in the U.S. that pain (psychological pain) is something to be relieved as quickly as possible, can actually interfere with normal grieving (Menand, 2010). Figure 7.1 (page 143) depicts the process of grieving that many people may want to avoid or shorten. The process of grieving takes time and is a way for the mind to adjust to the sorrow of the loss. Grieving has been described as acceptance of the finality of loss, experiencing the full range of feelings related to the loss, adjusting to life without the presence of the lost person or ideals, and acceptance of the loss (see Chapters 3 and 12).

Suicide While the majority of depressed persons do not commit suicide, some do. About one in 16 people diagnosed with depression die by suicide, and up to two-thirds of those who die by suicide have seen their primary care provider in the prior month (Swartz, 2006). The recognition of people at risk of suicide is an extremely important issue for primary care providers (see Chapter 4 for further information on suicide risk, assessment, depression as a risk factor, and approach to the suicidal patient).

Stigma Although the conditions that are included under the heading of mood disorders are currently considered to be biologically based mental illnesses and are covered by most insurances under parity laws, stigma is still an issue for people with depression and bipolar disease. Because of stigma, *more people with depression see primary care providers than mental health providers*. Labeling people, especially those with a severe mental illness, may have an effect on the healthcare these individuals receive for the rest of their lives (see Chapter 3 on labeling).

Stigma can have an effect on providers' screening for mental health issues, such as depression, if they are not aware of their own biases. A provider whose cultural belief does not allow for expressions of feelings of sadness or despair may not ask patients questions about their mood. Providers may need to examine and overcome some of their own attitudes and beliefs about depression in order to provide competent and compassionate care. Stigma also affects adherence to treatment regimens and may affect treatment response, especially if patients don't talk about the fact that they are not following treatment recommendations. An open and trusting relationship between patient and provider is essential in helping to overcome some of the difficulties that exist as a result of the stigma associated with mental illness.

Assessment Issues and Screening Tools

Failure to recognize the problem of depression in medical illness continues to be a major problem despite a growing body of evidence about medical co-morbidities with depression. Assuming that "anyone would be depressed with that condition" is a danger for providers, and can lead to inadequate assessment of a condition that is treatable. Failure to identify and treat depression associated with medical illness constitutes neglect, creates suffering for patients, and may affect the response to treatment of the medical illness.

Nearly all healthcare providers include some basic assessment of mood in an initial screening during a health visit. During the course of assessment, questions will be asked about mood, while observing the patient's emotional state, affective reactivity, temperament, and range of affect. The high prevalence of mood disorders with medical conditions, especially chronic conditions, alerts the primary care provider to the need to do a careful assessment if any general observations indicate a problem. Ruling out possible medical conditions that cause symptoms similar to depression is the first step, including syndromes associated with substance abuse such as intoxication and withdrawal from any substances (see Chapter 9 on substance abuse).

Relationship to Life Functioning as a Context for Assessment

A straightforward, matter of fact approach, similar to an assessment of a medical problem is important when asking questions about mood, vegetative symptoms, and suicidal thoughts and plans. The development of a trusting professional relationship with the primary care provider is of utmost importance in the assessment process.

The CMHA tool illustrated in Chapter 2 provides a context for linking questions about mood and suicide risk to basic life functions; for example, "Do you feel so down that you've had to miss work [or school]?" (Item 3) Or, "Since you've been depressed, have you been slowed down with your family life and usual social activities?" (Items 4 and 11). Ratings of 4 or 5 on Item 2 (self-concept and mood), suicide risk (Item 14) and basic life functions affected by depression should signal a referral for in-depth assessment and treatment by a mental health specialist—a next step greatly enhanced and more readily accepted by the client in the context of a trusting client/PCP relationship.

The next section is primarily the province of psychiatric specialists, except for those with *dual preparation*: e.g., a physician with a residency in primary care and psychiatry; a nurse practitioner in "adult primary care" and "psychiatric/mental health." Here psychiatric evaluation is reviewed briefly as background for PCPs to confidently make referrals; for example: "Mrs, Jones, I'm very concerned about what you're going through, and think you need more treatment than I can offer in these short appointments . . . I think an antidepressant drug could help, but it would be best if we do that with whoever you see for counseling."

Psychiatric Evaluation

When evaluating mood it is essential to assess for mood problems across the mood continuum. When symptoms of depression are elicited the clinician must also ask questions about the presence of symptoms of mania or hypomania and vice versa. There are tremendous implications for treatment in the assessment of mood. Initiation of treatment with antidepressant medication may precipitate a manic episode in a situation where only depression is assessed and a diagnosis of bipolar disease has been missed. This can result in needless suffering for the patient and a lack of trust in the providers' expertise.

Several screening tools to assist with assessment of mood disorders have been developed. The Cochrane Collaboration has published a review of "Screening and case finding instruments for depression" (Cochrane, 2008). The primary finding of the review was that the use of screening/case finding instruments had "little impact on the overall recognition of rates of depression" (p. 8). Despite such findings, many clinicians either rely on the use of screening tools as a time-saving mechanism, or use them as an adjunct along with a general assessment included in the review of systems. If used, rating scales scores should be interpreted in the context of the general history and physical and should not take the place of a more thorough assessment.

Clinicians who consider the use of various tools should note that the development of most of the tools was for research (not clinical) objectives, and because of their length cannot realistically and sensitively be utlilized in the limited 15–20 minute time frame of the average PCP visit. Furthermore, a depressed person who is also suicidal may feel even more alienated by the directive to "fill out a rating scale" outside of the context of a therapeutic relationship (see Chapter 2).

Many primary care clinicians use the mnemonic SIG E CAPS to assess for the presence of depression. This mnemonic developed by Liberman (2003) is a device utilized by many clinicians as a way of remembering some of the symptoms of MDD. The mnemnoic is:

Sex/sleep
Interest
Guilt
Energy
Concentration
Appetite
Psychomotor retardation or agitation
Suicide

There are several screening tools utilized to assess for the presence of depression including: the Beck Depression Inventory (BDI), Hamilton Depression Scale (HAM-D), Profile of Mood States, Geriatric Depression Screening Tool (GDS), Symptom Checklist 90-R, Zung Depression Scale, and Montgomery-Asberg Depression Rating Scale (MADRS). Rating scales to measure mania are: Mania Rating Scale (MRS), Bech-Rafaelsen Mania Rating Scale (BMRS), the Clinician Administered Rating Scale-Mania (CARS-M), the Altman Self-Rating Mania Scale (ASRM), and the Mood Disorders Questionnaire (MDQ). Only the most commonly used scales are cited here.

The Beck Depression Inventory (BDI) is probably one of the most widely used rating scales. It is a 21-item self-rating scale, which can be completed by the patient before the appointment and can be used in evaluation of depression and as a follow-up to measure response to treatment. The BDI does exclude some atypical neuro-vegetative symptoms.

The Hamilton Rating Scale for Depression (HAM-D) can be used for evaluating response to treatment for depression. It is a 17-item test that does not include depressive symptoms such as anhedonia (lack of interest in normal activities), favors somatic signs and symptoms of depression, and can miss some of the atypical symptoms such as overeating or oversleeping.

The Mood Disorders Questionnaire (MDQ) was developed by a team of providers, researchers, and consumers to come up with a quick and brief form for diagnosis of bipolar disorder. It is brief, takes about five minutes to complete and hopefully will shorten the time it takes for diagnosis of bipolar disorder (Hirschfeld, Williams, & Spitzer, 2000).

The Geriatric Depression Screening (GDS) tool is a self-rating screen frequently used for detecting depression in older adults who also have medical illness or mild to moderate cognitive impairments. It consists of 30 yes-or-no items, and a score of 10–11 warrants a more thorough assessment for depression in this population. The one drawback of the GDS is that there are no questions about suicidal ideation on the screening tool (Byrd, 2005).

Laboratory Tests

Routine laboratory testing including a complete blood count (CBC), liver function tests (LFTs), hormonal indices, and thyroid function tests should be included to assist in differentiating medical and psychological problems. Borderline thyroid function test results may require careful assessment and referral or collaborative care. Gender issues can affect treatment of women and mood disorders, and can occur across the lifespan with particular focus on changes in the menstrual cycle as well as a time of peri-menopause and menopause. Collaborative care or referral to a women's health or psychiatric provider specializing in women's mental healthcare may assist the primary care provider in delivering optimum care to the patient.

Special Populations

Depression in children and adolescents is covered in Chapter 11.

While postpartum depression is not the focus of this chapter, women with postpartum depression may present in some primary care settings. Its duration and debilitating effects on the mother, her ability to care for herself and/or bond with her baby, distinguish it from postpartum blues. About one in ten mothers may experience some degree of postpartum depression. Symptoms may present within days after the delivery and continue for up to a year later. Symptoms include fatigue, exhaustion, feelings of hopelessness or depression, sleep and appetite disturbances, confusion, uncontrollable crying, lack of interest in the baby, fear of harming the baby or oneself, and mood swings. It can be accompanied by anxiety or panic and/or intense or irrational fears about what they might do. Usually the woman feels isolated, guilty, and ashamed of these feelings.

Postpartum depression can present with or without anxiety or psychotic features. Infanticide is most often associated with postpartum psychotic episodes that include command hallucinations to kill the infant. The risk of postpartum episodes with psychotic features is increased for women with prior postpartum mood problems, and those with a history of mood disorder and/or family history of mood disorders. Women need to be evaluated for the presence of these symptoms and treated seriously when the symptoms occur.

Depression in elders is another group that bears additional attention, since 15–20% of older adults have significant depressive symptoms (Gallo & Liebowitz, 1999; Melillo & Houde, in press). The elderly are also at risk for increased suicide. Older patients often present with somatic complaints and often deny feeling sad or depressed. Complaints are often focused on pain, fatigue, weight loss, GI complaints, constipation and sleep difficulties. Assessment must include ruling out medical illness, drug interactions, delirium, and dementia in this population (see Chapter 12).

Treatment of Depressed Persons: Psychotherapeutic and Pharmacologic

Research about treatment outcomes in mental health suggests that the most successful treatment is a combination of talk therapy and psychotropic medication. Despite the findings of study after study, many people are not presented with this information and do not receive combined treatment. This may be due in part to the choice of the patient, stigma about mental health illness and care, lack of access to mental health professionals by the primary care provider, and inadequate reimbursement for therapy by the insurance companies.

Gonzalez and colleagues (2010) examined the prevalence and adequacy of depression care among ethnic groups in the U.S. and found that Mexican Americans and African Americans were least likely to receive depression care, especially care that followed the American Psychiatric Association guidelines for depression care. Awareness of the community and professional standards for treating depression is an important issue. Guidelines for depression treatment are widely available on the internet. Standards commonly used include the American Psychiatric Association guidelines and the U.S. government guidelines website (National Guideline Clearing House—www.guideline.gov). Guidelines for both major depressive disorder (MDD) and bipolar disease are included in these websites, are evidence-based, and include many sources and references for further information.

Treatments available for depressed persons includes: psychotherapy; psychotropic agents including antidepressants and mood stabilizers; light therapy; biologic therapies such as electroconvulsive therapy (ECT); new treatments under investigation; and patient self-management techniques, including herbal remedies. As already noted, many of these therapies are in the province of psychiatric specialists, with only an overview provided here.

Treatment guidelines include major recommendations for mild to moderate depression and separate guidelines for severe or chronic depression. The first step in treatment for mild to moderate depression states that either antidepressant medication or psychotherapy should be the first-line treatment (National Guideline Clearing House, www.guideline.gov). The first-line treatment for severe or chronic depression should be combined treatment of both medication and psychotherapy. The recommendation for patients with suicidal ideation is immediate referral to a psychiatric mental health provider.

Psychotherapeutic Modalities

In a therapeutic relationship the focus is on helping patients cope with troubling issues and feelings related to their condition, and to increase self-understanding and coping abilities. That is what therapy is about. It is one of the first-line treatments for mild to moderate depression, and part of the first-line treatment for those with more severe depression. The trusting relationship is the foundation of all psychotherapeutic treatment models.

Patients do not automatically understand what happens in psychotherapy. Understanding that improved mood is not necessarily an immediate outcome of psychotherapy, and that dealing with difficult personal issues requires a commitment on the part of the patient, is something that is discussed in early meetings with a therapist and can be reinforced by primary care providers. The bi-directional process of therapy (Figure 7.1) may assist in providing information that patients often experience pain and suffering while exploring these issues. The lack of acknowledgement of this process may lead to early discontinuation of therapy if the patient feels worse after exploring the difficult issues and does not understand that this may be a part of the process of therapy. The way through personal pain may be to feel it fully, rather than avoid it, to be able to heal and move on in one's life.

Several different therapy models have been effective in the treatment of depression, including interpersonal therapy, psychodynamic therapy, supportive therapy, behavioral therapy, and cognitive-behavioral therapy.

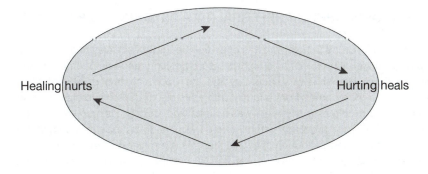

Figure 7.1 The Bi-directional Process of Psychotherapy

Supportive therapy helps people understand their illness and therefore assists in the setting of realistic goals for life. The focus is on the here and now and working on current relationship and life challenges, and developing new ways to face these problems and challenges. The therapy is goal oriented and the client and therapist set the goals together. Supportive therapy is a part of most all of the other types of therapy presented. Supportive therapy can be short- or long-term therapy, but is usually focused on an immediate problem and is usually short-term in nature.

Interpersonal therapy is most effective in the treatment of depression when the depression is precipitated by a life event such as the death of a loved one, job loss, or other life transition. The goal is to help the person cope with the situation by improving self-awareness, increasing coping skills, resolving conflicts, and making some behavioral changes. The focus is on the interpersonal connection and relationship with others. This model of therapy can be utilized in short- or long-term treatment.

Psychodynamic therapy focuses on past experiences as a way to understand current conflicts in the person's life. A crucial concept of psychodynamic therapy is the use of transference, which utilizes feelings about childhood figures as they are transferred onto the therapist. The therapist is able to help the patient analyze the feelings and work through past conflicts. This therapy is generally long-term in nature and helps people overcome destructive patterns in their lives.

Behavior therapy is based on the idea that people have learned destructive thought and behavior patterns that prolong their depression. Examination of these patterns helps with step-by-step changes in behavior, social skills, problem solving and self-control to change the way the person deals with life problems. The focus is not concerned with understanding underlying issues as in psychodynamic therapy, but is focused on behaviors that can be changed, and is usually short-term.

Cognitive-behavioral therapy (CBT) has been demonstrated to be effective in the treatment of depression in outpatients with mild to moderate depression, and when evaluated with the use of antidepressant medication, was found to be equally effective with the medication (Scott, 1996; Lynch, Laws, & McKenna, 2010). CBT examines errors in the patient's thinking that maintains negative distortions about oneself and the world one lives in. Homework assignments are utilized to help people apply the knowledge about their distortions and assumptions and correct negative thinking. Cognitive therapy can be conducted in individual and group settings and can be short- or long-term.

Most therapists will utilize several different techniques borrowed from these therapy models in their approach to an individual patient. Use of the supportive and cognitive-behavioral models are most often cited as effective in dealing with depression.

CASE EXAMPLE: APPROPRIATE REFERRAL TO A PSYCHIATRIC PROVIDER

Debra is a 57-year-old divorced female who has one adult daughter who lives nearby. Debra is a CPA for a major accounting firm, has a high-pressure position, and has been promoted by the firm several times. Her job is very sedentary and she reports her lack of movement as a problem as she ages. She comes from a family with a history of depressive disorder and some substance abuse problems (her mother was hospitalized for depression once, and her father's three siblings all have problems with alcohol). Debra is 35 pounds overweight and has been unable to lose weight, although she says that this is a major goal in her life.

Debra had her first episode of depression at age 23 and has been on antidepressant medications on and off since that time. She is followed by an MD psycho-pharmacologist every three to four months; she has been referred to a psychotherapist a number of times, but either does not make an appointment or does not continue in therapy for a variety of reasons. She has been followed by her family nurse practitioner for the last 12 years, and although she does not have any major medical problems, she has several medical appointments a year for a variety of physical complaints, which have been worked up, but no findings have indicated a medical problem.

Debra presents today with vague complaints of a feeling of fatigue, joint aches, and difficulty with concentration. Her last medical visit was two months ago with similar complaints. At that time after a negative physical exam and blood work her FNP suggested an exercise regime of walking daily, as a way to lose weight, improve mood, and possibly decrease her joint pain. Today Debra reports that she has not attempted to walk more than a couple of days following her last medical appointment. She reports increasing depression and thinks that her antidepressant medication is no longer working. The option of not continuing to provide care to Debra and referral to another primary care provider is something the FNP has been considering, since she finds it quite frustrating to work with this patient who follows none of her recommendations.

Instead, the FNP consults with a psychiatric clinical nurse specialist (CNS) colleague on how to proceed with this patient.

The psychiatric CNS validates that the FNP has been attempting to treat this patient alone when she needs additional care, and that the patient is not really participating in her own treatment other than to take her medications (we assume that she is taking the medication). The addition of psychotherapy to assist with depression, lack of motivation, negative thought processes, and resistance to making life changes is essential; the FNP is the person who has the most consistent relationship with Debra and is therefore probably the best person to insist that her treatment is incomplete without this additional psychotherapeutic modality. The FNP anticipates that the patient will once again not respond to this recommendation and the FNP and Psychiatric CNS discuss ways to deal with the patient's resistance.

Antidepressant Medications

Treatment with antidepressant medications is one of the major approaches utilized by primary care providers. One of the major difficulties in the use of antidepressant medications is that most of these medications do not take effect for up to four to six weeks. When a patient is suffering from depression, this month can be a crucial period of time. Simply prescribing medication without providing some other relief of suffering may alienate patients who are desperate for help and relief.

With the use of any antidepressant medication a thorough assessment of suicidal ideation should be included (see Chapter 4). Providers should also discuss the fact that sometimes after initiation of treatment suicidal thoughts may increase (especially with use of SSRIs in a child or adolescent population), and that the provider should be informed immediately if this happens. Frequent follow-up appointments, prescriptions with only a small number of pills, and family involvement in care are a few ways to assist PCPs in dealing with this risk. Development of collaborative relationships with mental health professionals who can also provide psychotherapy for patients is an important way for the PCP to assure that patients have access to additional support during this time of initial treatment of depression.

Treatment guidelines described above (from National Guideline Clearing House and APA) include a recommended follow-up schedule that includes at least one follow-up appointment within a month of initiation of medication treatment and a second appointment during the next four to eight weeks. An adequate acute trial of medications is considered to be about 12 weeks. If there has not been an adequate response by 12 weeks, consideration of maximizing the dosage, augmentation of medication, or change to a different medication are the options to be explored. An overall adequate trial, in which the goal is symptom remission, should be 6–12 months. The importance of symptom remission should be underscored since many patients only achieve partial symptom remission. Acceptance of partial remission is no longer acceptable, and close follow-up along with the use of rating scales may help both clinicians and patients focus on symptom relief that has not yet been fully successful. If the patient does not respond to the treatment, referral to a psychiatric mental health specialist is recommended.

Determining which antidepressant medication will be useful depends on several factors. Any class of antidepressant medication may be effective. A recent broad-based research study, the Sequenced Treatment Alternatives to Relieve Depression (STAR*D) concluded that no treatment for depression was clearly superior to any other (Rush, Trivedi, & Wisniewski, 2006). The factors to be considered in choosing an antidepressant medication include:

- prior response to a specific antidepressant by patient or first-degree relative;
- fit between profile of medication and presenting symptoms;
- patient or clinician preference;
- potential side effects;
- cost of medication.

Antidepressant medications include several classes of medications: Selective Serotonin Reuptake Inhibitors (SSRIs), Tricylcic/tetracyclic antidepressants (TCAs), Monoamine Inhibitors (MAOIs) Buproprion, Mirtazapine, Selective Norephinephrine Reuptake Inhibitors (SNRIs), psychostimulants, and others. Box 7.3 lists the SSRI Medications and dosing ranges and Box 7.4 lists the Tricyclic/tetracyclics and dosing ranges.

BOX 7.3 SSRI Antidepressants and Dosage Ranges

Fluoxetine (Prozac)	20–80 mg.
Sertraline (Zoloft)	50–200mg.
Citalopram (Celexa)	20–60 mg.
Escitalopram (Lexapro)	5–20 mg.
Paroxetine (Paxil)	20–50 mg.
Fluvoxamine (Luvox)	100–200 mg.

BOX 7.4 Tricyclic/Tetracyclic Antidepressants and Dosage Ranges

Amitriptyline (Elavil)	100–300 mg.
Nortriptyline (Pamelor)	75–150 mg.
Imipramine (Tofranil)	100–300 mg.
Desipramine (Norpramin)	100–300 mg.
Clomipramine (Anafranil)	100–300 mg.
Doxepin (Sinequan)	100–300 mg.
Protriptyline (Vivactil)	15–60 mg.
Maprotiline (Ludiomil)	100–225 mg.

SSRIs are most commonly used to treat anxious depression, depression with panic and obsessive/compulsive features, irritable depression, and depression with features of social phobia. SSRIs are used with a variety of medical co-morbid conditions, however dosage adjustments may be necessary due to P450 inhibition. The major side effects that are problematic and can lead to discontinuation or non-adherence to the medication regimen are sexual dysfunction, weight gain, and sleep difficulties. SSRIs have low toxicity. Use of medications in this class with a longer half-life lowers the risk of a discontinuation syndrome. SSRIs and MAOI should never be used together since serotonin syndrome can occur (see below). SSRIs have been associated with tachyphyllaxis, which is described as ineffectiveness of the drug after a period of time.

Two particular problems have been associated with SSRIs as well as the SNRIs: Discontinuation syndrome and serotonin syndrome. Discontinuation syndrome occurs following abrupt discontinuation of the drug and includes symptoms such as: dysphoric mood, irritability, agitation, paresthesias such as electric shock sensations, anxiety, insomnia, emotional lability as well as headache, nausea and vomiting, and dizziness and vertigo. Patients should be advised to *taper the medication under medical supervision* rather than abruptly stopping the medication to avoid these problems.

Serotonin syndrome is a *potentially life-threatening situation* that can occur with SSRIs and SNRIs with concomitant use of serotoneric drugs including triptans and drugs that impair metabolism of serotonin, such as MAOIs, cold or allergy preparations, cocaine, lithium, ginseng, or St. John's wart. Symptoms include mental status changes such as agitation, hallucinations, or coma, tachycardia, labile blood pressure and hyperthermia, GI symptoms such as nausea, vomiting and diarrhea, neuromuscular changes such as hyperreflexia, and incoordination (Hagerty & Patusky, 2008).

Tricyclic/tetracyclic antidepressants are commonly used for anxious depression. Some specific drugs in this class have been used for specific syndromes:

- Amitriptyline—sleep deprived depression
- Imipramine—depression and panic
- Amitriptyline—depression and pain
- Nortriptyline—depression and migraine
- Doxepin—depression and GI symptoms
- Clomipramine—depression with obsessive/compulsive symptoms.

This class of medications has a *much higher toxicity potential and a two-week supply of medications can be lethal.* There are also many P450 interactions common with this class of drugs so when used with other medications drug interactions must be considered. Serum level monitoring may be done with several tricyclics (imipramine, desipramine, and nortriptyline), so that adherence and drug interactions may be monitored. Side effects that may contribute to discontinuation or non-adherence include weight gain, sedation, anticholinergic effects, sexual dysfunction, and orthostasis.

Buproprion (Wellbutrin) is a dopamine/norepinephrine reuptake inhibitor and has been used effectively in hypersomnolent depression and patients who have cognitive cloudiness with depression. It may have less effect on sexual dysfunction and weight gain than other antidepressants. There is a greater risk of seizures with this medication than other antidepressants. Buproprion is a P450 2 D6 inhibitor and has a 14-hour half-life. Side effects that may lead to discontinuation or non-adherence include headache, dry mouth, jitteriness, insomnia, and irritability. Buproprion dosing begins with 150 mg. once a day for the initial dose with an increase to 300 mg. a day in divided doses.

Mirtazapine (Remeron) is an effective treatment for depression with appetite problems, psychotic features, sleep disturbance, difficulty or inability to tolerate nausea, or sexual dysfunction caused by other antidepressant medications. It has a safe toxicity level, but has been associated with higher lipid levels. Dose ranges are 15–45 mg. per day. Weight gain can be a problem and sedation may increase with higher doses of the medication. Mirtazepine has strong antihistamine action and is a 5HT2 and 5HT3 antagonist and alpha 2 antagonist.

Venlafaxine (Effexor) and *Duloxetine* (Cymbalta) are included in a class of drugs called Selective Norephinephrine Reuptake Inhibitors (SNRIs). Venlafaxine is a 5HT and NE reuptake inhibitor and is effective for anxious depression. The dose ranges are 75–225 mg. Many people have fewer difficulties with side effects with this medication. It cannot be used with MAOIs, and has a safe toxicity profile. This medication may have an effect of increasing blood pressure, more commonly with men than women. It is essential to taper this medication when discontinuing it due to the risk of discontinuation syndrome and rebound depression. It can be given once a day, however if side effects are problematic it can be given in divided doses. The side effects that contribute to discontinuation or non-adherence include: nausea, constipation, dizziness, and sexual dysfunction. Duloxetine has been used in treating depression with anxiety as well as pain associated with fibromyalgia and diabetic peripheral neuropathy. The dose ranges are 40–60 mg. a day; higher doses have not been shown to be associated with increased effectiveness. Side effects include hyponatremia, urinary retention, abnormal bleeding, and orthostatic hypotension.

Psychostimulants, *methylphenidate*, and *dextroamphetamine* have been used to treat depression in medical settings for decades. They may be used alone or in combination with other medications. Research studies about their use in patients with HIV/AIDS, stroke, and cancer have reported to improve mood and energy as well as initiative of the patients. Their effect is important due to the rapid onset of action and the resulting increase in mood, appetite, and decrease of fatigue. This benefit as compared to the four to six week waiting time for the effect of many antidepressants makes psychostimulants an attractive option in many settings. Side effects include agitation, nausea, and insomnia, and rarely psychotic symptoms, tachcardia, or hypertension (Benton, Staab, & Evans, 2007).

Trazdone and *Nefazadone* are considered antidepressants. However, most often these two drugs have been used as sleeping medications and clinical efficacy with depression has been associated with higher doses. *Monoamine Inhibitors* (MAOIs), including Phenelzine (Nardil), Tranylcypromine (Parnate), and Isocarboxazid (Marplan), are not used often since there are so many dietary and medication restrictions, with higher toxicity levels than other drugs. MAOIs have been used with patients who are treatment-resistant with other medications or those who have had a positive response in the past to use of an MAOI.

The STAR*D findings presented information about the treatment of depression that allows providers to look at treatment of depression in a familiar way. The findings suggest that depression treatment can be viewed as similar to treatment for other chronic illnesses such as hypertension, asthma, and diabetes. Patients need close monitoring after treatment has been initiated. Dose changes and switching and/or combining drugs will be common issues and monotherapy will be insufficient for many patients (Kroenke, 2007). When one antidepressant does not work another should be tried. Primary care providers may initiate a trial of a second antidepressant medication after maximizing the dosage of the first medication. Most often, after failure to reach remission following the second medication trial, referral to a psychiatric provider for therapy and/or further medication management is appropriate.

Mood Stabilizers These agents are used in treatment of acute mania in bipolar disorder and include lithium, carbamazepine, divalproex, and lamotrigine. For the treatment of acute bipolar mania the FDA has also approved atypical antipsychotics, while Olanzapine has been indicated for the treatment of acute bipolar depression (Fortinash & Holloday Worret, 2008). Antidepressants are typically used in treatment of bipolar disease only in combination with mood stabilizers to prevent switching from depression to mania as already noted. Benzodiazepines such as Clonazepam may also be used as adjunct therapy for treatment of acute mania.

Lithium carbonate (Lithotabs, Eskalith, Lithobid) is a salt that requires drug monitoring to prevent toxicity. A therapeutic range of serum level should be maintained of 0.6–1.2 mEq/L. A toxic level is anything greater than 1.5 mEq/L. Symptoms of toxicity include vomiting, diarrhea, drowsiness, confusion and lack of coordination, presence of a coarse hand tremor, and muscle twitching. *Lithium toxicity can also cause seizures, oliguria, circulatory failure, coma, and death.* Certain herbal preparations that include dandelion, goldenrod, juniper, and parsley can increase the effects of lithium and/or cause toxicity. Changes in sodium intake can alter lithium excretion and diruetic fluids such as tea and coffee may decrease lithium levels.

Carbamazepine (Tegretol), valproic acid (Depakene), and divalproex sodium (Depakote) are second-generation anticonvulsants that are used in treating bipolar disease. They require therapeutic serum levels in the 50–100 mcg/ml range; toxic levels are considered >100 mcg/ml. These medications are not to be used in conjunction with MAOIs and may cause seizures or hypertensive crisis if used together. Toxic reactions can include blood dyscrasias. Third generation anticonvulsants such as topiramate (Topamax), lamotrigine (Lamictal), and oxacarbazepine (Trileptal) have also been used as mood stabilizers. Abrupt stopping of these drugs may increase the seizure threshold. Lamotrigine has been associated with a life-threatening rash called Stevens-Johnson syndrome. Slow titration of lamotrigine is recommended to minimize this problem. Clonazepam has also been utilized in treatment of bipolar disease (see Chapter 6 on anxiety).

Light and Electroconvulsive Therapy

Phototherapy has been demonstrated to lessen the symptoms of Seasonal Affective Disorder (SAD). Phototherapy is believed to work by regulating rhythms that promote sleep and wakefulness. There are several methods of delivery of light therapy: light boxes, light visors, dawn simulators, and other devices. Delivery of a minimum of 2,500 lux is administered in the morning. Examples of lux for comparative purposes are: 300 lux in an ordinary office space, 4,000 lux on a cloudy morning and 10,000 lux on a clear morning. Patients sit in front of the box for 30 or more minutes (depending on the strength) a day, in the morning. Treatment effects are noticeable after two to four days and maintenance treatment is 30 minutes a day. Side effects are rare but include irritability, headaches, or insomnia. Use of photo therapy can potentially trigger hypomania or mania in people with bipolar disease. Although the potential for eye damage is uncertain, people with retinal problems or those who are thinking about cataract surgery should consult with their eye doctor before using light therapy (Swartz, 2006).

Electroconvulsive therapy (ECT) is described as the use of electrically induced seizures to treat severe depression and less frequently to treat intense mania. It is a safe and effective treatment for people who have not responded to psychotherapy and/or antidepressant medication. Between 60% and 80% of study participants in clinical trials were shown to have a response to antidepressant medications. Of those who do not respond to medications approximately 70% will respond to ECT (Saddock & Saddock, 2003). Often ECT is utilized when patients have failed at trials of psychotherapy and psychopharmacology.

The mechanism of action of ECT is not well understood. The treatment also has a poor reputation due to some early methods of treatment delivery and media portrayal of the treatment. Patient education including family discussion is an important issue in ECT treatment.

Referral to an inpatient psychiatric program that performs ECT is necessary when the patient has not had previous ECT treatment. Some patients may require maintenance therapy and/or repeated series of ECT treatments. Use of ECT for older adults may be indicated when side effects of antidepressant medications are considered too risky for the person's overall health.

The side effects of ECT include headaches, nausea, muscle ache, soreness, confusion, and disorientation (Swartz, 2006). Problems with recent memory may be seen but usually resolve within a few weeks.

New Treatments under Investigation

Transcranial magnetic stimulation is a new treatment under investigation for its efficacy in treating MDD. An electromagnet is placed on the scalp and electric current is generated, and depolarizing cortical neurons. The intervention has been shown to increase monoamine concentrations in the brain and it appears that the treatment is effective with unipolar depression. It is noninvasive and does not cause generalized seizures (Saddock & Saddock, 2003).

Vagal Nerve Stimulation is conducted by implanting a stimulator in the left chest wall, under the collarbone, that electrically stimulates the vagus nerve. In studies this treatment has shown promise for the treatment of MDD. Deep brain stimulation is currently being researched in the treatment of treatment-resistant depression. It involves insertion of an electrode into the brain and then delivering an electrical current to stimulate the brain.

Patient Self-management, Family, and Alternative Therapy Approaches

Self-management approaches have become more and more important in this era of cost containment. Additionally, the use of self-management approaches in chronic illnesses such as asthma and cardiac disease have improved long-term health outcomes. Research about wellness incorporating self-management strategies in chronic mental illness is in the early stages, but this is an area where advanced practice nurses and other primary care providers can play a major role in discussing self-care with patients and developing research studies (Morgan, 2007).

Presenting chronic MDD in discussions with patients as a challenging disease that requires our full and best efforts can help enhance patient involvement in their care. Relapse prevention, psycho-education, close follow-up care with consistent providers, and development of a trusting relationship can improve patient adherence and follow-up with care plans. Involvement of family and significant others in treatment and relapse prevention is important. Support groups for family and significant others provide education as well as a place to discuss the effects of living with a family member who has mental illness. The National Alliance of Mentally Ill (NAMI) provides patients, family, and others with an organization dedicated to education and advocacy for those with mental illness. Clinicians can inform patients and their families about this organization as well as become involved in the organization themselves.

Actively eliciting patient information about what improves the condition and what makes it worse, and encouraging the positive efforts, is the way to begin to engage around self-management strategies. Regular exercise has been demonstrated to improve mood. Use of relaxation techniques, bibliotherapy, peer support, and problem solving are all self-management approaches that can be taught to patients in a group format. Improving self-esteem and self-efficacy can also be enhanced through group sessions.

Use of alternative and complementary therapies has exploded in the U.S. in the last two decades. Use of treatments such as massage, acupuncture, and relaxation therapies is common in those with either medical or mental illnesses. Herbal treatments are also common with use of St. John's wart, SamE (S-adenosylmethionine), and fish oil being used in the self-management of depression. These substances are not necessarily benign, and patients should be questioned about use of herbal remedies in the initial assessment. Concerns about quality control in the preparation of these remedies in terms of purity and dosing accuracy exist, since production is not regulated. Patients need to be informed that providers need to know about how they utilize these treatments since there are possible drug–drug interactions that can affect their care (see Chapter 13).

In summary, treatment of depression should utilize the model of chronic disease management. Utilizing a wide variety of treatment modalities including self-management approaches allows providers to take a fresh look at the need for collaborative models of care between primary care and mental health providers. Development of model programs will provide the blueprint for needed changes to a healthcare system that separates the mind from the body in treatment models. Patients and providers alike will benefit from the merging of care systems.

References

American Psychiatric Association (APA). (2000). *Diagnostic and statistical manual of mental disorders* (4th Edition Text Revision) DSM-IV-TR. Washington, DC: American Psychiatric Association (www.psych.org).

Benton, T., Staab, J., & Evans, D. L. (2007). Medical co-morbidity in depressive disorders. *Annals of Clinical Psychiatry*, 19 (4), 289–303.

Byrd, E. H. (2005). Nursing assessment and treatment of depressive disorders in late life. In Melillo, K. & Houde, S. (Eds.). *Geropsychiatric and mental health nursing*. Sudbury, MA: Jones and Bartlett Publishers.

Center for Disease Control (CDC). http://www.cdc.gov/nchs/data/databriefs/db07.htm (accessed on 2 July 2010).

Cochrane (2008). Screening and Case Finding Instruments for Depression. www.thecochranelibrary.com (accessed July 12, 2010).

Fortinash, K. M., & Holoday Worret, P.A. (2008). *Psychiatric mental health nursing* (4th Ed.). St. Louis: Mosby.

Gallo, J. J., & Liebowitz, B. D. (1999). The epidemiology of late life mental disorders in the community: Themes for a new century. *Psychiatric Services*, 50(9), 1158–1166.

Gonzalez, H. M., Vega, W. A., Williams, D. R., Tarraf, W., West, B. T., & Neighbors, H. W. (2010). Depression care in the United States: Too little for too few. *Archives of General Psychiatry*, 67(1), 37–46.

Greden, J. F. (2001). *Recurrent depression*. Washington, DC: American Psychiatric Publishing.

Hagerty, B. M., & Patusky, K. L. (2008). Mood disorders and adjustment disorders. In Fortinash, K. M. & Holoday Worret, P. A. (Eds.) (2008). *Psychiatric mental health nursing* (4th Edition) (pp. 208–248). St. Louis, MI: Mosby.

Hirschfeld, R., Williams, J. B., & Spitzer, R. L. (2000). Development and validation of a screening instrument for bipolar spectrum disorder: The mood disorder questionnaire. *American Journal of Psychiatry*, 157, 1873–1875.

Hirschfeld, R. M. A., Keller, M. B., Painco, S. The National Depressive and Manic-depressive Association consensus statement on the undertreatment of depression. *Journal of the American Medical Association*, 277, 333–340.

Kessler, R. C., McGonagle, K. A., Zhao, S., Nelson, C. B., Hughes, M., Eshleman, S., Wittchen, H., & Kendler, K. S. (1994). Lifetime and 12-Month prevalence of DSM-III-R psychiatric disorders in the United States: Results from the National Comorbidity Survey. *Archives of General Psychiatry*, 51(1), 8–19.

Kessler, R. C., Bergland, P., Demler, O., Jin, R., Koretz, D., Merikangas, K. R., Rush, A. J., Walters, E. E., & Wang, P. S. (2003). The epidemiology of major depressive disorder: Results from the National Comorbity Survey replication (NCS-R). *Journal of the American Medical Association*. 289(23), 3095–105.

Kroenke, K. (2007). Efficient and effective care of depression in medical settings. *2007 Medical Director Colloquy, Managed Care Supplement*, Supplement 2, 17(3), 15–21.

Lesperance, F., & Fraser-Smith, N. (2000). Depression in patients with cardiac disease: A practical review. *Journal of Psychosomatic Research*, 48, 379–391.

Liberman, J. A. (2003). The differential diagnosis of fatigue and executive dysfunction in primary care. *Journal of Clinical Psychiatry*, 64(14), 40–43.

Lin, E. H., Katon, W., & Von Korff, M. (2003). Effect of improving depression care on pain and functional outcomes among older adults with arthritis: a randomized controlled trial. *Journal of the American Medical Association*, 290, 2428–2429.

Lin, E. H. B., Katon, W., Von Korff, M., Rutter, C., Simon, G. S., Olive, M., Ciechanowski, P., Ludman, E. J., Bush, T., & Young, B. (2004). Relationship of depression and diabetes self-care, medication adherence, and preventive care. *Diabetes Care*, 27(9), 2154–2160.

Lynch, D., Laws, K. R., & McKenna, P. J. (2010). Cognitive behavioural therapy for major psychiatric disorder: Does it really work? A meta-analytical review of well-controlled trials. *Psychological Medicine*, 40, 9–24.

Mathers, C. D., & Loncar, D. (2006). Projections of global mortality and burden of disease from 2002 to 2003. *PLos Medicine*, 3(11), e442.

Melillo, K. D., & Houde, S. C. (In Press) *Geropsychiatric and mental health nursing* (2nd Ed.). Sudbury, MA: Jones and Bartlett Publishers.

Menand, L. (2010). Head case: Can psychiatry be a science? March 1. New York: *The New Yorker*.

National Institute of Mental Health (NIMH) (2009). www.nimh.nih.gov (accessed on July 12, 2010).

Polsky, D., Doshi, J. A., Marcus, S., Oslin, D., Rothbard, A., Thomas, N., & Thompson, C. L. (2005). Long-term risk for depressive symptoms after a medical diagnosis. *Archives of Internal Medicine*, 165(11), 1260–1266.

Reiger, D. A., Goldberg, I. D., & Taube, C. A. (1978). The defacto U.S. Mental Health Services Systems. *Archives of General Psychiatry*, 35, 685–693.

Robins, L. N., Helzer, J., Weissman, M. M., Orvaschel, H., Gruenberg, E., Burke, J. D., & Reiger, D. A. (1984). Lifetime prevalence of specific psychiatric disorders in three sites. *Archives of General Psychiatry*, 41, 949–958.

Rush, A. J., Trivedi, M. H., & Wisniewshi, S. R. (2006). Acute and longer term outcomes in depressed outpatients requiring one or several treatment steps: A STAR*D report. *American Journal of Psychiatry*, 163, 1905–1917.

Saddock, B. J., & Saddock, V. A. (2003). *Kaplan and Saddock's synopsis of psychiatry: Behavioral sciences/clinical psychiatry* (9th Ed.). Philadelphia, PA: Lippincott Williams & Wilkins.

Stewart, W. F., Ricci, J. A., Chee, E., Hanhn, S. R., & Morganstein, D. (2003). Cost of lost productivity work time among US workers with depression. *Journal of the American Medical Association*, 289(23), 3135–3144.

Styron, W. (1990). *Darkness visible: A memory of madness*. New York: Random House.

Swartz, K. L. (2006). *The Johns Hopkins White Papers: Depression and anxiety*. Baltimore, MD: Johns Hopkins Medicine.

World Health Organization (WHO). (2001). The world health report 2001: Mental Health: New understanding, new hope. Geneva, Switzerland: WHO.

Young, A. S., Klap, R., Sherbourne, C. D., & Wells, K. B. (2001). The quality of care for depressive and anxiety disorders in the United States. *Archives of General Psychiatry*, 58, 55–61.

8 The Person with Schizophrenia

With Mary Linda O'Reilly

- Schizophrenia: A Serious but Treatable Illness
- Functional Assessment and Diagnosis of Schizophrenia
- Treatment of Persons with Schizophrenia
- Co-morbidities
- Medication-induced Movement Disorders
- Family/Caregiver Issues
- Collaborative Practice: Patient/Family and Health/Mental Health Provider
- Appendix 1
- Appendix 2
- References

"Your daughter has schizophrenia," I told the woman.

"Oh, my god, anything but that," she replied. "Why couldn't she have leukemia or some other disease instead?"

"But if she had leukemia she might die," I pointed out. "Schizophrenia is a much more treatable disease."

The woman looked sadly at me, then down at the floor. She spoke softly. "I would still prefer that my daughter had leukemia."

Torrey, 2001, p. xxi

Schizophrenia: A Serious but Treatable Illness

Schizophrenia is notorious for being the most frightening, disabling, and misunderstood of mental illnesses, historically sentencing the sufferer to an existence of terrifying experiences such as hearing voices, and thwarting hopes and dreams for the future. Family and caregivers of the individual with schizophrenia also experience stigma associated with this cruel illness, coupled with the burdens of uncertainty about the future, lack of social support, and coping with symptom relapses as best they can. Persons with schizophrenia are also at increased risk of morbidity and early mortality, the mortality rate being three times that of the general population (Saha, Chant & McGrath, 2007; Brown, Inskip & Barraclough, 2000). While it is unclear if the genetic mutations that predispose the individual to schizophrenia also contribute to the early development of cardiovascular and metabolic syndromes, numerous studies have established that schizophrenia can trigger a cascade of socioeconomic and lifestyle factors that culminate in adverse physical health outcomes (Lumby, 2007; Saha, Chant & McGrath, 2007; Capasso, Lineberry, Bostwick, Decker & St. Sauver, 2007).

With newly emerging information about the etiology of schizophrenia, the availability of newer generation antipsychotic medications or neuroleptics, and recognition of the critical importance of community-based interventions for patient and family, there is hope for control of symptoms and reintegration of the individual into society. While the pharmacologic management of schizophrenia remains in the purview of the mental health expert, the primary care provider (PCP) plays an essential role in providing ongoing education about symptom management and relapse prevention. A PCP's collaborative relationship with the mental health provider who prescribes the neuroleptic regimen provides a safety net for the patient in terms of monitoring for a multiplicity of medication side effects. The PCP can also act as coach for adherence, supportive listener for the emotional struggle to incorporate schizophrenia into the life plan, and an informational resource about community services. The PCP who provides care for the entire family is in an excellent position to support healthy family dynamics and coping mechanisms, and to encourage the caregivers to meet their own needs.

The PCP has an important role to play regarding the concept of psychological recovery. This describes a process that includes the development of hope, establishment of an identity beyond that as a patient with schizophrenia, finding meaning in life, and accepting responsibility for control of the illness (Anderson, Oades & Caputi, 2003). It views as possible a belief in the patient's ability to meet life goals, to be self-sustaining, and to assume control over his or her life. The PCP, as part of the mosaic of care that comprises the patient, caregivers, and mental health provider, can confirm the reality of life with schizophrenia and intervene either directly or through collaboration in promoting a successful outcome for the individual with schizophrenia.

This chapter provides an overview of schizophrenia, including patient evaluation and diagnosis, approaches to treatment, and clinical monitoring and supportive interventions to maximize social functioning. It stresses the PCP's role in working collaboratively with the patient and his or her family, and with the patient's mental health provider, to ensure the best possible outcomes in the realms of both physical and mental health.

Scope of the Problem

Schizophrenia is a severe, chronic, debilitating mental illness associated with abnormalities of brain structure and function and alterations in brain neurochemistry (NIMH, 2007; Picchioni & Murray, 2007). Individuals with schizophrenia experience disorders of thought rather than of mood; between exacerbations of symptoms, there is a tendency toward lower levels of social and vocational functioning (Glick, Suppes, DeBattista, Hu & Marder, 2001).

The sex ratio in schizophrenia in the United States, Canada and Western Europe is 1.2:1, with males being affected slightly more often than females. Males have an average age of onset between ages 18–25, where females have two peaks of onset: one between ages 25 and 35 and a second peak after age 45. Many women with schizophrenia are initially diagnosed as having an affective disorder, because women with schizophrenia appear to have more difficulties with emotional regulation than men. Women may also have higher levels of pre-symptom functioning than men.

Current estimates of the incidence of schizophrenia in the United States reveal that between 1 and 1.5% of the population is affected, representing approximately three million people (NIMH, 2007). This general incidence has remained stable since the collection of statistical information became standardized and it appears to be stable across cultures. While the incidence appears low in comparison to affective disorders, the cost to the healthcare system is disproportionately high, accounting for 2.5% of all healthcare costs or $40 billion dollars per year in the United States. The severity and recidivism of the symptoms of schizophrenia, and the resultant risk to the safety of the patient and others may require increased use of acute care psychiatric services, including hospitalization, until symptoms can be stabilized. Additionally, there is increasing recognition of significant physical co-morbidities associated with schizophrenia. These include, but are not limited to, cardio-vascular disease, metabolic syndrome, pulmonary disease and neoplastic disease (Lumby, 2007). Unrecognized and therefore poorly controlled cardiovascular disease, diabetes, and emphysema contribute significantly to the drain on available healthcare resources.

The cost in terms of loss of productive participation in society and in human suffering is not as easily quantified. Disappointed hopes and plans for the future affect the family as well as the individual with schizophrenia. Major financial readjustments may have to be under-taken, if the patient was the major wage-earner, or if childcare demands make it difficult for a partner to subsidize family income through inability to take on more employment. If aging parents are the major caregivers, their own increasing physical needs may make it impossible for them to assist an adult child with a severe and marginally controlled illness (Tsang, Person, & Yuen, 2002).

With deinstitutionalization in the 1960s, large numbers of individuals with severe mental illness were released into the community; their needs for assistance with housing, self-care, and symptom management easily overwhelmed programs designed to support integration into society (Hoff, 1993; Johnson, 1990). Many disappeared into the correctional system when their symptoms resurfaced and they engaged in either self-soothing by using illegal substances, or they acted on the commands issued by their voices or by the dictates of their paranoia. Others remain visible but invisible, representing a significant proportion among the ranks of the chronically homeless.

Major Symptoms

Schizophrenia is characterized by symptoms that suggest a disconnection between what exists in reality and what is experienced as reality by the individual with schizophrenia. There are several subtypes of schizophrenia, and the illness may be best understood as a family of related disorders in which symptoms evolve over time; not all patients share the same symptoms. Symptoms of schizophrenia fall into three broad categories: positive symptoms, negative symptoms, and cognitive symptoms. The cognitive and negative impairments are often the greatest deterrents to regaining interpersonal and vocational normalcy.

Positive symptoms (primarily cognitive dysfunction) are the most easily recognized and refer especially to those that have responded more quickly to neuroleptic medications. Positive symptoms can be further characterized as perceptual (hallucinations), beliefs (delu-sions), behavioral, and speech:

- Hallucinations: sensory perceptions that are experienced without evidence of stimuli, with auditory hallucinations the most common.
- Delusions: fixed false beliefs that are not shared by others in the person's community; persist in the face of overwhelming evidence to the contrary; for example, the conviction that one is being persecuted, or victimized by a plot or threat.
- Speech is distorted or illogical.

These symptoms are usually first noted by a family member who may seek help from a PCP stating, for example: "I'm afraid something's really wrong with my son . . . He thinks people on the TV are talking directly to him . . . He's just not like himself."

Negative Symptoms (primarily behavioral and emotional) Negative symptoms involve a withdrawing from participation in life and from engaging in contact with others; they represent a loss of or reduction in normal functioning. These have responded less well to typical or first-line antipsychotic medications. Negative symptoms are less easily recognized and may be mistaken for evidence of depression or laziness; they appear to be less troubling to the patient, but may be more distressing to family or caregivers. The most common are:

- Alogia: or "poverty of speech"; an inability to express or expand upon thoughts.
- Blunted or flattened affect: the face may be unresponsive or expressionless, and speech is lacking in emotionality.
- Avolition: little motivation to initiate or continue goal-directed or group activities; also expressed in self-neglect with regard to grooming.
- Anhedonia: a loss of capacity for enjoyment or appreciation of life's pleasures.

Cognitive Symptoms   Cognitive symptoms include problems with attention, memory, and executive functions:

- Planning and organization deficits: difficulty with activities that support independent functioning, such as managing a budget and paying bills.
- Limited appreciation about the symptoms of schizophrenia, effects on independent and interpersonal functioning.
- Denial that he or she has a chronic, severe mental illness (NIMH, 2007, Picchione & Murray, 2007).
- Anosognosia: lack of insight about the severity of the illness; associated with higher rates of poor treatment adherence, increased risk of recurrent psychotic episodes and poorer prognosis for recovery.

The presence of severe positive symptoms usually precipitates an urgent mental health evaluation and treatment in an inpatient setting in order to protect the patient and others. Symptoms may be minimally present after discharge, but should not exert an influence that is distressing or disruptive to the patient or the environment. For example, patients may acknowledge the continued presence of auditory hallucinations, but find ways of reducing them to background noise, such as by playing music or engaging in physical activity.

Once discharged and/or referred to primary care for follow-up, the PCP may observe continued presence of negative symptoms in the restricted emotionality of the patient's responses, in the limited mobility of facial features, and the difficulty in eliciting an elaboration of responses to questions. Caregivers may remark on difficulty in motivating the patient to maintain personal hygiene or frustration in attempts to engage the patient in social activities. The cognitive and negative impairments are often the greatest deterrents to regaining interpersonal and vocational normalcy.

The PCP plays a significant role in ongoing education about the diagnosis of schizophrenia, especially regarding its chronicity and the breadth of the areas of self care it affects. Being able to refer to community resources that support the patient's independent functioning contributes to maintaining care in an ambulatory setting and may assist caregivers in coping while symptoms come under control.

Etiology: Genetic, Environmental, and Neurobiological Factors

Ethnographic studies have revealed that schizophrenia has been present in all cultures throughout the ages. Trepanation, the boring of holes into the skull to release evil spirits, was practiced as early as 10,000 BC (Korn, 2001). Understanding of the disease etiology has evolved from beliefs in possession by demons, to an imbalance of bodily humors, to impaired and destructive family dynamics, to the current acceptance of abnormal neurobiological underpinnings. Schizophrenia is now considered to result from multiple factors.

Genetic Risk The greatest risk is a positive family history of schizophrenia (Picchioni & Murray, 2007; Glick, Suppes, DeBattista, Hu, & Marder, 2001). The lifetime risk increases from just about 1% in the general population to 6.5% in the first degree relatives of those with schizophrenia, and it rises to more than 40% in the identical twin of the affected person. Other genetic research has revealed that a disorder known as the 22q deletion syndrome poses a 25% risk of developing schizophrenia (Bassett, O'Neill, Murphy, *et al*., 2001). There is some evidence to suggest that having a father older than 50 at the time of conception could increase the risk for schizophrenia up to three times the expected risk (Malaspina, 2006).

Environmental Factors Environmental events associated with increased risk for schizophrenia include maternal factors, such as exposure to starvation, influenzas during the second trimester of pregnancy, and RH incompatibility in a second or third pregnancy. It is unclear if environmental stressors such as separation from family of origin in late adolescence may trigger the onset of schizophrenia in individuals with genetic or psychological vulnerabilities. Research on possible links between schizophrenia and substance abuse reveal that substance abuse is prevalent among individuals with schizophrenia. A New Zealand study showed that early cannabis use increases the future risk of schizophrenia fourfold, even after controlling for any effect of self-medication (Arseneault, *et al*., 2002). An Italian study indicated that cannabis use may precipitate the onset of schizophrenia at an earlier age (Mauri, *et al.*, 2006). However, only a small proportion of people who use cannabis develop schizophrenia. This may reflect a gene–environment interaction in individuals who are genetically vulnerable. Social factors, such as the experience of racial discrimination or having a marginalized identity within one's ethnic group, have been posited as risk factors for schizophrenia and other psychotic disorders (Chakraborty & Mckenzie, 2002; Veling, Hoek, Wiersma, & Mackenbach, 2009).

Neurobiological Factors Abnormalities in brain structure, including increased ventricular size and diminishing grey matter over time have been found in some, but not all, individuals with schizophrenia. In 2002, research demonstrated a connection between two abnormalities of brain functioning in schizophrenia. High levels of dopamine and dopamine transmission abnormalities are linked to the delusions and hallucinations of psychosis, the positive symptoms. Negative symptoms are seen as consequences of gross structural brain abnormalities and ventricular enlargement (Andreasen & Olsen, 1982). Positron Emission Tomography revealed that reduced activity in the prefrontal cortex was associated with abnormally elevated levels of dopamine in the striatum in individuals with schizophrenia. This finding suggests that treatment might be targeted specifically at the prefrontal cortex.

Functional Assessment and Diagnosis of Schizophrenia

The *Diagnostic and statistical manual of mental disorders* emphasizes the presence of positive symptoms and social and vocational impairment. However, there is growing appreciation of the negative symptoms and cognitive impairment frequently seen among persons with schizophrenia, as it is felt that these symptoms have a greater impact on long-term prognosis (Glick, Suppes, DeBattista, Hu, & Marder, 2001). Primary care providers who do not follow these clients with an already established diagnosis of schizophrenia according to DSM criteria may initially identify this serious illness through use of the Comprehensive Mental Health Assessment (CMHA) tool described in Chapter 2—specifically, Item 8 that screens for thought disorders such as schizophrenia (see online descriptions for rating of this basic life function.)

Initial manifestations of schizophrenia may include nebulous symptoms such as anxiety, social problems, or changes in behavior such as becoming withdrawn, and difficulties in concentrating (Picchioni & Murray, 2007). Few individuals with schizophrenia present either to psychiatric specialists or to PCPs with a sudden onset of florid psychotic symptoms without prodomal subtle shifts and deteriorations in other areas of cognitive and interpersonal functioning that typically are observed first by family members. The rapid development of new hallucinations, delusional thinking, and disorganized behavior and speech must be evaluated against other organic causes, such as metabolic imbalance, substance use, seizures disorder, or neoplasms (Powell, Heckers, & Bierer, 1998).

CASE EXAMPLE: EARLY SYMPTOMS

Ben was nineteen years old when his family approached their PCP for assistance with behavior changes that were becoming increasingly problematic. Their concern was that Ben was using illegal substances. After some reflection, the family described changes that had slowly become noticeable and had increased over a three year period. Ben had become increasingly withdrawn from the family and spent his time alone in his room, had discontinued his community activities, and his previously average grades were failing. He did not bring friends to visit, and was not out socializing as had been his pattern in the past. He was not showering and was dressing in the same clothing for days at a time; he also had taken to wearing a knitted wool cap day and night. Matters came to a head when he tried to give his grandmother's cat boiling water.

Ben was a pale young man with slowed speech and significant difficulty in answering questions without digressing into stories that had shed no appreciable light on the information being requested. He was dressed, on a warm autumn day, in a wool coat and cap; it was evident once he was persuaded to remove the coat that he had not bathed in many days. Ben described to the PCP that neighbors were spying on him and that the hat was to keep them from putting dirty pictures into his head. His action towards the cat was intended to eliminate one more spy who could see into his mind. The PCP's action was to arrange for an immediate referral for a psychiatric evaluation and Ben was admitted to an inpatient facility for further evaluation and treatment.

Ben's case demonstrates the subtlety of onset that is characteristic of schizophrenia. His initial behaviors were initially interpreted by his family as adolescent moodiness. As symptoms progressed, worry about experimentation with substances of abuse, then outright concern about addiction was in the forefront of his family's mind. Ben's parents were shocked and grieved when given the diagnosis, and saddened that addiction, which they viewed as "curable" was not the root of their son's deterioration (see Chapter 9: Substance Abuse, Addiction, and Mental Health).

Diagnostic Criteria

Diagnostic criteria listed in the *Diagnostic and statistical manual of mental disorders* revised fourth edition (DSM-IVTR, 1994) includes the following:

*   Presence of positive and negative symptoms: There must have been two or more of the following symptoms during a one-month period: delusions, hallucinations, disorganized speech, disorganized or catatonic behavior, negative symptoms.

- Decline in social, interpersonal or occupational functioning, including personal hygiene or self-care
- Duration: the symptomatic behavior must last for at least six months.

Treatment of Persons with Schizophrenia

Past treatment of the severely mentally ill reflected the incomprehensibility of the symptoms as well as the fear and disgust that the symptoms engendered in society. These approaches included the inhumane such as exorcism, ice baths, and sequestering (imprisoning!) the mentally ill in subhuman conditions, as well as sensory deprivation and early efforts at convulsive therapy. The gentler intervention of psychoanalytic treatment proved ineffective in controlling psychotic symptoms, and may pose a risk for greater distress during probing of long-suppressed subconscious thoughts that may be competing with current hallucinations and delusions (Malmberg & Fenton, 2001; Torrey, 2001).

The Therapeutic Relationship as Context for Treatment

All health professionals are already grounded in basic principles of the therapeutic relationship as a premise for successful treatment. It is now well established that the best outcomes of psychotropic drug treatment occur when combined with psychotherapeutic approaches. But the challenges of an illness like schizophrenia—for patient, family, and health providers alike—and relational approaches to treatment are great, in that the essence of the illness is a breakdown in normal cognitive, emotional, and behavioral functioning. As Dubovsky and Dubovsky (2007, p. 7) note: The widespread marketing of psychotropic drugs "helped move psychiatry into the 'brain based' era and away from a true 'biopsychosocial' model, or as some have said, from the brainless psychiatry of the past to the mindless psychiatry of the present."

We therefore offer the following vignettes that suggest some helpful relationship points in the care of people with schizophrenia (Hoff, 2008). They affirm the principles of interpersonal psychiatry and psychiatric nursing propounded decades ago by these pioneers in the field: Psychiatrist Harry Stack Sullivan (see Evans, 1996), and Hildagarde Peplau (1993).

The Brief Session in Primary Care

After listening to a brilliant scientific lecture on schizophrenia, a primary care physician remarked: "You know, I quite like working with these patients . . . They seem glad to see me . . . I ask how things are going, see if there are any troubling side effects from medications, check any laboratory results, and just chat a bit. They thank me for the help and that's about it. But it seems like I should be doing more? I sure don't have time or skills for any kind of psychotherapy. What do you think?" The mental health consultant replied: "You seem to be doing just what's recommended for these folks . . . In-depth probing can actually induce anxiety, based on the social psychology concept of 'the strength of weak ties.' That is, people with schizophrenia need to know that someone cares and takes an interest in their welfare, but typically, they don't easily tolerate getting too close, as in a psychotherapy relationship. Usually, though, they are keenly sensitive in detecting sincerity or a judgmental attitude in human interaction of any kind." The physician seemed reassured by this brief exchange.

"Checking out Reality" vs. Hallucinations with a Health Provider

Jonathan, age 22, was hospitalized for an acute psychotic episode in a facility deeply committed to the concept of "therapeutic milieu" in which everything in the setting holds the potential for therapeutic outcome of exacerbation of patients' anxiety, fear, and other symptoms. In the morning Jonathan freely shared with the nurse that he "had been to Paris during the night," he then went over to a window and asked the nurse: "Do you see that bulldozer out there?" The nurse replied: "No, Jon, I don't see any bulldozer," to which Jon responded: "Well, I guess it must have been another hallucination." Jon then asked the nurse to check out the walls in his room that he said were marked up with "directions." The nurse thought ". . . maybe visual hallucinations connected to his 'trip to Paris'...". But sure enough, there were pencil marks on the wall depicting North, South, East, and West. Jonathan said he did not put them there, the nurse noted that most likely another patient was just getting oriented to the hospital environment, and Jonathan said: "Well, I thought maybe it was one of my hallucinations."

Obviously, this kind of reality-checking by a person with schizophrenia, trying to understand and deal with his illness, could not easily have taken place without the trust and compassion implicit in therapeutic relationships. In essence, it means a lot to such a patient who senses that the provider is trying to understand what "going crazy . . . losing one's mind" feels like. It also contributes to the patient's adherence to the treatment program. In such context, the PCP inquiring about medication side-effects might also ask, for example: "How about the troubling voices . . . What kind of effect has the medication had on them? Are they better, worse or about the same?"

Medications

Medications, specifically the neuroleptics, are the mainstay for treating the symptoms of schizophrenia. Antipsychotic medications are selected empirically, that is, chosen for their ability to control target symptoms (Glick, Suppes, DeBattista, Hu, & Marder, 2001). Treatment goals are stage specific. In the acute phase, the primary goal is to relieve the most serious symptoms, which typically include hallucinations, delusions, disorganized behavior, and agitation. This is most usually done in an inpatient or other restricted-milieu setting for the protection of the patient and others. It is vital that treatment is initiated quickly, as delays may result in worsening of subsequent episodes and poorer social outcomes in terms of persistent negative symptoms (Melle, Larsen, Haahr, Friis, Johannesen, *et al.*, 2008). In the maintenance phase, the goal is to reduce the risk for relapse and improve functional capacity and quality of life (Ghaemi, *et al.*, 2005; Glick, Suppes, DeBattista, Hu, & Marder, 2001). The PCP has greater involvement with patients in this phase, acting as a coach for medication adherence and observing behaviors in an ambulatory setting.

Symptom reduction occurs over a period of several weeks, and symptoms respond in different time frames. In general, agitation and sleep and appetite symptoms often respond during the first two weeks of treatment. Personal hygiene and basic interpersonal socialization may be slower to begin resolving, taking two to three weeks. However, not all patients return to their baseline level of social and vocational functioning. If response to medications is inadequate after four to six weeks, plasma levels of medication should be checked. If the medication level reveals that the drug is being taken, the dose may be increased or a switch may be made to another neuroleptic. An adequate trial is considered to be four weeks with an atypical antipsychotic medication. Clozapine trials may last for up to three months. Full effectiveness of selected medications should be in evidence by 12 weeks of treatment (Argo *et al.*, 2008; Glick, Suppes, DeBattista, Hu, & Marder, 2001).

Since recurrent psychotic episodes facilitate future and more severe episodes, it is important to prevent relapse. In the maintenance phase, antipsychotic medications are dosed at the lowest effective level, and long-term injectable formulations may be considered if treatment adherence seems problematic. Intermittent treatment with antipsychotic medications for episodic control of symptoms has been shown to be ineffective in preventing symptom relapse, and may potentiate episodes of psychosis that occur with increasing frequency and severity (Picchioni & Murray, 2007).

Selection and dosing of antipsychotic medications is a complex process and preferentially is managed by mental health professionals in collaboration with PCPs who manage co-morbid medical conditions so prominent among these vulnerable clients. Symptoms may change and evolve over time and medications must be titrated carefully to maintain a balance among efficacy, safety, and tolerability (Ghaemi, et al., 2005).

There does not appear to be a significant advantage of first generation agents or typical antipsychotic medications (chlorpromazine and haldoperidol) over second generation with regard to control of positive symptoms. The effectiveness of the newer medications on quality of life and social and vocational function appears to be associated with a lower incidence of involuntary movement (Swartz, Perkins, Stroup, Davis, Capuano, et al., 2007). The second generation medications, including risperidone (Risperdal®) and ziprasidone (Geodon®) are associated with fewer extrapyramidal symptoms (EPS) but may elevate prolactin levels. The third generation class is prolactin sparing and associated with fewer EPS and less tardive dyskinesia, and has a broader spectrum of efficacy for both positive and negative symptoms; medications in this class include clozapine (Clozaril®), olanzepine (Zyprexa®) and quetiapine (Seroquel®) (Maguire & Yu, 2001).

The Texas Medication Algorithm Project (TMAP) guidelines recommend the use of atypical agents in patients with first-time episodes of schizophrenia and in those who have previously failed to respond to one or two trials with typical neuroleptics (Argo, et al., 2008). Aripiprazole (Abilify®) and ziprasidone appear to be more metabolically neutral than olanzepine quetiapine , or risperdone (Ghaemi, et al., 2005). Risperdone has a higher incidence of extrapyramidal and prolactin-related side effects than aripiprazole or ziprasidone (Stahl, 2005). Clozapine (Clozaril®) has been associated with agranulocytosis, especially among children, adolescents, and the elderly (Wahlbeck, Cheine, & Essali, 1999). It is generally considered to be a third-line agent.

Medications are initiated at the lowest recommended dose, and *safety monitoring is critical for early intervention if side effects arise or other symptoms emerge*. Initial starting doses are recommended as follows: airpiprazole 10–15mg daily, olanzepine 5–10mg daily, quetiapine 50mg dosed twice daily, risperadone 1–2mg daily and ziprasidone 40–80mg dosed once or twice daily (Argo, et al., 2008).

It is important to stress that mental health professionals are the best prepared to perform an in-depth evaluation of symptoms and to initiate and manage antipsychotic medications. Many PCPs, however, work in resource-poor settings where access to specialized psychiatric consultations are difficult to arrange and may be logistically near impossible for patients and family caregivers to attend. It would be essential in these situations for the PCP to develop a close collaborative relationship with a prescribing mental health provider in order to receive ongoing consultation, support, and clinical supervision.

Adjuvant Interventions

Schizophrenia requires a long-term integrative treatment strategy. The provider, patient, and family must agree on goals and work collaboratively towards control of symptoms and maximizing function and quality of life. Besides empiricism in selection of neuroleptic medications, other treatment principles emphasize interventions to maximize adherence to medications, integrating psychosocial approaches to improve social and vocational function, and involving family and significant others as well as a consumer organization (Glick, *et al.*, 2001).

Development of a long-term collaborative relationship with a primary care provider is as important as promoting trust and assisting patients to take back some of the control that has been lost during the acute phase of the illness. Patients value kindness, patience and ability to inspire confidence in their interactions; being treated as an equal partner in the therapeutic relationship promotes personal empowerment (Lester, Tritter, & England, 2003).

Psychosocial interventions refer to nonpharmacologic interventions designed to decrease symptom severity, avoid hospitalizations, improve social and vocational functioning, and improve satisfaction with life (Mueser, Bond, & Drake, 2002). Among these are cognitive behavior therapy (CBT) that may benefit patients in early stages of schizophrenia, and Assertive Community Treatment (ACT) indicated for those with long-standing symptoms or who have not responded well to early intensive treatment.

Cognitive Behavioral Interventions

Cognitive behavior therapy (CBT) has been used to reduce the distress associated with persistent symptoms and improve insight and management of these events. This approach involves exploring, evaluating, and challenging clients' thought and beliefs about psychotic phenomena, and actively engages patients in their treatment. Mueser, Bond, and Drake (2002) compared four studies in which clients were provided with between five weeks and nine months of CBT, with follow-up ranging between six and 18 months. Clients who received the intervention experienced a more rapid resolution of psychotic symptoms and had lower overall levels of these symptoms. A more recent meta-analysis by Lynch, Laws, and McKenna (2010) concludes that CBT is no better than non-specific control interventions, such as befriending and supportive counseling, in reducing the symptoms of schizophrenia or in preventing relapse. It may have some effectiveness in assisting to cope with the symptoms of depression that are often present in individuals with schizophrenia.

Assertive Community Treatment

The Assertive Community Treatment (ACT) model evolved to address the needs of those patients with schizophrenia who, through sub-optimal adherence to medications and mental health services, are at increased risk to utilize high cost services such as inpatient care and emergency room visits (Mueser, Bond, & Drake, 2002). In the ACT model, there is a low client to case manager ratio, often as low as ten to one, rather than thirty or more to one. Clinicians share caseloads, 24-hour coverage is provided through an on-call system, there is close attention paid to illness management, and there is high frequency of client contact. Services are provided in community settings, rather than in clinics. The process involves daily contact with clients, monitoring and support for adherence to medications, follow-up visits, and active case management to enable clients to participate in community programs— including jobs commensurate with their skills and health/illness status. The most prominent effects of ACT have been observed in reducing the amount of time spent as an inpatient and improved housing stability. It did not seem to have a consistent effect on social adjustment or vocational functioning, but there was improvement for those patients employed in positions supported by rehabilitation programs (Mueser, Bond, & Drake, 1998).

The PCP's role with both ACT and CBT is to support the patient's ongoing participation in the process by discussion about the use of community supports and counseling. By valuing the interventions as important adjuvants to medication, the PCP can promote these as being critical in adherence to medication regimens and to maintaining control of symptoms.

Co-morbidities

Schizophrenia contributes significantly to the global burden of disease (Ustun, 1999). Besides the association with elevated risks of suicide, schizophrenia is linked to premature death related to numerous co-morbid somatic conditions (Saha, Chant, & McGrath, 2007). Individuals with schizophrenia are at higher risk for a number of health-related problems, including diabetes, coronary artery disease, hypertension, and emphysema. The lifestyles of people with serious mental illnesses are often associated with poor dietary habits, obesity, high rates of tobacco consumption, and the use of alcohol and street drugs. Thus, co-morbidities result from effects of the illness itself, treatment with antipsychotic medications, and lifestyle factors, coupled with the stigma of living with a severe mental illness (Marder, *et al.*, 2004).

Substance Use: Tobacco, Alcohol, Street Drugs

The neurobiologic effects of nicotine, through its interaction with dopaminergic circuits, may ameliorate some negative symptoms of schizophrenia such as amotivation, social isolation, and anhedonia (Combs & Advocat, 2000; Lyon, 1999). Compared with 20% of the general public, over 70% of people with schizophrenia smoke cigarettes, and tend to smoke more cigarettes per day than people without serious mental illness (Hennekens, Hennekens, & Hollar, 2005). This leads to higher incidence of chronic bronchitis and chronic obstructive pulmonary disease among individuals with schizophrenia than is found in the general public. Other tobacco related illnesses may include neoplasms of both the upper and lower airways and cardiovascular disease.

Yet, people with schizophrenia are less likely to receive smoking cessation counseling (Himmelhoch, Lehman, Kreyenbuhl, *et al.* (2004). Use of tobacco also potentiates the metabolism of antipsychotic medications through activation of the cytochrome P450 pathway, and this may result in plasma levels of medication that are inadequate to control symptoms. If higher doses of neuroleptics are required, there is increased risk of medication side effects and adverse events (Compton, 2006). Individuals with schizophrenia are also less likely to receive ongoing and regular preventive care, so that when a diagnosis of tobacco-related illness is made, it may be well advanced and require significant medical interventions and lifestyle adjustments.

With regard to assisting patients with schizophrenia to relinquish use of tobacco products, the PCP may take advantage of numerous publically funded initiatives. The "5 As" (ask, advise, assess, assist, and arrange) provide a framework for providers to approach the subject and find strategies to assist patients to stop tobacco use (Compton, 2006). Nicotine replacement therapies including patches and gum may be useful. Varencycline (Chantix®), a nicotine drive suppressant, has been associated with the development of neuropsychiatric symptoms such as depression, anxiety, and thoughts of suicide. Patients taking varencycline require careful monitoring for increase in existing neuropsychiatric symptoms or development of new ones (FDA, 2008). Because tobacco potentiates the excretion of antipsychotic medications, once tobacco use has ceased, additional monitoring is necessary to identify medication side effects.

Approximately 47% of people with schizophrenia have a co-occurring substance use disorder (Owen, Fischer, Booth, & Cuffel, 1996). The presence of a co-occurring substance abuse disorder with schizophrenia, i.e., a dual diagnosis, is associated with many unfavorable outcomes, including symptom relapse and re-hospitalization, housing instability, violence directed toward self or others, family conflict, and legal problems (Mueser, Bond, & Drake, 2002; (Batki, Leontieva, Dimmock, & Ploutz-Snyder, 2008). The substances most usually abused by individuals with schizophrenia include alcohol, marijuana and cocaine (Argo, *et al.*, 2008). Batki, Leontieva, Dimmock, & Ploutz-Snyder's study (2008) also found that there was less alcohol craving and alcohol-related euphoria when there was a predominance of negative symptoms, specifically social withdrawal, blunted affect, and difficulty with abstract thinking. It appears that control of positive symptoms may play a significant role in assisting the person with schizophrenia to achieve and maintain sobriety from alcohol.

Cocaine use among individuals with schizophrenia has risen, with some estimates as high as 40%. It is believed that cocaine use may serve to relieve some of the negative symptoms and feelings of dysphoria. However, cocaine use worsens hallucinations and delusions and deepens anxiety and depression (Copersino & Serper, 1998).

There are two traditional treatment approaches for individuals with dual diagnosis: sequential and parallel. In sequential treatment, one disorder, e.g., the psychiatric disorder, is treated before beginning interventions on the second disorder, substance abuse. In parallel treatment, both disorders are treated simultaneously, but by different clinicians, usually working for different agencies. Typically there are high rates of treatment failure with these approaches, which is based on ineligibility criteria, poor service coordination, and dropout (Mueser, Bond, & Drake, 2002). Integrated programs have been found to be more successful at engaging and keeping patients in treatment for both the mental health problem and the substance abuse disorder (Drake, Mercer-McFadden, & Mueser, 1998).

While the PCP usually does not try to play a direct role in the work of sobriety, expressions of interest, support, and compassion for the struggle can do much towards accompanying the client on his or her journey to abstaining from abuse of substances. Knowledge of community resources and how to mobilize them are valuable tools in the PCP's armamentarium. By engaging the client in ongoing discussion about the issues surrounding substance use and the use of community agencies and programs, the PCP communicates concern and supports all efforts made by the client.

Other interventions that patients can be supported to participate in include opiate substitution programs such as those for methadone and buprenorphine, 12-step programs, and day programs. Much of the success of these programs will depend on the degree of collaboration among clinicians that provide the service and the support that the patient receives to enable participation. Control of symptoms appears to be important in promoting the discontinuation of substance abuse. There is evidence to suggest that clozepine has the most significant and positive outcomes when patients have schizophrenia and substance abuse as co-morbidities (Argo, *et al.*, 2008) (see Chapter 9 on substance abuse).

Depression

Since much substance use appears to be related to co-morbid depression, it is essential to screen for this illness in patients with schizophrenia. Prevalence of depression among those with schizophrenia is estimated to be about 60% (Maguire & Yu, 2001). As in non-schizophrenic populations, depression can be lethal if unrecognized and untreated. Part of the difficulty in diagnosing depression among patients with schizophrenia is the assumption that social withdrawal, anhedonia, and feelings of indifference represent only the negative symptoms of schizophrenia. Further questioning of subjective reports of feeling sad, worthless, or demoralized may reveal that the person suffers from an affective disorder (Weiden, 2005). Two third generation antipsychotics appear to improve depression, olanzepine and clozepine (Maguire & Yu, 2001). Other appropriate interventions include supportive counseling and use of a serotonin reuptake inhibitor once the positive symptoms have been stabilized (Kane, Leucht, Carpenter, & Docherty, 2003) (see Chapter 7 on depression).

Metabolic Disease

With the introduction of second-generation antipsychotic medications, individuals with schizophrenia enjoy a better quality of life, including reduced incidence of movement disorders, better control of negative symptoms, and increased possibility of avoiding relapse. However, concern arises because several of the medications in this newer class are likely, as is the case with the first generation antipsychotic medications, to cause weight gain and result in metabolic syndrome.

Metabolic syndrome is a constellation of findings that may culminate in the development of Type 2 Diabetes and cardiovascular disease (Lumby, 2007). A diagnosis of metabolic syndrome is made when abdominal obesity (a waist size of 35 inches or more for women and 40 inches or more for men) combines with two of the following four criteria: elevated triglyceride level, reduced high-density lipoprotein, elevated blood pressure (or previously elevated blood pressure that is currently controlled by medication), or elevated fasting plasma glucose. Allison, *et al.* (1999) found that 42% of individuals with schizophrenia met the criteria for a diagnosis of obesity as defined by a Body Mass Index of 27 or higher, whereas 27% of the control population met the criteria. Among older women with schizophrenia, 71% are overweight or obese as compared to 38% of aged matched women in the general population (Dickerson, Pater, & Origoni, 2002).

Type 2 Diabetes has a high incidence among those with schizophrenia. It is estimated that impaired glucose metabolism is present at two to three times the rate of the non-schizophrenic population (Ryan & Thakore, 2002). This places individuals with schizophrenia at increased risk of both microvascular and macrovascular disease. Factors that accumulate to increase the relative risk of developing Type 2 Diabetes in this population include poor diet, sedentary lifestyle, and use of antipsychotic medications (Lumby, 2007).

Besides the risk of other obesity-associated illness, including osteoarthritis, gallbladder and liver disease, and certain neoplastic illnesses such as colon cancer, obesity has significant psychosocial consequences. Individuals may suffer from low self-esteem, be reluctant to continue taking the medication and experience increased difficulty with readjusting to living in society.

Monitoring Symptoms and Treatment Outcomes

An important collaborative role for the PCP is in ongoing observation for undesirable medication side effects. These include, but are not limited to: monitoring for metabolic abnormalities, changes in cognition, and involuntary movements caused by antipsychotic medications. Discussion about medication adherence provides an opportunity for ongoing surveillance of medication side effects, education about disease process, and early intervention for the development of new symptoms or relapse of pre-existing ones.

Because of the risk of cardiovascular disease, Type 2 diabetes, and early death, ongoing surveillance of metabolic markers should be discussed with patients and both physical and laboratory markers monitored regularly. These include personal and family history, both at baseline and repeated annually, so as to include new findings in other family members. Patients should be weighed and body mass index calculated at the time of medication initiation, then at four, eight, and 12 weeks into the regimen, and then quarterly. Waist circumference should be measured at baseline, then annually. Blood pressure, fasting glucose and fasting lipid profile should be measured at baseline, at 12 weeks and yearly (Lumby, 2007; Marder, *et al.*, 2004).

Table 8.1 Metabolic Monitoring

	Baseline	4 weeks	8 weeks	12 weeks	Quarterly	Annually
Personal/family history	X					X
Weight/BMI	X	X	X	X	X	
Waist	X	X	X	X	X	X
Blood pressure	X			X		X
Fasting glucose	X			X		X
Fasting lipids	X			X		X

Patients and their families or caregivers can be encouraged to monitor weight on a monthly basis at home. If taking a waist measurement is not possible at home, the patient can monitor his or her comfort level around the waist when wearing trousers or a skirt, and note if a larger size is needed when buying new clothing. Patients can learn the symptoms of hyperglycemia and can be encouraged to report visual blurring, increased urination, increased thirst, and numbness or tingling in the fingers or toes.

Other Side Effects of Neuroleptic Medications

Some antipsychotic medications, especially when given in conjunction with antidepressants, can result in a prolongation of the QTc interval and *torsade de pointes,* a ventricular arrhythmia. Additional risk factors for this problem include known cardiovascular disease, history of syncope, family history of sudden death before the age of 40, or congenital long QT syndrome (Marder, *et al.*, 2004). Ziprasidone was found to be the atypical antipsychotic agent most commonly associated with prolongation of the QTc interval (FDA, 2000). Recommendations for monitoring for arrhythmias include assessing risk and doing a baseline EKG, and repeating it at 12 weeks and then annually (Lumby, 2007).

Hyperprolactinemia is associated with all first generation antipsychotic medications, as well as risperidone. This may result in menstrual irregularities including amenorrhea, and galactorrhea in women, and in gynecomastia and sexual dysfunction in men. Suppression of estrogens or testosterone may result in osteopenia (Lumby, 2007). Taking a sexual history and asking about sexual function may provide early identification of problems and may help to prevent symptom relapse if medications are discontinued because of sexual side effects. There may also be a need to initiate bone density studies at a younger age.

Clozapine has been associated with myocarditis. Signs of myocarditis include unexplained fatigue, tachypnea or dyspnea, or palpitations. Patients should be educated to report these symptoms promptly to their healthcare provider. If there is evidence of myocarditis found on evaluation of EKG, white blood cell count, or serum troponin level, patients should immediately stop the clozapine and be referred to an internist.

Medication-induced Movement Disorders

Movement disorders may arise secondary to treatment with antipsychotic medications. Neuroleptic medications that block the action of dopamine at dopamine receptor sites impair communication between neurons. This precipitates abnormal movements and lack of movement coordination in different parts of the body.

Early onset movement disorder, occurring within the first week of treatment with neuroleptics, is known as neuroleptic-induced acute dystonia. It is characterized by abnormal contractions of muscle groups, resulting in spasm or twisting of the head, neck, jaw, lips, tongue, and eye muscles, and abnormal movement and posturing of the limbs and trunk. It occurs most commonly in young males, and is associated with the typical, conventional antipsychotic medications. Incidence is about 15–20% with typical neuroleptics, and drops to less than 5% with the newer atypical antipsychotics.

Intermediate-onset types of movement disorders usually develop within the first three months of treatment, and are known as neuroleptic-induced Parkinsonism and akathisia. Signs associated with Parkinsonism include difficultly in initiating movements and, once begun, the movements are very slow. Other characteristics include tremor and muscle rigidity. Akathisia is associated with uncontrollable restlessness and a sense of inner tension that may find expression in compulsive rocking, foot tapping or pacing. Older patients are more likely to experience neuroleptic-induced Parkinsonism, with about 30% being affected. Acute akathisia is not age-related and occurs in about 20% of patients being treated with neuroleptics.

Late-onset type of movement disorder is known as tardive dyskinesia, and may appear months to years after starting the neuroleptic medication. It is manifested as grotesque, repetitive, and involuntary movements, usually seen in the mouth and face. The incidence is related to total lifetime treatment with antipsychotics, with a cumulative incidence of about 5% per year. The probability of developing tardive dyskinisia is therefore about *50% per ten years of cumulative neuroleptic treatment.*

Medication-induced postural tremor is characterized by a regular, rhythmic oscillation of hands, finger, head, mouth, or tongue, most easily observed when the affected part is in a sustained position.

Finally, severe muscle rigidity accompanied by fever (ranging from 100F–106F), tremor, changes in level of consciousness (from confusion to coma), acute tachycardia and hypertension are features of neuroleptic malignant syndrome (NMS). It usually develops within four weeks after starting neuroleptic medications, and *two-thirds of cases develop within the first week.* Incidence of NMS is about 0.5%, but it is *fatal in 20–30% of cases.*

Current monitoring recommendations for neuroleptic-related movement disorders include doing a patient movement examination using the Abnormal Involuntary Movement Scale (AIMS) *before any medications are initiated*. There should be weekly monitoring until the medication dose has been stabilized for at least two weeks, and for the two weeks following any significant dose increase. Those patients receiving typical antipsychotics should be *examined for tardive diskinesia every six months, and annually for those receiving an atypical medication* (Marder, Essock, Miller, Buchanan, *et al.*, 2004). The examination and scoring procedures are detailed in Appendices 1 and 2 (Munetz, 1988).

Symptom Monitoring and Medication Adherence Promotion

Patients should be asked about the presence of symptoms of schizophrenia at each visit. Causes of non-response to medications include non-adherence, substance abuse, medication side effects, psycho-social stressors, and uncorrected medical problems such as thyroid disease, anemia, and diabetes (Argo, 2008).

Questions to ask about the presence of positive symptoms cover the areas of suspiciousness, unusual thought content, and hallucinations, as well as observation of speech disorganization. This must be evaluated in relation to unpleasant or dangerous side effects of medications—keeping in mind that, for some patients, the original symptoms may outweigh medication side effects for their tolerance level. Sample questions may include:

- "Do you feel uncomfortable in public because others are watching you or giving you a hard time? Do you feel as though others are gossiping about you?"

- "Are you receiving special messages or seeing references to yourself through the radio, internet, or television?"
- "Do you feel as though you are under the control of another person?"
- "Do you ever hear your name being called or hear voices when others are not around?"

Negative symptoms may be observed as an unusually long delay before a question is answered (alogia), or an expressionless face or verbal expression which is much less than the emotional content of the conversation would indicate (flattening or blunting of affect). There may be diminished attention to grooming and personal hygiene (amotivation). Questions to ask may include:

- "Do you have any desire to socialize with others? If not, what seems to be holding you back? How have you spent your time in the last week?"
- "How often did you bathe and change your clothing in the last week?" (Argo, *et al.* 2008)

Observe the patient's speech for confusion, sudden shifts in topic, inclusion of irrelevant detail and difficulty getting to the point, and use of words whose meaning is known only to the patient. If the PCP has a solid, caring, and trusting relationship with the patient, honest answers to these questions are very likely.

Adherence to Treatment

Treatment adherence encompasses a variety of areas: taking medications, attending follow-up appointments, attending scheduled appointments with other providers, exhibiting behaviors that respect the structure of the community, and participating in recommended treatment modalities such as cognitive behavior therapy and adherence to Assertive Community Treatment (Compton, 2006). Here, adherence focuses on active collaboration in the treatment process in two areas: clinical follow-up and medications.

Between 30% and 60% of patients do not attend their first outpatient appointment after hospitalization. Risk factors for non-adherence to follow-up include younger age, male gender, Hispanic culture, concomitant substance abuse, living alone, poorly controlled symptoms, and having a complex medication regimen. Compounding factors include poor accessibility of treatment services; long intervals between appointments, especially post-hospitalization, and family factors such as lack of knowledge about schizophrenia or its treatment, and attitudes that do not validate the illness or support treatment (Compton, 2006). Adherence to treatment is promoted by attention to these important factors:

- Since a longer interval from hospital discharge to first appointment is a predictor of follow-up non-adherence, schedule the first outpatient appointment as soon as possible after release.
- Involve the patient and family in the follow-up plan.
- Negotiate for a mutually convenient time and date before discharge to promote col-laboration in the outpatient care plan.

The most important predictor for medication non-adherence is impaired insight into the seriousness of the diagnosis and importance of ongoing control of symptoms (Compton, 2006). Other significant risk factors include concomitant substance abuse, higher levels of positive symptoms, including suspiciousness and hostility and environmental factors such as low level of family support, housing instability and limited access to transportation (Kozuki & Schepp, 2005). Patients and family members should therefore be engaged in a discussion of these risk factors in the context of a trusting patient/provider relationship.

Questioning about symptoms provides an opportunity to assess adherence and to either applaud the person's efforts in taking the regimen or to work collaboratively with patients to improve adherence strategies. At each visit, patients should be asked how many doses of medications they believe they have missed in the preceding two weeks, and what interfered with taking their medications. For example: "How is it going with your medications?" Answer: "I missed a few times." PCP: "Can you tell me what was happening when you missed? Did you just forget, or was it maybe because of the side effects?"

By phrasing the question as a possible expectation of missed doses, the provider gives permission for disclosure of less than perfect adherence and removes shame and humiliation from the admission. Questions about the reasons for poor medication adherence may reveal that the patient is suffering from unpleasant side effects, has a cognitive impairment that interferes with the organization required to take medications, such as that imposed by lack of insight, delusional thinking or substance use, or has other reasons for not taking medications. The PCP could ask questions such as: "What happens when you go to take your medicine? In the past your voices have told you that it is poison; are you still getting that message from them? For the times that you succeed in taking your medication, how do you work around what the voices are telling you?"

CASE EXAMPLE: ADHERENCE STRATEGIES

Bob's symptoms were well controlled on the regimen he had been taking for several years. He lives by himself and works in an established and secure community-based program. During a follow-up visit he described listening to the voice of God on the radio all night. Further questioning revealed that Bob had begun to taper off his antipsychotic medications with the intent of stopping them entirely. He had disclosed to a young woman in whom he was romantically interested that he was taking antipsychotic medications and she had broken off the budding relationship. His experience led to fears of never being able to have another relationship. After a discussion of the risks of being off medications versus the perceived benefit of being off them, Bob agreed to begin a medication titration to a level that controlled his symptoms, and to contact his prescribing mental health provider.

Table 8.2 presents a model for patient and provider discussion of the risks and benefits of medication.

The primary care provider asked questions based on CMHA (item #8) regarding cognitive functioning: "Bob, in the past you've been troubled by hearing voices. You look a little distressed now, like you did before? Has this become an issue for you again?" An important consideration in this example is that Bob had a trusting relationship with his PCP and felt respected and welcomed into the provider–patient relationship.

Adherence can be aided by two general approaches: educating the patient and family about the symptoms and chronicity of schizophrenia, and adjusting medications so as to minimize

Table 8.2 Risks and Benefits of Medication

	Off medication	*On medication*
Risk	Hurt self related to command hallucinations Lose housing and job	"Scare off" girlfriends Feel like a "normal" guy
Benefit	No one will guess I'm sick	Keep job and housing Look for another girlfriend

side effects (Glick, *et al.*, 2001). Active collaboration among the PCP, mental health provider, and community service organizations supports patient and family to be full partners in the plan of care. Motivational interviewing explores the value that patients place on health promoting activities, the readiness to make necessary changes and the devising of a personal plan to achieve desired goals (Rollnick, Mason, & Butler, (2005). This can be a useful technique in helping patients to take their medications and has been shown to be effective in promoting adherence (Mueser, Bond, & Drake, 2002). Other important considerations to promote adherence to treatment include:

- removing impediments to accessibility such as transportation;
- assisting with housing stability and promoting vocational activities;
- instituting case management services that encourage participation in the process of treatment;
- supporting self-efficacy in the community through jobs, etc.

Together, these strategies enable adherence to both medications and partnership in other treatment modalities.

Family/Caregiver Issues

As patients with schizophrenia began to be released during the wave of de-institutionalization, family members played an increasingly important role as caregivers. It is estimated that between 30% and 60% of those with a serious mental illness live at home (Mueser, Bond, & Drake, 2002). Families who provide ongoing care for their loved one with schizophrenia face a high degree of stress that, unchecked, will result in personal health issues and caregiver burnout (Mittelman, 2005). The initial responses, which may include fear and embarrassment, may progress to a sense of overwhelming burden of care as the family struggles with the chronicity of the illness and uncertainty about what the future may hold (Brady & McCain, 2005).

With the increase in personal stress and perceived burden of care, caregivers may find themselves less able to support the person with schizophrenia and to enable the plan of care. Lack of personal support will likely result in the patient's inability to adhere to medications and treatment follow-up; this results in increased use of high-cost psychiatric services, in inpatient or emergency settings. It is essential, therefore to provide support for the caregivers of persons with schizophrenia for both fiscal and humane reasons.

CASE EXAMPLE: LIZ AND ERIC

Liz approached her PCP about sleeping medication and "something for stress." She was pale and tired looking, and seemed at the end of her rope. Her husband, Eric, had recently been discharged from an inpatient psychiatric unit when his symptoms of schizophrenia had begun to reassert themselves. He had stopped taking his medications following the suicide of his brother. While hospitalized, he had taken medications, but had apparently discontinued them shortly after discharge at which time he had also resumed alcohol use. Liz described a recent night in which Eric had returned home drunk and threatened to harm her. He accused Liz of plotting against him and had heard "evidence" of her treachery on the television. Liz was able to break free and locked herself and their son in the bedroom while he smashed everything breakable in the kitchen before passing out. Liz had no phone in the bedroom but called the police the next day to report the incident; Eric had since fled the home and was staying with a relative. Liz blamed herself for not making sure that Eric took his medication; she also felt that she could never trust Eric again and made plans for obtaining a restraining order to prevent him from re-entering the home.

The PCP's role in this situation was to evaluate, first, the safety of Liz and her son. Questions from CMHA (items #13 and #19) included: Have there been other times when you were frightened or intimidated by Eric? Often emotional abuse is accompanied by physical or sexual abuse; has this ever happened to you? Do you feel safe at home at this time? Do you have a plan for what to do in the event that Eric returns before this situation is straightened out? The PCP's other priority was to assist Liz to contact Eric's mental health provider to apprise him of the relapse of both symptoms and alcohol use.

Education: Medications, Symptoms, Relapse Recognition, Interventions

Effective family intervention programs provide the family and patient with information about psychiatric illness, including causes, symptoms, and treatment plan. The focus should be on a collaborative approach to treatment of the symptoms, including adherence to medications and recognition of symptoms to permit early intervention (Mueser, Bond, & Drake, 2002; Truman, 2005). This approach permits an active role in decision-making, and enables individuals to make choices and have control over life decisions.

Involvement of the family at the earliest possible stage, preferably during the initial hospitalization, provides opportunities for the family to process the shock and grief of having a family member diagnosed with this devastating illness. Issues such as stigma and misinformation can be addressed and ongoing education about the plan of care provided. Current family dynamics, such as ways of dealing with disagreements, can be evaluated and support provided to incorporate ways of coping that will nurture the family unit in the face of the new challenges it will face, once the person with schizophrenia is released into the family's care.

Education about symptoms is vital to ensure that relapse is identified early so as to initiate the plan for continued treatment. Positive symptoms are most easily observable once the family knows what to look for. Living with a family member with negative symptoms, however, continues to be the most distressing aspect of care for caregivers (Brady & McCain, 2005). The family requires ongoing education and support to cope with under-responsiveness and lack of purposeful activity, which may be perceived as laziness or designed to annoy or provoke others.

Stress management is an important consideration for all family members. While education assists in determining a plan of care, the ongoing sense of responsibility and a sense of existential aloneness contribute greatly to the emotional burden carried. The burdens can be objective, such as financial setbacks if vocational obligations cannot be fulfilled, or as curtailment of normal social activities. Subjectively it is expressed as the sense of carrying a burden, and experienced as guilt, shame, denial, helplessness, and worry about the future (Tsang, Pearson, & Yuen, 2002). From the beginning, families can be assisted to understand that they are not responsible for the diagnosis of schizophrenia. Any genetic links within the family should be acknowledged, but it is important to stress that nothing that was said or unsaid, done or not done "caused" the cascade of neuro-biological events that culminated in the development of symptoms. The source of stress may not necessarily be altered, but the sense of being able to manage the additional responsibilities and life changes may be enhanced through compassionate support.

Families can benefit from being connected with consumer agencies such as the National Alliance on Mental Illness (NAMI), to broaden their understanding of the illness and to learn to advocate for both their family member and themselves to gain better support and access to services. Referral to local support groups may assist in alleviating some of the existential aloneness that many experience when caring for a loved one with a chronic mental illness.

Collaborative Practice: Patient/Family and Health/Mental Health Provider

The PCP is uniquely positioned to provide integrated care for the whole individual, including ongoing monitoring for recurrence of symptoms of schizophrenia, metabolic and cardiovascular status, and working collaboratively with client and family to promote health maintenance practices.

CASE EXAMPLE: LIZ AND ERIC (CONTINUED)

Liz was successful in obtaining a restraining order and was able to persuade Eric's relative to contact the police who brought Eric back to be re-hospitalized; during this hospitalization, he agreed to begin receiving an injectable form of his antipsychotic. On release, Eric went to live with his father but continues to binge on alcohol on occasion. He has not had another psychotic break. When he is sober, he is able to have supervised visits with his and Liz's son. Liz continues to resist pressure from Eric's family to have him move back in with her, and she has seen their interest and concern for her dwindle. She is now very worried that her son will someday be diagnosed with schizophrenia.

   Liz's PCP played a significant role in validating her concerns, and in assisting her to get information to Eric's mental health provider who was in the best position to help Eric. Ongoing assessment for Liz, who is now a single parent, will include assessing her level of support from her family. Using the CMHA questions on Immediate Family (item #4) the PCP may ask who Liz can turn to, or who would be most likely to come in an emergency to get an understanding of her resources and ability to mobilize them. It will be important to work with Liz and to be vigilant about evaluating her son for evidence of the subtle changes that might signify early symptoms of schizophrenia.

Appendix 1

AIMS Examination Procedure (Munetz & Benjamin, 1988)

Definitions
Athetoid: slow, irregular, complex, serpentine movements
Choreic: rapid, objectively purposeless, irregular, and spontaneous movements
Tremor: repetitive, regular, rhythmic movements

Observe the patient unobtrusively at rest, while he or she is waiting to be seen.
   The chair in which the patient sits for this examination should be a firm one, without armrests.

1. Ask the patient whether there is anything in his or her mouth and if so, ask for it to be removed.
2. Ask about the current condition of the patient's teeth and if there is any mouth discomfort. If the patient wears dentures, ask if they are bothersome or uncomfortable.
3. Ask if the patient notices any movements in his or her mouth, face, hands, or feet. If so, ask the patient to describe them and the extent to which they are currently bothersome.
4. Have the patient sit in the chair with hands on knees, legs slightly apart, and feet flat on the floor. Look at the entire body for movements while the patient is in this position.
5. Ask the patient to sit with hands hanging unsupported, e.g. hanging over his or her knees or between the legs. Observe the hands and other body areas.

6. Ask the patient to open his or her mouth. Observe the tongue at rest within the mouth, repeating the action and observation twice.
7. Ask the patient to protrude his or her tongue. Observe any abnormalities of tongue movements, repeating the action and observation twice.
8. Ask the patient to tap his or her thumb with each finger as rapidly as possible for 10 to 15 seconds, starting with the dominant hand. Observe facial and leg movements.
9. Flex and extend the patient's right and left arms, one at a time.
10. Ask the patient to stand up. Observe the patient in profile, in all body areas, hips included.
11. Ask the patient to extend both arms out in front, palms down. Observe the trunk, legs, and mouth.
12. Have the patient walk a few paces, turn, and walk back to the chair. Observe hands and gait, repeating the action and observation twice.

Appendix 2

Scoring Procedure

0 = none, minimal   1 = minimal   2 = mild   3 = moderate   4 = severe

Table 8.3 Appendix 2

Area Facial and Oral Movements	**Muscles of facial expression** Movements of forehead, eyebrows, periorbital area, cheeks. Include frowning, blinking, grimacing of upper face.	Score
	Lips and perioral area Puckering, pouting, smacking.	
	Jaw Biting, clenching, chewing, mouth opening, lateral movement.	
	Tongue Increase in movement in and out of mouth, **not** inability to sustain movement.	
Extremity Movements	**Upper (arms, wrists, hands, fingers)** Include movements that are choreic or athetoid. Do **not** include tremor.	
	Lower (legs, knees, ankles, toes) Lateral knee movement, foot tapping, heel dropping, foot squirming, inversion and eversion of foot.	
Trunk Movements	**Neck, shoulders, hips** Rocking, twisting, squirming, pelvic gyrations, diaphragmatic movements.	
Global Judgments 0 = no awareness 1 = aware, no distress 2 = aware, mild distress 3 = aware, moderate distress 4 = aware, severe distress	**Severity of abnormal movements** Based on highest single score 0-4. Incapacitation due to abnormal movements. Patient's awareness of abnormal movements. Total	

References

Allison, D., Fontaine, K., Hero, M., Mentore, J., Cappeleri, J., & Chandler, L. (1999). The distribution of body mass index among individuals with and without schizophrenia. *Journal of Clinical psychiatry*, 60, 215–220.

American Psychiatric Association (1994). *Diagnostic and statistical manual of mental disorders.* (4th ed.). Washington, DC: American Psychiatric Association.

Andreasen N., & Olsen, S. (1982). Negative vs. positive schizophrenia. *Archives of General Psychiatry*, 39(7), 789–94.

Anderson, R., Oades, I., & Caputi, P. (2003). The experience of recovery from schizophrenia: Towards an empirically validated stage model. *Australia and New Zealand Journal of Psychiatry*, 37, 586–594.

Argo, T., Crismon, M., Miller, A., Moore, T., Bendele, S., & Suehs, B. (2008). Schizophrenia treatment algorithm. In *Texas medication algorithm project procedure manual.* Texas Department of State Health.

Arseneault, L., Cannon, M., Poulton, R., Murray, Capsi, A., & Miffitt, T. (2002). Cannabis use in adolescence and risk for adult psychosis: longitudinal prospective study. *British Medical Journal*, 325, 1212–1213.

Bassett, A., O'Neill, S., & Murphy, J. (2001). Expression of schizophrenia symptoms in 22q deletion syndrome. *American Journal of Human Genetics*, 69, 287.

Batki, S., Leontieva, L., Dimmock, J., & Ploutz-Snyder, R. (2008). Negative symptoms are associated with less alcohol use, craving and "high" in alcohol dependent patients with schizophrenia. Schizophrenia bulletin. August 12. (Epub ahead of print) (accessed on August 28, 2008).

Brady, N., & McCain, G. (2005). Living with schizophrenia: a family perspective. *Journal of Issues in Nursing*, (10)1, http://www.medscape.com/viewarticle/499269 (accessed on August 15, 2008).

Brown, S., Inskip, H., & Barraclough, B. (2000) Causes of excess mortality of schizophrenia. *British Journal of Psychiatry*. 177, 217–221.

Capasso, R., Lineberry, T., Bostwick, M., Decker, P., & St. Sauver, J. (2007). Mortality in schizophrenia and schizoaffective disorder: An Olmsted County, Minnesota cohort: 1950–2005. *Schizophrenia Research*, 98, 287–294.

Charkaborty, A., & McKenzie, K. (2002). Does racial discrimination cause mental illness? *British Journal of Psychiatry*, 180, 475–477.

Combs, D., & Advocat, C. (2000). Antipsychotic medication and smoking prevalence in acutely hospitalized patients with chronic schizophrenia. *Schizophrenia Research*, 24, 120–137.

Compton, M. (2006). Cigarette smoking in individuals with schizophrenia. *Medscape Psychiatry and Mental Health*, (25)10, http://www.medscape.com/viewarticle/516304_print (accessed on August 16, 2008).

Copersino, M., & Serper, M. (1998). Comorbidity of schizophrenia and cocaine abuse: Phenomenology and treatment. *Medscape Psychiatry and Mental Health eJournal*, 3(2), http://www.medscape.com/viewarticle/430756_print (accessed September 3, 2008).

Dickerson, F., Pater, A., & Origoni, A. (2002). Health behaviors and health status of older women with schizophrenia. *Psychiatric Services*, 53(7), 882–884.

Drake, R., Mercer-McFadden, C., & Mueser, K. (1998). Review of integrated mental health and substance abuse treatment for patients with dual disorders. *Schizophrenia Bulletin*, 24, 589–608.

Dubovsky, S. L., & Dubovsky, A. N. (2007). *Psychotropic drug prescriber's guide: Ethical mental health treatment in the age of Big Pharma.* New York: W.W. Norton.

Evans, F. B. (1996). *Harry Stack Sullivan: Interpersonal theory and psychotherapy.* London: Routledge.

Food and Drug Administration (FDA) (2008) FDA issues public health advisory on Chantix. http://www.fda.gov/bbs/topics/NEWS/2008?NEW1788.html (accessed on August 27, 2008).

Food and Drug Administration (FDA) (2000). *Briefing document for Zeldox Capsules (ziprasidone).* New York, Pfizer, Inc. July 18.

Ghaemi, N., Schneider, L., Barbee, J., Marder, S., McIntyre, R., Buckley, P., McEvoy, J., Cutler, A., & Masand, P. (2005). Expert consensus roundtable: A focus on the new atypical antipsychotics. psychCME (9): RP-009-091505-08.

Glick, I., Suppes, T., DeBattista, C., Hu, R., & Marder, S. (2001). Psychopharmacolgic treatment strategies for depression, bipolar disorder and schizophrenia. *Annals of Internal Medicine*, (134)1, 47–60.

Hennekens, C., Hennekens, A., & Hollar, D. (2005). Schizophrenia and increased risks of cardiovascular disease. *American Heart Journal*, 150(6), 1115–1121.

Himmelhoch, S., Lehman, L., Kreyenbuhl, J., Daumitt, G., Brown, C., & Dixon, L. (2004). Prevalence of chronic obstructive pulmonary disease among those with serious mental illness. *American Journal of Psychiatry*, 161, 2317–2319.

Hoff, L. A. (2008). Personal communication.

Hoff, L. A. (1993). Review essay: Health policy and the plight of the mentally ill. *Psychiatry*, 56(4), 400–419.

Johnson, A. B. (1990). *Out of bedlam: The truth about deinstitutionalization*. New York: Basic Books.

Kane, J., Leucht, S., Carpenter, C., & Docherty, J. (2003). The expert consensus guideline series: optimizing pharmacologic treatment of psychotic disorders. *Journal of Clinical Psychiatry*, (64)12, 1–100.

Korn, M. (2001). Historical roots of schizophrenia. *Medscape Portals, Inc.* June 21. www.medscape.com (accessed on August 16, 2008).

Kozuki, Y., & Schepp, K. (2005). Adherence and nonadherence to antipsychotic medications. *Issues in Mental Health Nursing*, 26, 379–396.

Lester, H., Tritter, J., & England, E. (2003). Satisfaction with primary care: The perspective of people with schizophrenia. *Family Practice*, (20)5, 508–513.

Lumby, B. (2007). Guide schizophrenia patients to better physical health. *The Nurse Practitioner*, 32(7), 30–37.

Lynch, D., Laws, K., & McKenna P. J. (2010). Cognitive behavioural therapy for major psychiatric disorder; does it really work? A meta-analytical review of well-controlled trials. *Psychological Medicine*, 40, 9–24.

Lyon, E. (1999). A review of the effects of nicotine on schizophrenia and antipsychotic medications. *Psychiatric Service*, 50, 1346–1350.

Maguire, G., & Yu, B. (2001). Solutions for recovery and wellness. Medscape portals, Inc. http://www.medscape.com/viewarticle/418618 (accessed on September 3, 2008).

Malmberg L., & Fenton, M. (2001). Individual psychodynamic psychotherapy and psychoanalysis for schizophrenia and severe mental illness. *Cochrane Database of Systematic Reviews*. Issue 2. Article No.: CD001360. DOI: 10.1002/14651858.CD001360.

Malaspina, D. (2006). The influence of paternal age on schizophrenia: An expert interview with Dolores Malaspina MD, MPH. *Medscape Psychiatry and Mental Health*, (11) 1, posted January 11, 2006, Article 520009.

Marder, S., Essock, S., Miller, A., Buchanan, R., Casey, D., Davis, J., Kane, J., Lieberman, J., Schooler, N., Covell, N., Stroup, S., Weissman, E., Wirshing, D., Hall, C., Pogach, L., Pi-Sunyer, X., Bigger, J., Friedman, A., Kleinberg, D., Yevich, S., Davis, B., & Shon, S. (2004). Physical health monitoring of patients with schizophrenia. *American Journal of Psychiatry*, 161, 1334–1349.

Mauri, M., Volonteri, L., De Gasperi, I., Colasanti, A., Brambilla, M., & Cerruti, L. (2006). Substance abuse in first-episode schizophrenia patients: A restrospective study. *Clinical Practice and Epidemiology in Mental Health*. 2: 4 doi: 10.1186/1745-0179-2-4 (accessed on August 28, 2008).

Melle, I., Larsen, T. K., Haahr, U., Friis, S., Johannesen, J. O., Opjordsmoen, S., Rund, B. R., Simonsen, E., Vaglum, P., & McGlashan, T. (2008) Prevention of negative symptom psychopathologies in first-episode schizophrenia: Two-year effects of reducing the duration of untreated psychosis. *Archives of General Psychiatry*. June, 65, 634–640.

Mittelman, M. (2005). Taking care of the caregivers. *Current Opinions in Psychiatry*. (18)6, 633–639.

Mueser, K., Bond, G., & Drake, R. (1998). Models of community care for severe mental illness: A review of research on case management. *Schizophrenia Bulletin*, 24, 37–74.

Mueser, K., Bond, G., & Drake, R. (2002). Community-based treatment of schizophrenia and other severe mental disorders: Treatment outcomes. *Medscape General Medicine*, (3)1, http://www.medscape.com/viewarticle/430529 (accessed on August 15, 2008).

Munetz, M. R., & Benjamin, S. (1988) How to examine patients using the Abnormal Involuntary Movement Scale. *Hospital and Community Psychiatry*, 39(11), 1172–1177.

National Institute of Mental Health (NIMH) (2007). *National Institutes of Health: Schizophrenia.* January, 2007. www.nimh.nih.gov/health/publications/schizophrenia/schiophreniabooklet (accessed on 16 August 2008).

Owen, R., Fischer, E., Booth, B., & Cuffel, B. (1996). Medication noncompliance and substance abuse among patients with schizophrenia. *Psychiatric Services*, (47)8, 853–857.

Peplau, H. (1993). *Interpersonal relations in nursing.* New York: Springer.

Picchioni, M., & Murray, R. (2007). Schizophrenia. *British Medical Journal*, 335, 91–95.

Powell, A., Heckers, S., & Bierer, M. (1998). Approach to the patient with hallucinations and delusions. In T. stern, J. Herman, & P. Slavin (Eds.) *The MGH Guide to Psychiatry in Primary Care* (pp. 231–238). New York: Mcgraw-Hill.

Rollnick, S., Mason, P., & Butler, C. (2005). Health behavior change: A guide for practitioners. London: Churchill Livingstone.

Ryan, M., & Thakore, J. (2002). Physical consequences of schizophrenia and its treatment: The metabolic syndrome. *Life Sciences*, 71, 230–257.

Saha, S., Chant, D., & McGrath, J. (2007). A systematic review of mortality in schizophrenia: Is the differential mortality gap worsening over time? *Archives of General psychiatry*, 64(10), 1123–1131.

Stahl, Stephen. (2005). *Essential psychopharmacology: The prescriber's guide.* New York: Cambridge University Press.

Swartz, M., Perkins, D., Stroup, T., Davis, S., Capuano, G., Rosenheck, R., Reimherr, R., McGee, M., & Keefe, R. (2007). Effects of antipsychotic medications on psychosocial functioning in patient with chronic schizophrenia: findings from the NIMH CATIE study. *American Journal of Psychiatry*, (164) 3, 428–436.

Torrey, E. F. (2001). *Surviving schizophrenia.* (4th Ed.) (pp. xxi) New York: HarperCollins.

Tsang, H., Pearson, V., & Yuen, C. (2002). Family needs and burdens of mentally ill offenders. *International Journal of Rehabilitation Research*, 25, 25–32.

Truman, C. (2005). The autonomy of professionals and the involvement of patients and families. *Current Opinions in Psychiatry*, (18)5, 572–575.

Ustun, T. B. (1999). The global burden of mental disorders. *American Journal of Public Health*, 88(1), 12–14.

Veling, W., Hoek, H., Wiersma, D., & Mackenback, J. (2009). Ethnic identity and risk of schizophrenia in ethnic minorities: a case control study. *Schizophrenia Bulletin doi: 10.1093/schbul/sbp032.*

Wahlbeck, K., Cheine, M., & Essali, A. (1999). Clozapine vs. typical neuroleptic medications for schizophrenia. *Cochrane Database of Systematic Review*, 4, CD000059, (accessed on August 21, 2008).

Weiden, P. (2005). Moving beyond positive symptoms: the importance of addressing cognitive and affective symptoms in the treatment of schizophrenia. *Medscape Psychiatry and Mental Health.* (10)2, http://www.mesdcape.com/viewarticle/511186_print (accessed on September 3, 2008).

9 Substance Abuse, Addiction, and Mental Health

People have been using substances over millennia to alter their state of being. Substance abuse, however, is a major health and social problem in the United States and many other societies. Addiction is a chronic progressive illness with a predictable pattern and outcomes. People with addictive disorders exchange short-term pleasure or relief at the expense of long-term effects. There are significant health, social, and interpersonal risks associated with addictive disorders, while self-destructive behaviors are a major component of the disorder. As an addictive disorder progresses, the patients' behavior narrows around the use and procurement of the substance. The disease is maintained by denial, projection, and rationalization of the behaviors.

The care of patients with addictive disorders is a challenge for most primary care providers. Many providers feel ill equipped to deal with the complex chronic problems that people with addictive disorders present. Educational programs for healthcare professionals continue to provide only brief lectures regarding alcohol and drug use and tend to focus on the identification of drug use and withdrawal syndromes related to the specific drugs of abuse. Discussion of how to build a therapeutic relationship and provide motivation for engagement in treatment is usually left to the addiction professional. However, most people in the early stages of alcohol or drug addiction have no contact with addiction professionals. The role of primary care providers is therefore essential in the early intervention and/or prevention of addictive disorders.

This chapter provides information on the prevalence of addictive disorders, definitions related to drug use and abuse, the drugs of abuse and co-morbid problems of addictive disorders, and associated mental health problems. Assessment issues, including screening tools, methods and philosophies of treating addictive disorders, as well as pharmacological treatment, are included. Finally, primary care treatment approaches are discussed.

Prevalence

Studies are conducted each year in the United States to monitor the prevalence of addictive disorders in the country. The leading studies are the National Survey on Drug Use and Health (NSDUH) sponsored by the Substance Abuse and Mental Health Services Administration (SAMHSA) and Monitoring the Future (MTF) conducted by the University of Michigan's Institute for Social Research. Additionally, the Center for Disease Control and Prevention conducts a biannual survey, National Youth Risk Behavior Survey, and the Drug Abuse Warning Network provides annual information on drug-related emergency department visits and drug-related deaths.

The NSDUH estimated that in 2007 19.9 million Americans aged 12 or older were current illicit drug users (had used illicit drugs in the month prior to the survey). This number is approximately 8.0 % of the U.S. population over age 12. It is important to note that the survey excludes people in institutions such as hospitals, shelters, and prisons where many people with addictive disorders are housed. Illicit drugs included in the survey were marijuana/hashish, cocaine, heroin, hallucinogens, inhalants, or prescription-type psychotherapeutics used non-medically. Marijuana was the most commonly used illicit drug, with 14.4 million users in the month before the survey (NSDUH, 2007). Prevalence rates in other countries are available at www.who.org.

Alcohol, a legal drug, is also included in the NSDUH survey. Slightly more than half of the participants reported being current drinkers in 2007 (51.0 %), which translates to 126.8 million Americans; 23.3 % reported engaging in binge drinking (defined as having five or more drinks on the same occasion on at least one day in the month prior to the survey). Heavy drinking (binge drinking on at least five days in the past month) was reported by 6.9 % of the population age 12 and over in 2007 (NSDUH, 2007).

Treatment for illicit drugs and alcohol is also included in the survey. 22.3 million people, or 9.0 % of the population aged 12 and over, were classified with substance dependence or abuse based on criteria in the *Diagnostic and statistical manual of mental disorders* (DSM-IV-TR) (APA, 2000); 15.5 million of these people abused or were dependent on alcohol alone, 3.7 million on illicit drugs alone, and 3.2 million on both alcohol and drugs. Of these people who met the criteria for alcohol/substance dependence or abuse, 3.9 million received treatment in the year prior to the survey and over half of that number (2.2 million) received treatment in a self-help group. 21.1 million people in the U.S. were estimated to need treatment for drug or alcohol problems but did not receive such treatment (NSDUH, 2007).

One of the major concerns over the past decade has been the use/misuse of prescription pain relievers. In 2007, 2.1 % of people age 12 and over (5.2 million people) reported using prescription pain relievers for nonmedical reasons in the month prior to the survey. This number has been fairly stable since 2002 and the rate for females has been stable, but there was an increase in the rate for males between 2002 and 2007 (NSDUH, 2007).

Co-morbid Drug Abuse and Mental Illness

The National Institute on Drug Abuse (NIDA) estimates that six out of ten people with a substance abuse problem also have mental health problem. Issues such as stress, trauma, including physical and sexual abuse, and early exposure to drugs are some of the common issues that can increase the risk of developing mental illness and/or substance abuse. Patients with mood disorders or anxiety disorders are twice as likely to have a substance abuse problem and vice versa (NIDA, 2010). NSDUH identified 24.3 million adults aged 18 and older with serious psychological distress (SPD) or 10.9 % of adults in the country. Of those with SPD, 22.3 % were dependent on or abused illicit drugs or alcohol (NSDUH, 2007). Patients with both disorders often exhibit more severe symptoms and are in need of specialized treatment programs.

The person who abuses substances is engaging in a chronic form of self-destructive behavior. We can assume that when self-destructive people experienced a crisis at earlier points in their lives, they lacked the social support and coping skills for healthy crisis resolution. People who abuse alcohol and other drugs commonly avoid getting help for their problem until another crisis occurs, often as a result of the addiction itself. For clients suffering from depression, post traumatic stress disorder (PTSD), bipolar disorder, or other psychiatric conditions, substances often serve as a buffer to provide emotional distance from the source of their psychic pain. Abstinence will not resolve the underlying mental health issues; many patients will experience a surge of emotional and cognitive pain once substance use is discontinued. Vulnerability to the re-experience of past trauma and the emergence of psychiatric symptoms impedes the ability of these patients to reduce substance use. An increase in the affective or cognitive symptoms may concomitantly increase the frequency and amount of substances consumed.

Definitions

Substance Abuse   The terms substance abuse, chemical dependency, or addictive disorder are used interchangeably and are defined as "the use of a substance or substances in an uncontrolled, compulsive and potentially harmful manner" (Savage, 1993, p. 265). The DSM-IV-TR criteria for a diagnosis of substance abuse includes a maladaptive pattern of substance use. This pattern leads to clinically significant impairment or distress resulting in a failure to fulfill major role obligations at work, school, or home, and continued use despite consequences such as legal, medical, social, or interpersonal problems (APA, 2000). Often a pattern of taking the drug in larger amounts over time, unsuccessful attempts to stop or quit drug use, and spending more and more time in the procurement of the drug will accompany the other types of impairment seen with substance abuse (APA, 2000).

Substance Dependence   Dependency can be physical and/or psychological. Physical dependency refers to the development of a withdrawal syndrome following abrupt cessation of the drug (Savage, 1993). Often people with a substance dependency will take a related substance to avoid withdrawal symptoms. Physical dependence may be accompanied by *tolerance* to the substance, which is a pharmacological property of opioid and other drugs, and occurs when the effects of the same dose of drugs are diminished or an increased dose is required to sustain the same effects of the drug (APA, 2000).

Addiction   The term addiction is not defined or used by the DSM-IV-TR. Addiction is characterized by the psychological dependence and "preoccupation with obtaining or using a substance, loss of control over the use of the substance and continued use despite adverse consequences" (Savage, 1993, p. 266). Another definition of addiction is provided by the American Society of Pain Management Nurses (ASPMN) as based on definitions by the American Society of Addiction Medicine (ASAM), the American Academy of Pain

Management (AAPM) and the American Pain Society (APA). Addiction is: "A primary, chronic, neurobiologic disease with genetic, psychosocial, and environmental factors influencing its development and manifestations. It is characterized by behaviors that include one or more of the following: impaired control over drug use, compulsive use, continued use despite harm, and craving" (ASPMN, 2003, p.1).

Intoxication   The state of being poisoned; usually intoxication is thought of as occurring with alcohol but it may be caused by any drug.

Cross-tolerance   Cross-tolerance is defined as the development of tolerance to all drugs within a class. The concept of cross-tolerance is utilized when someone needs to be detoxified from drugs such as alcohol or benzodiazepines to prevent a medical crisis. A drug within the same class as the abused drug (usually a medication with a short half-life) is substituted and then a schedule for tapering the dosage is developed.

Pseudo-addiction   A term most often used when dealing with the co-morbid problems of pain and addiction. Pseudo-addiction is an iatrogenic syndrome created by the under-treatment of pain. It is characterized by patient behaviors such as anger and escalating demands for more or different medications and results in suspicion and avoidance by staff. Pseudo-addiction can be distinguished from true addiction in that the behaviors resolve when pain is effectively treated (Weisman & Haddox, 1989).

Drugs of Abuse

Alcohol   In terms of numbers affected and costs to society, alcohol is the number one problem in North America (Allen, 2001). The U.S. Department of Health and Human Services defines a standard drink as 12 oz. of beer, 5 oz. of wine, 8 oz. of malt liquor, and 1.5 oz. of 80 proof spirits as all containing 15 grams of alcohol. Knowledge of the standard size of a drink is important to accurately assess a person's intake of alcohol. Heavy drinking is defined as more than 2 drinks/day for men and more than one drink/day for women. Binge drinking is defined as drinking 5 or more drinks on any occasion for men or 4 or more drinks on any occasion for women (CDC, 2010). From 2001–2005 there were approximately 79,000 deaths annually due to excessive drinking, and excessive alcohol use is the third leading lifestyle-related cause of death in the US each year (CDC, 2010). Since drinking is widely accepted in U.S. society it is important for clinicians to know how to differentiate between social drinking and excessive or problematic drinking and alcoholism.

The multiple effects of alcohol use on the neurological system, liver, gastrointestinal tract, nutrition, cardiovascular system, immune system, and effects on the hormonal system and sleep disturbance are well known to primary care providers, who most often see the long-term effects of alcohol abuse on the body. The rate of automobile accidents associated with alcohol in the U.S is documented yearly. Many studies have linked alcohol and/or drug use to violent acts. Alcohol abuse also significantly contributes to accidents at home and at work. Alcohol is frequently used by cocaine users to prevent or ease the "crash" or depression after cocaine use. Use of alcohol in the form of NyQuil (an over-the-counter cold medicine) is common among cocaine users.

Estimates of the prevalence of hospitalized patients with a problem with alcohol range from 12.5–30 % (Moore, Bone, & Geller, 1989). Management issues of alcohol withdrawal syndrome, hallucinations, withdrawal delirium, and withdrawal seizures are medical issues that require accurate assessment and immediate intervention. Long-term problems such as

Wernicke-Korsakoff psychosis and encephalopathy are most often accompanied by malnutrition and require medical treatment. Alcohol affects memory in up to 50% of those with a chronic alcohol problem, but the impairment may be subtle and may be accompanied by/or underlie the denial of any problem with alcohol.

Cannabis or Marijuana   Cannabis is the most commonly used illicit drug in the United States (Allen, 2001; NIDA, 2010; NSDUH, 2007). The active ingredient is tetrahydrocannabinol (THC). Data about the long-term effects of marijuana use are conflicting; the development of pulmonary problems has been documented with prolonged use. Marijuana is often used with other drugs to either extend or potentiate a high, to prevent a crash, or to decrease the anxiety associated with cocaine or other stimulants. Medical use of marijuana in the form of marinol has been used for appetite stimulation as it relates to chemotherapy and wasting from HIV/AIDS, and for treatment of glaucoma.

Stimulants   This category includes amphetamines (benzedrine), dextroamphetamines (dexedrine), cocaine, methamphetamines (Desoxyn), and methylphenidates (Ritalin). Amphetamines were used medically in the 1950s and 1960s for problems such as depression, fatigue, and weight problems, as well as use as a bronchodilator. They are currently used in the treatment of narcolepsy, attention deficit disorder (ADD), and attention deficit hyperactivity disorder (ADHD) (Armstrong, 2008; NIDA, 2010). Stimulants are also currently used to treat depression in the medically ill, particularly geriatric patients and people with HIV/AIDS (Keltner & Folks, 2001). Impairment in decision-making and psychotic reactions can occur with the use/abuse of stimulants, which can lead to hostile and violent behavior, especially when combined with alcohol.

Cocaine   Cocaine is available in several forms: white powder for intranasal use (snorting), or dissolved and injected intravenously, or smoked, or freebased in the form of "crack" (rocks of cocaine base). Cocaine can also be used orally. Cocaine provides an immediate high or rush, with a short duration, so that repeated and frequent use becomes a major problem. Cocaine can result in improved sexual desire and a euphoric feeling that is followed by a moderate to severe depression or "crash" that reinforces the desire for further use. Cocaine and crack are the most costly illicit drugs to society in terms of crime, morbidity, and mortality (Allen, 2001). A cocaine-induced psychosis may occur with chronic use and resembles the psychosis produced by amphetamine use, but is usually of shorter duration (NIDA, 2010).

Amphetamines   Methamphetamine and crystal meth are addictive stimulants that are taken orally, intra-nasally (by snorting), smoking, or intravenously. Studies have demonstrated that chronic methamphetamine use shows severe structural changes in areas of the brain associated with memory and emotion, motor performance, and verbal learning (NIDA, 2010). A paranoid psychosis can occur with methamphetamine intoxication that may be difficult to distinguish from an acute schizophrenic episode. The psychosis presents with paranoia, visual and auditory hallucinations, and delusions. Transmission of HIV and hepatitis B and C may be the consequences of intravenous methamphetamine use.

Club Drugs   MDMA or ecstasy, GHB, and ketamine are the most commonly used "club drugs." MDMA has hallucinogenic and amphetamine like effects and can produce perceptual distortions, confusion, hypertension, hyperactivity, and hyperthermia that can be fatal. GHB (known as the "date rape" drug) is a depressant used in the treatment of narcolepsy but can produce a coma and be fatal in overdoses. Ketamine has been used as an anesthetic and in overdoses can result in delirium, amnesia, and respiratory depression. Other hallucinogens that are not considered club drugs are lysergic acid diethylamide (LSD) and phencyclidine (PCP). The herb Salvia divinorum has been marketed as an herbal high or an hallucinogenic (NIDA, 2010).

Inhalants   These volatile substances can produce mind-altering effects when inhaled. Many drugs can be inhaled but drugs classified as inhalants are rarely taken any other way. Common products in the home and workplace can be used to get high. Children and adolescents are more likely to use these substances. Volatile solvents such as gasoline, paint thinners, dry-cleaning fluids, lighter fluids, correction fluids, and glue make up one category of inhalants. Aerosols that contain propellants and solvents (as found in spray paints, hair or deodorant sprays, and cleaning products) are another category. Gases found in butane lighters and propane tanks or whipped cream aerosol dispensers are also inhalants. Nitrites are a class of inhalants that are used as sexual enhancers; because of their use as sexual enhancers there is a risk associated with HIV disease and hepatitis.

Inhalants are breathed in through the nose or mouth by sniffing or snorting fumes, spraying directly into the nose or mouth, or by huffing which means placing an inhalant-soaked rag in the mouth. Intoxication is brief, lasting only a few minutes, reinforcing the need to inhale repeatedly. The effects of inhalants are similar to the effects of alcohol, but air is displaced in the lungs resulting in hypoxia and cell damage, especially brain cell damage. Addiction to inhalants can occur but is not common. Sudden sniffing death can occur from use of butane, propane, and other chemicals in aerosols (NIDA, 2010).

Nicotine   This is one of 4,000 chemicals found in the smoke from tobacco in cigarettes, cigars, and pipes, and is the component of tobacco that acts on the brain. It is a highly addictive substance. Nicotine physical withdrawal symptoms peak within one to three days, but can last four to six weeks, while cravings and weight gain can last even longer. Smoking cessation programs improve success rates if the person stays in the program. Relapse rates are high without medical assistance.

Caffeine   Although caffeine is abused or misused by all age groups, caffeine abuse will not be considered substance abuse for the sake of this chapter as it does not result in the same consequences encompassing all spheres of life as the other substances described in this section.

Prescription Drug Abuse

Use of psychotherapeutic drugs for non-medical purposes has been an area of increased use/abuse in the past decade. This increase may be due to direct advertisement to consumers about these drugs, less concern about the danger of such drugs due to the fact that they do have legitimate uses, and a decline in the number of street drugs over the last decade. Prescription drugs that are abused include stimulants, sedative-hypnotics, opioids, anabolic steroids, and laxatives. Laxative abuse is seen primarily with eating disorders and will not be described in this section, as a referral for mental health follow-up therapy is indicated.

Stimulants   Drugs such as Ritalin and Concerta are prescribed for people with ADHD and are also used for treating narcolepsy. These drugs have a calming and focusing effect for those with ADHD but because of their stimulant properties they have become an abusable substance for those without ADHD. Stimulants have been abused for both "performance enhancement" and "to get high." They suppress appetite (resulting in weight loss), increase wakefulness, and increase focus and attention. The euphoric effects of stimulants usually occur when they are crushed and then snorted or injected (NIDA, 2010).

Stimulants can cause increased blood pressure, heart rate, body temperature, and decrease sleep and appetite, which can lead to malnutrition and its consequences. Habitual use of stimulants can lead to hostility and paranoia. They can also lead to serious cardiovascular complications, including stroke.

Sedative-hypnotics   Drugs in this class are commonly prescribed for a variety of medical problems. Included in this category are barbiturates such as Seconal, Nembutal, Amytal, Tuinal, and Phenobarbital, barbiturate-like drugs (Quaaludes), and benzodiazepines (Valium, Librium, Xanax, Klonopin, Halcion, and Ativan).

Barbiturates are used in headache preparations, for sleep, and as anticonvulsants. Benzodiazepines are used to treat anxiety and panic disorders, sleep disorders, have anti-seizure properties, and are used as muscle relaxants. A loss of inhibition, drowsiness, emotional instability, ataxia, decreased aggressiveness, and memory loss can occur. Both barbiturates and benzodiazepines can be lethal if taken in an overdose and can produce physical and psychological dependence that has a severe, life-threatening withdrawal syndrome (Allen, 2001; Armstrong, 2008; Morgan, White, & Wallace, In Press; NIDA, 2010). Benzodiazepines are often used by people with an addictive disorder, especially with opioids to boost or potentiate the effects of the opioid. They may also be used with alcohol to prevent withdrawal or to prevent the crash related to cocaine or stimulant use. Polysubstance use is common for these reasons.

Opioids   Opioid refers to opiates and their derivatives, both natural and synthetic, and includes both legal and illicit drugs. Natural opiates include opium and morphine. Heroin is a semi-synthetic narcotic and is an illicit drug in the United States. These drugs can be taken orally, smoked, snorted, injected into soft tissue (skin-popping) or used intravenously (Allen, 2001; NIDA, 2010). Opiates have both sedative hypnotic and analgesic effects and can produce physical and psychological dependence (Morgan, *et al.*, In Press).

In the last two decades there has been an increase in the medical use of opiates. In the past opiate use was primarily reserved for cancer and terminal care; recently opiates have been prescribed for nonmalignant chronic pain conditions as well. This increase in prescriptions, combined with new drug formulations such as Oxycontin, may have contributed to the increased abuse of legal opiates.

Anabolic Steroids   These drugs are prescribed legally to treat hormone deficiency and body wasting in diseases like AIDS. Steroids can be abused by athletes and others to enhance physical performance and appearance. Some people combine several types of steroids and this is called "stacking." Anabolic steroids do not produce a high as most other drugs of abuse do; however, long-term use of these drugs can affect mood and behavior and have an impact on the same brain chemicals (dopamine, serotonin, and opioid systems) as other drugs. Aggression, mood swings, paranoid jealousy, extreme irritability, delusions, and impaired judgment can be seen with long-term use of steroids. Use of steroids is seen to be reinforcing; many users spend much energy procuring the drugs, with negative effects on their social relations, as is seen with abuse of other drugs that are addicting.

There are serious and irreversible effects on health with steroid use, such as liver damage, high blood pressure, and increases in LDL and decreases in HDL. There is little known about treatment other than supportive therapy, and education about possible withdrawal can be helpful (NIDA, 2010).

Gambling Addiction

Problem gambling is behavior that causes disruptions in any major area of life: psychological, physical, social, or vocational. The term "problem gambling" includes, but is not limited to, the condition known as "pathological", or "compulsive" gambling, a progressive addiction characterized by increasing preoccupation with gambling, a need to bet more money more frequently, restlessness or irritability when attempting to stop, "chasing" losses, and loss of control manifested by continuation of the gambling behavior in spite of mounting, and serious, negative consequences.

Gambling addiction is referred to as the "hidden illness" because there are no obvious physical signs or symptoms as in drug or alcohol addiction. Problem gamblers typically deny or minimize the problem. They also go to great lengths to hide their gambling; they often withdraw from their loved ones, sneak around, and lie about where they've been and what they've been up to, neglect work and family, gamble with money needed to pay bills, and steal to get money for gambling.

Treatment for gambling can include cognitive behavioral therapy and Gamblers Anonymous groups. Naltrexone, a drug used to treat alcoholism and opiate addiction has been used with gamblers to cut down the craving to gamble (National Council on Problem Gambling, 2009: www.ncpgambling.org).

Assessment

The presentation of alcohol and/or other substance abuse may be non-specific and atypical and may be mistaken for other medical problems. Routine primary care appointments should always include questions about alcohol use and illicit drug and non-medical use of prescribed drugs. Providers are comfortable asking routine questions about tobacco use; questions about alcohol, illicit substances, and prescription use should follow this format. Item number 16 in the CMHA tool illustrated in Chapter 2 offers a screening question for such routine inquiry. Utilizing a non-judgmental approach when asking about substances will help patients feel comfortable discussing these issues.

When a provider gets a positive response to a question about substances, further assessment is indicated (as with the CAGE tool discussed below) either by the primary care provider or through referral to an addiction or mental health specialist. Additionally, use of other information elicited as part of the routine history or physical exam may indicate the need for a more detailed assessment even if the patient is not acknowledging drug or alcohol use. Table 9.1 lists some of the cues that substances may be a problem in the social, psychological, behavioral, employment, legal, and family realms. The effect of substances on a patient's ability to function in these realms is important in helping define the difference between social use and problems with the substance.

Medical consequences that may be attributed to alcohol and substance use should also highlight the need for further assessment. Listed below are some of the medical consequences of alcohol or drug abuse. Any one of these issues alone is not necessarily cause for concern. Primary care providers who follow people over years should be alert to changes from the usual presentation of a patient. "Holding up the mirror" of the effect of drugs on the physical well-being of the person, and drawing conclusions about how these consequences are a result of the drug/alcohol use, is a useful technique for primary care providers. Statements like "I'm concerned that all of the bruises you keep getting are not caused by any medical condition that we can determine. I wonder if you've been bruising yourself because of using too much alcohol and have not been aware of these injuries" can be presented in a nonjudgmental way to open the door for further discussion.

Table 9.1 Factors Related to Substance Abuse Problems

Social—any change in social behavior	*Psychological—any change*
Reclusive, withdrawal from social contacts	Mood swings, erratic mood
Frequent conflicts with family/friends	Acute or chronic depression
Change of friends	Suicidal thoughts
Change of activities	Evasive or manipulative
Accidents, driving arrests	Impulse control problems
Frequent drug/alcohol use of friends	Sexual dysfunction
Life revolves around drug/alcohol use	Frequent or chronic anxiety or distress
	Preoccupied with alcohol or drugs

Behavioral—any change in behavior	*Employment or school patterns*
Complains that life is out of control	Frequent absences or tardiness
Changes in school or work performance	Frequent unexplained job changes
Blames others for problems	Job performance diminished and productivity is low
Denial and minimization of problems	
Frequent lateness or cancellation of appointments	Frequent complaints about job, employer, coworkers
Drinking during pregnancy	High incidence of on the job accidents and injuries

Family	*Legal*
Family history of drug and alcohol abuse	Drunk driving arrests
Family complaints about patient's drinking/ drug use	Arrests and/or incarceration
Family history of mood disorder	Legal problems related to financial situation
Continued use of alcohol or drugs despite family conflict over use	Divorce
Unexplained change in family system such as divorce, separation, abandonment	
Rejection or absence of involvement of family	
High level of family conflict	
Secretiveness	
Less responsible at home	
Reports of financial difficulties	

Medical consequences of alcohol and drug abuse can include:

- frequent trauma;
- unexplained injuries or accidents;
- malnourishment in an otherwise healthy adult;
- signs of a withdrawal syndrome;
- excessive complaints of gastritis or heartburn with no physical findings of GI problems;
- unexplained bruises and burns;
- frequent infections such as cellulitis or abscesses;
- deterioration in personal hygiene;
- sleep disturbances;
- disturbances in motor function;
- jaundice, enlarged liver;
- decreased sensation in hands or feet (peripheral neuropathy);
- presence of needle tracks.

Assessment of addictive disorders is best thought of as a process and not an event or one-visit issue. Gaining trust and developing a working relationship with a patient with an addictive disorder is the first step in the process that can help patients acknowledge and begin to understand their disease. Often people with addictive disorders are in denial about the problems that drugs or alcohol have caused in their lives and are also filled with shame about the havoc that substances have created for them. The stigma associated with addictive disorders can make patients reluctant to divulge their histories in the primary care setting. Most patients with addictive disorders have experienced a negative interaction with a healthcare provider that has discouraged their involvement with the healthcare system.

Questions about alcohol and each class of drugs of abuse should be included if screening reveals the need for a more in-depth assessment. Review of each class of drugs with questions about the amount used in the past day, past week, past month, or ever should be addressed. Further questions about the frequency of use, withdrawal symptoms experienced, the presence of blackouts or seizures with alcohol or benzodiazepine use, and any legal, social, or medical problems related to use/abuse should be part of the in-depth assessment. Questions about most recent use are of utmost importance with all drugs, but specifically alcohol and benzodiazepine use, to prevent a medical emergency in the case of a withdrawal syndrome.

Assessment should also include an assessment of the patient's readiness to change, since motivation to change is essential in the success of any plan of care for alcohol or substance addiction. Prochaska, DiClemente, and Norcross developed the Readiness for Change Model based on nicotine addiction and include five stages in their model (Prochaska, DiClemente, & Norcross, 1992). The stages include:

1. precontemplation—the person does not see a problem;
2. contemplation—person does acknowledge that there is a problem and has vague thoughts about change;
3. determination—a decision is made that a change is needed;
4. action—the person is ready to make the change;
5. maintenance—continued work on the problem.

Relapse has been added as a step in the process, since relapse is a part of the change process and must be planned for to prevent treatment dropout.

CASE EXAMPLE: READINESS TO CHANGE ALCOHOL USE/ABUSE

Going back to the example of Fred from Chapter 3: The assessment indicated that Fred is not in crisis and is not currently suicidal, but reacting to the fact that his wife has just asked for a divorce. He refused to come into the clinic because he needed to go to work and was fearful about losing any more time at work. Fred is clearly being presented with a number of consequences of his drinking behavior, but may still not be able to acknowledge these consequences as a direct result of his alcohol abuse. He does acknowledge that he needs help with his drinking at this point which is a positive sign.

Since he is not currently in the clinic and values his continued ability to work, it would make sense to agree with him about the importance of keeping his job and talk about a time when he could come for an appointment. Letting Fred know that you think he definitely needs some help and could benefit from seeing a healthcare provider would be important at this point. Since he is talking to the intake nurse at that point s/he might offer to set up an appointment for him to see a primary care provider to have a physical, to talk more about the alcohol problem, and to coordinate care with a mental health or addictions professional. This might be less threatening than simply setting up an appointment with a counselor. If this primary care practice would allow the intake nurse to do some follow-up s/he might call Fred to remind him about the appointment, or if he misses the appointment, to reschedule another appointment. Fred would most accurately be assessed as being in the contemplation stage at this point and his contact with the providers at this clinic can help move him further into contemplation about change as it relates to his drinking problem.

Primary care providers probably encounter people who are in the precontemplation and contemplation stages, and can contribute significantly to moving people through these initial stages with simple interventions. Planting seeds for thought and making connections about how the substance is causing health, social, or relational problems are important techniques for the primary care provider. Presentation of this information in a nonjudgmental, factual manner can be done in a brief encounter. The expectation is not that the person will accept this information and agree with the provider, but the information has been presented and can be reinforced in subsequent appointments. Highlighting discrepancies is another useful technique. For example: "You say that you don't have a problem with drugs, but your liver enzymes are elevated and in the absence of any other problem, I think this is due to your continuing drug use." It is very important to not use an accusing tone of voice, but to simply state the information and then move on in the overall discussion of health assessment and plan of care.

Screening Tools

Several screening tools are available and useful in the overall assessment of alcohol and drug use. These screening tools should be used in addition to a thorough history and physical examination. The CAGE questionnaire is one of the most widely used and reliable screens of alcohol use. It consists of four questions about use:

1. Have you ever felt that you should **C**ut down on your drinking?
2. Have people **A**nnoyed you by criticizing your drinking?
3. Have you ever felt bad or **G**uilty about your drinking?
4. Have you ever had a drink first thing in the morning to steady your nerves or get rid of a hangover? (**E**ye-opener) (Ewing, 1984, p. 1905).

A score of two or more (one or more for elders) to these questions is generally considered a positive response and indicative of the need for further assessment. Fingerhood (2000, p. 987) suggested the use of lead-in questions prior to the use of the CAGE such as "We have talked about your usual diet and your smoking. Can you tell me how you use alcoholic beverages?" and " Has your use of alcohol caused any kinds of problems for you?" or "Have you ever been concerned about your drinking?" Clinicians have expanded the use of the CAGE and replaced the word alcohol with drugs to assess for drug use.

Other screening tools include the Drug Abuse Screening Test (DAST) (Gavin, Ross, & Skinner, 1989) and the Alcohol Use Disorders Identification Test (AUDIT) (Babor, Higgins-Biddle, Saunders, & Monteiro, 2001) that are useful for identifying both alcohol and drug abuse disorders.

Urine drug screens help detect the presence of drugs or alcohol and are used in conjunction with blood tests, which are most often in emergency departments. These tests are also used in monitoring drug use in long-term drug treatment settings or in pain management clinics when diversion or abuse is a problem.

Treatment Issues

The National Institute of Drug Abuse (NIDA, 2009, pp. 2–5) has set forth principles of drug addiction treatment, briefly summarized in the box below. As described in these principles, the need for readily available treatment designed to meet the needs of the individual with both counseling and psychopharmacological approaches is of utmost importance. Providers must recognize that relapse is an expected part of treatment and that mental disorders are common and need attention. This helps to deliver the message that the treatment is complex and requires the work of several disciplines together. Primary care providers play a key role in assessment and identification of these disorders. Development of a network of addiction providers for referral is very important since primary care providers cannot provide the necessary care in their busy settings.

Treatment Philosophies and Methods of Treatment

Most primary care providers are familiar with the acute treatment or detoxification programs and protocols to prevent sudden withdrawal states. As stated in the principles of drug addiction treatment, medical detoxification is only the beginning step in treatment and does little to change the more complex behavioral changes needed to occur in long-term cessation of drug use. Despite this clear statement and principle, most of the available treatment in the United States is focused on this first step of treatment, with referral to self-help groups such as Alcoholics Anonymous (A.A.) or Narcotics Anonymous (N.A.) as the only follow-up

---

BOX 9.1   Principles of Effective Treatment

1. Addiction is a complex but treatable disease that affects brain function and behavior.
2. No single treatment is appropriate for everyone.
3. Treatment needs to be readily available.
4. Effective treatment attends to multiple needs of the individual, not just his or her drug abuse.
5. Remaining in treatment for an adequate period of time is critical.
6. Counseling—individual and/or group—and other behavioral therapies are the most commonly used forms of drug abuse treatment.
7. Medications are an important element of treatment for many patients, especially when combined with counseling and other behavioral therapies.
8. An individual's treatment and services plan must be assessed continually and modified as necessary to ensure that it meets his or her changing needs.
9. Many drug-addicted individuals also have other mental disorders.
10. Medically assisted detoxification is only the first stage of addiction treatment and by itself does little to change long-term drug abuse.
11. Treatment does not need to be voluntary to be effective.
12. Drug use during treatment must be monitored continuously, as lapses during treatment do occur.
13. Treatment programs should assess patients for the presence of HIV/AIDS, Hepatitis B and C, tuberculosis, and other infectious diseases as well as provide targeted risk-reduction counseling to help patients modify or change behaviors that place them at risk of contracting or spreading infectious diseases.

Source: From Principles of Drug Addiction Treatment (NIDA, 2009, pp. 2–5)

upon discharge from detoxification units. In addition to detoxification programs and self-help programs, long-term residential programs, short-term residential programs, individual and group outpatient therapy are other modalities used to treat persons with addictive disorders.

There are several different philosophies of longer term drug and alcohol treatment. A brief review of these philosophies will help primary care clinicians to refer or recommend a treatment program that may best meet the needs of their patient, where such treatments are available.

Abstinence

Many programs—including inpatient units, halfway houses and self-help groups—maintain a philosophy that abstinence from any mind-altering substances is the only way to achieve recovery. This philosophical approach can present a problem for people with mental health or medical conditions. Use of medications for depression and anxiety as well as pain or sleep medications are contraindicated in treatment programs with an abstinence focus, and use of such medications could result in discharge from the program.

SBIRT: Screening, Brief Intervention, and Referral to Treatment

SBIRT represents a new approach to treatment for people with a substance abuse problem. The focus of treatment in the past has been for those with an identified problem and/or dependence on substances. This new approach seeks to identify those at risk for substance related problems. Screening determines the severity of the problem and identifies which level of intervention is appropriate for the individual.

Brief intervention provided in a community or primary care setting can provide immediate attention to the problem, and early intervention will have a preventive impact on the numbers of people going on to develop more serious problems with substances. Also, providing care in primary care settings will help reduce the stigma associated with substance abuse treatment.

Motivational Interviewing (MI)

Motivational interviewing is a well-established approach to treating addictions. It is defined as a client-centered, directive method for enhancing the individual's motivation to change by exploring and resolving ambivalence (Miller & Rollnick, 1991). It meets patients at the level they are in terms of recognizing their problem and motivation for change. There are four basic principles in MI:

1   expression of empathy;
2   developing the discrepancy;
3   supporting self-efficacy;
4   rolling with the resistance.

The active involvement of the client in MI is a key strategy for clinicians working with addicted patients.

Dual Diagnosis Treatment

Since the mid-1980s the recognition that many people with an addictive disorder also have psychiatric problems has grown. Since that time inpatient psychiatric programs have developed dual diagnosis programs that focus on integrating the care of these two disorders in one setting with the belief that one is not adequately treated without paying attention to the treatment of the other disorder. Outpatient programs also may focus on the dual problems; however, an adequate supply of professionals educated to provide care for those with addictive disorders is a major problem in the U.S.

Harm Reduction

Harm reduction meets the patient at his or her own level in terms of desiring change in harmful behavior. The techniques utilized in harm reduction assist in helping the person decrease exposure to risky behaviors and adopt behaviors leading to a healthier lifestyle. Needle exchange programs to decrease HIV transmission are an example of a harm reduction program. The following case example demonstrates the use of a harm reduction model in a more complex situation.

CASE EXAMPLE: REDUCING HARM FROM ALCOHOL

Jim is a 39-year-old Caucasian male with HIV disease (with a high CD4 count) and chronic Hepatitis C who is being followed in the HIV clinic. He was referred for treatment of his continuing substance abuse to the psychiatric clinical nurse specialist connected with the HIV clinic after several car accidents related to his alcohol and substance use (he was not arrested for these accidents). These accidents resulted in major medical problems.

His medical providers were so worried about his addiction that they told him he would not be able to continue treatment at the clinic unless he engaged in drug treatment and/or other therapy; he chose to be in therapy. He acknowledged using cocaine and alcohol but had no interest in stopping his drug or alcohol use. He was not very interested in treatment for about the first six months but consistently came to scheduled appointments and talked about his concerns about his girlfriend who also had HIV disease and was much sicker than he was. He and his girlfriend had a very tumultuous relationship that often resulted in physical abuse (they were both perpetrators and victims of the abuse).

He continued to have no interest in drug treatment or stopping his drug use. After about six months of treatment he was willing to talk more about drug use and eventually began to work on harm reduction strategies. One day he identified peppermint schnapps as the alcohol that made him crazy and that he thought was the cause of his accidents and worst fights with his girlfriend. He agreed to stop using that one drug. Weekly check-ins about his use (or non-use) of the peppermint schnapps was a helpful technique and he was able to contract on a week-to-week basis to not use this type of alcohol. He was honest about continuing to drink mostly beer (up to two six-packs a day on some occasions) during this time. He did not get into any additional car accidents and his fights with his girlfriend decreased.

He got involved with an AIDS organization and started educating himself about his disease and more specifically about his Hepatitis C, which was the more urgent issue medically and in his mind as well. Desire for treatment of his Hepatitis C brought him to another level of harm reduction and he began educating himself about the liver and effects of alcohol use. He set up a goal of gradually weaning himself from all alcohol that he was able to be successful with, and after a period of six months of sobriety he began Interferon treatment for his Hepatitis C. He remained in counseling to monitor any problems with depression as a result of the treatment. He successfully completed Interferon treatment with good results and only at the end of treatment did he have some symptoms of depression that were managed with therapy.

Recovery Model

The recovery model focuses on learning to avoid environmental cues that would stimulate desire or craving for drugs and access to drugs or alcohol. The goals of this model are to reassert self-control, end preoccupation with the substance in order to repair life goals and relationships, and connect to others. Often peer support is an important piece of the recovery model so that patients can see a person who has been successful in dealing with their problems.

Relapse Prevention

Most models of care utilize some relapse prevention strategies since relapse is widely accepted as a part of the disease process of addiction. Assisting the patient in the identification of cues or "triggers" (people, places, and things) associated with drug use that could lead to craving and relapse is the main focus of this work. Practice of alternative ways of dealing with the cravings to expand patients' coping mechanisms is a practical focus of the model. Additionally, telling patients to come to treatment even when they relapse reinforces the idea that it is an expected outcome and that staying away from treatment due to shame, and at a time when they most need the treatment, is not a helpful response.

Primary care providers are familiar with relapse as it relates to medical conditions, yet providers' frustration with those who have an addictive disorder and relapse has resulted in turning patients away from care, or refusing to care for people "until they are ready to participate." Comparing relapse rates in addictive disorders to relapse rates in other medical conditions highlight the inappropriateness of this behavior by providers. NIDA (2009) published data comparing relapse rates in the following illnesses:

- Diabetes: 30–50%
- Drug Addiction: 40–60%
- Hypertension: 50–70%
- Asthma: 50–70% (NIDA, 2009, p. 11).

Behavioral Therapy

Often behavioral therapy is used in combination with other treatment approaches. Use of relaxation or biofeedback can help patients learn to identify and manage stressful situations (see Chapter 13). Aversive conditioning may be used in nicotine dependent patients and is also used in alcohol dependence in the form of disulfiram (Antabuse), which will be discussed under medications.

Trauma Informed Care

Trauma informed care is a philosophy of care that takes into account that up to two-thirds of men and women in substance abuse treatment report childhood abuse and neglect, 90% of public mental health clients have been exposed to trauma, and 50% of women in substance abuse treatment have a history of rape or incest (National Executive Training Institute, 2005). Trauma informed care incorporates an understanding of the effects of such trauma on the individual and identifies ways of providing care that are collaborative rather than using coercive interventions that cause traumatization and re-traumatization. This model looks at the traditional way of delivering care in US institutions, including practices that are re-traumatizing to many patients. The goal is to minimize the power and control issues inherent in systems and work towards a collaborative partnership with patients, where labeling behavior is eliminated and improved sensitivity and knowledge of the staff are a focus (see Chapter 5).

Support Groups

For decades, 12-step support groups such as A.A. and N.A. were the only treatment modalities available for addictive disorders. These groups provided care and support to hundreds of thousands of people. They are still very effective in providing support and reinforcing the principles of recovery for many people. Some people have not liked the "God focus" of A.A./N.A. and as a result other self-help recovery programs, such as Rational Recovery and SMART Recovery, were developed. SMART recovery focuses on enhancing motivation, coping with urges, problem-solving and maintaining lifestyle balance. Finally, Al-Anon and Al-a-Teen self-help groups have assisted family members of those with addictive disorders in dealing with the problems they encounter when living with a family member who has an addictive disorder.

Spiritual care can be an essential part of the care that is needed by those recovering from an addictive disorder. Patients who express hopelessness and powerlessness, and whose life lacks meaning are at risk for use of escalating or lethal doses of substances to numb the pain and meaninglessness of their lives. They may no longer associate their substance use with pleasure, but are powerless to stop responding to the craving for continued drug use. They may also feel unworthy of love or compassion, that their addiction is a punishment from God, and that the pain they feel is deserved for their past behavior that was associated with the addiction. Spiritual support from A.A., N.A., sponsors, or pastoral counselors as well as psychiatric support and assessment of suicidality may be crucial at crisis points in the treatment (see Chapter 4).

Medications Used in Treating Addictive Disorders

Medications are used to detoxify patients from substances. Most primary care providers are familiar with detoxification protocols and thus these drugs are discussed only briefly here. Observation and a thorough history and physical examination are key in determining whether or not someone is at risk for a withdrawal syndrome. Use of rating scales such as the Clinical Withdrawal Assessment Scale (CIWA) will assist in rating the severity of an alcohol related withdrawal and help determine treatment response. Benzodiazepines utilizing the concept of cross-tolerance is the primary method of providing a safe medically assisted withdrawal from alcohol.

The rest of this section includes medications used in the longer-term treatment of addictive disorders. Primary care providers should be familiar with these drugs as a foundation for referral to addiction specialty services, and for monitoring outcomes in relation to an addicted patient's overall medical condition.

Medications can aid recovery by reducing cravings, reducing psychological preoccupation with substances, improving impulse control, and reducing isolation by connecting the patient with a prescriber. Two categories of medications are utilized: Agonist replacement therapies, such as buprenorphine, methadone, and nicotine replacement and abstinence-promoting therapies, such as naltrexone, acamprosate and disulfarim. Medications with demonstrated safety and efficacy are:

* Alcohol dependence

    – Disulfarim
    – Naltrexone
    – Acamprosate

- Nicotine dependence

    – Nicotine replacement therapy (NRT)
    – Buproprion
    – Chantix

- Opioid dependence

    – Methadone
    – Buprenorphine
    – Naltrexone

Medications Used in the Treatment of Alcoholism   Disulfarim (Antabuse) has been used for treatment of alcoholism for many years and may be indicated when other therapies have failed, for people who are at risk for an immediate job loss or loss of custody of their children related to alcohol, or in other high risk situations such as vacations, holidays, or travel. The use of this drug makes alcohol psychologically unavailable (due to the severe reaction if combined with alcohol) and decreases craving. Dosing of Disulfarim ranges from 125–500 mg daily. Even small amounts of alcohol, such as is found in vinegar, mouthwash, hand sanitizers and cologne when used while taking Disulfarim may result in flushing, feelings of heat in face and upper body, hypotension, dizziness, blurred vision, palpitations, nausea and vomiting, air hunger, and numbness of the upper extremities. The consequences of this kind of reaction make any patients that are not in good health poor candidates for this treatment. It is contraindicated for patients who have cardiac disease and fulminant hepatotoxicity can occur in one in 50,000 people. Impulsive heavy drinking while taking Disulfarim may be fatal (Williams, 2005).

Naltrexone (Revia) is an antagonist at the mu receptor and interferes with the euphoric effects of alcohol and opiates. For some people it may reduce the intensity and frequency of cravings to drink or use opiates. It can improve the chance that a patient who drinks can interrupt a "slip" and not continue to relapse. It has resulted in fewer drinking days for patients and an altered experience of intoxication. It is contraindicated in patients who may need opioids for pain, and those with cough or GI motility problems. Side effects can include nausea, fatigue, headache, anxiety, and muscle and joint pain. There is an FDA black box warning about the risk of hepatotoxicity that is dose dependent (higher risk is most often with higher doses, 100–300mg/day) and mostly reversible with discontinuation of the drug. Dosage ranges are 25–100 mg. daily (Williams, 2005).

Acomprosate (Campral) decreases the symptoms associated with early abstinence such as dysphoria, irritability, anxiety, insomnia, and restlessness. It is used following detoxification and improves the patient's ability to remain sober. The side effects are primarily GI problems, but side effects can be minimized by titrating the dosage by 333 mg. tid once a week (up to 666 mg. tid). Patients are instructed to take the medication with meals to improve adherence. Acomprosate is contraindicated in patients with abnormal renal function (Williams, 2005).

Medications Used in the Treatment of Nicotine Addiction   Nicotine replacement therapies (NRT) include the over the counter nicotine patches, gum and lozenges, and the prescription inhalers and nasal spray. Nicotine replacement is calculated by averaging the number of ciga-rettes or packs of cigarettes per day. Each cigarette is thought to have approximately 1 mg. of nicotine and each pack has 20 cigarettes = 20 mg. of nicotine/pack of cigarette. The aim of replacement therapy is to replace the current daily amount or decrease by no more than 25% initially with a gradual decrease in the amount of nicotine. Patches are available in 7–28 mg.

Patches may cause skin irritation or nightmares, and removal at night may decrease the night-mares. Patches also can come off with heavy sweating. They may be combined with gum/lozenges for breakthrough cravings. Nicotine gum is available in 2–4 mg. and is utilized by the "chew and park" method since the nicotine is absorbed through the mucosa of the cheek. The lozenges are available in candy form. If the lozenges are chewed they can cause gastric reflux and gastritis. The lozenges may be irritating to teeth, gums, throat, and stomach. Both the NRT inhalers and nasal spray require a prescription and are more expensive than the other forms of NRT. The inhaler looks like a cigarette and delivers nicotine to the mouth, not the lungs. IT takes approximately 80 puffs to equal the amount of nicotine delivered by 1 cigarette. Mouth irritation can be problematic with the inhaler. The nasal spray has the highest peak of nicotine delivery and may be appropriate for highly dependent smokers. The dosage is 2 puffs per nostril that delivers the equivalent of the nicotine in one cigarette. Nose and throat irritation may be problematic with the nasal spray (Pbert, Ockene, & Reiff-Hekking, 2004).

Buproprion (Zyban, Wellbutrin) is an antidepressant medication that has shown effec-tiveness for smoking cessation. Treatment should begin one to two weeks before the date the patient quits smoking, with a starting dose of 150 mg. a day for three days, then increase as tolerated to 150 mg. bid. It is contraindicated for use in patients with seizure disorders. Side effects include insomnia and a jittery feeling. Buproprion can be used in combination with NRT (Pbert, Ockene, & Reiff-Hekking, 2004).

Chantix is the newest medication used for nicotine addiction. It is a partial agonist at the nicotinic receptors and provides mild activation while blocking exogenous nicotine from activating the receptors. Abrupt discontinuation of Chantix can cause a mild withdrawal syndrome. Chantix should be started one week before the quit date. Treatment from days one to three should be dosed at 0.5 mg. once a day, days four to seven at 0.5 mg twice a day and day eight through end of treatment at 1 mg. twice a day. Treatment can last from 12–24 weeks. Common side effects include nausea, insomnia, and headache. In February 2008 the FDA issued a warning about the links between Chantix and suicidal thoughts and behavior (Smoking Cessation Health Center).

Medications Used to Treat Opiate Addiction   Medications used to treat opiate dependence include the opiate agonist replacement therapy such as methadone and buprenorphine, and opiate antagonist therapy such as naltrexone.

Methadone is a full agonist that works at the mu opiate receptor site. It has been in use for decades and it costs only pennies to make. Federal guidelines about dispensing methadone are very strict and methadone maintenance may only be provided at a licensed clinic, and not in a primary care practice. Methadone has a long half-life (24–36 hours) and this makes it ideal for once a day dosing for patients. Routine drug screens and counseling are part of the program that patients agree to when admitted to a methadone program. Methadone treatment does require that patients go to a clinic on a regular basis, daily, and take the dose while being observed by a nurse. Patients who have been stable in their treatment may apply to receive take-home doses, but depending on the clinic, patients may have to go to the clinic daily for months or longer before this is allowed. This puts constraints on patients who might need to travel a distance away from the clinic. For working people there is often an early morning time for dosing to ensure that patients can get to work on time. For those who are medically ill, there usually is a "medical line" that requires less time on one's feet waiting to get the methadone dose. There is a stigma attached to going to the clinic, and patients may still be told by addiction treatment providers, and other people in recovery, that they are not really sober if they are using methadone.

Most methadone related deaths occur during the first few weeks of maintenance therapy, and are probably related to a rapid escalation of the dose and to the risk of respiratory depression. There have been cardiac problems associated with methadone, and methadone alone or in combination with other drugs or cardiac problems may result in the development of prolongation of the QT interval resulting in a severe arrhythmia called torsades de pointe. For this reason, careful medical screening is done by clinic staff even if the person is referred for treatment by a primary care provider who has just done a complete history and physical exam (NIDA, 2010; Schottenfeld, 2004).

Buprenorphine (Subutex) is a partial agonist at the mu receptor site. Like methadone, it relieves craving for the drug but does not induce euphoria. As with all opiates there is a risk of respiratory depression and patients should be advised about combining this buprenorphine with other CNS depressants. Buprenorphine also has a competitive antagonist effect at the mu receptor sites and this results in blocking the effects of heroin or other opiates; this can also induce a withdrawal syndrome if the buprenorphine is given after heroin. Most buprenorphine is administered in combination with Naloxone, an opiate antagonist, (Suboxone) to prevent diversion. The Naloxone component is mostly inactive when taken as prescribed (sublingually) but is active when the pill is crushed and injected. Despite these precautions there is now evidence that Suboxone is being diverted and has street value as a detoxification tool. Dose ranges of Suboxone are 6–24 mg. daily taken sublingually (NIDA; O'Brien & Kampaman, 2004).

There are several advantages of Suboxone over methadone. It is a safe drug, and it is well tolerated. Side effects include a cold or flu-like syndrome, difficulty sleeping, nausea, constipation, sweating, mood swings, and fatigue. The greatest benefit is that it is office-based treatment and can be prescribed by M.D.s who have completed a training session; to date other primary care providers are not able to prescribe this medication. The fact that it is office-based rather than clinic-based treatment with a prescription for a week or two, reduces the stigma associated with having to go to a treatment program daily, and has resulted in increased retention in treatment. The number of patients per provider has been restricted so far in the U.S., so finding a prescriber can be a challenge in some areas of the country. If patients require opiate pain medications on a long-term basis Suboxone treatment is not appropriate.

Naltrexone (described under medication treatments for alcoholism) may be an important maintenance option following detoxification from opiates and stabilization. There is some risk that patients will try to overcome the antagonism and accidentally overdose or develop sensitivity to opiates, discontinue treatment, and then accidentally overdose (NIDA, 2010; O'Brien & Kampman, 2004).

Primary Care of Patients with Addictive Disorders

Primary care providers are not going to be providing the bulk of addiction treatment for individuals. However, a thorough assessment and frank discussion of the long-term effects of addiction are the first step towards treatment. Helping people stay in treatment and providing encouragement to do so will have major benefits for most people. Development of ongoing collaboration with addiction and psychiatric providers will enable the primary care provider to facilitate access to specialized care for their patients when it is needed.

Maintaining a respectful relationship with the patient will enhance adherence with treatment suggestions. Approaching patients with an attitude that they are coping as best they can with the resources that they have allows providers to engage around ways to increase these resources for their patients. Remembering that long-term change takes a long time and that relapse is a part of the disease of addiction is essential in providing care. Having a trusted colleague with whom you can discuss difficult cases and "blow off steam" may be especially important when dealing with people who have the complex problems associated with addictive disorders.

References

Allen, L. (2001). Drugs of abuse. In N. L. Keltner & D. G. Folks (Eds.) *Psychotropic drugs* (3rd Ed.). St. Louis, MI: Mosby.

American Psychiatric Association (APA). (2000). *Diagnostic and statistical manual of mental disorders* (4th Ed.). (DSM-IV-TR). Washington, DC: APA.

American Society of Pain Management Nurses. (2003). *ASPMN position statement: Pain management in patients with addictive disease*. Pensacola, FL: Author.

Armstrong, M. (2008) Substance-Related Disorders. In Fortinash, K. M., & Holoday Worret, P. A., *Psychiatric mental health nursing* (3rd Ed.) (pp. 304–341), St. Louis, MI: Mosby.

Babor, T. F., Higgins-Biddle, J. C., Saunders, J. B., & Monteiro, M. G. (2001). *AUDIT: The Alcohol Use Disorders Identification Test: Guidelines for use in primary care* (2nd Ed.). Geneva: World Health Organization, Department of Mental Health and Substance Dependence.

Center for Disease Control and Prevention (CDC). (2010). Alcohol and public health. www.cdc.gov/alcohol (accessed on 5 July 2010).

Ewing, J. (1984). Detecting alcoholism: The CAGE questionnaire. *Journal of the American Medical Association*, 252(14), 1905–1907.

Fingerhood, M. (2000). Substance abuse in older people. *Journal of the American Geriatrics Society*, 48(8), 985–995.

Gavin D. R., Ross H. E., & Skinner, H. A. (1989) Diagnostic validity of the Drug Abuse Screening Test in the assessment of DSM-III drug disorders, *British Journal of Addiction*, 84(3): 301–307.

Keltner, N. L., & Folks, D. G. (2001). *Psychotropic drugs* (3rd Ed.). St. Louis, MO: Mosby.

Miller, W. R., & Rollnick, S. (1991). *Motivational interviewing: Preparing people to change addictive behavior*. New York: The Guilford Press.

Moore, R., Bone, L., & Geller, G. (1989). Prevalence, detection and treatment of alcoholism in hospitalized patients. *JAMA*, 261, 403–407.

National Executive Training Institute (NETI). (2005). Training curriculum for reduction of seclusion and restraint. Draft curriculum manual. Alexandria, VA: National Association of State Mental Health Program Directors (NASMHPD), National Technical Assistance for State Mental Health Planning (NTAC).

National Institute on Drug Abuse (NIDA). (2010). www.nida.nih.gov/Drugpages/ (accessed on July 12, 2010).

National Institute on Drug Abuse (NIDA). (2009). Principles of Drug Addiction Treatment: A research based guide. National Institute of Health Publication #00– 4180.

National Council on Problem Gambling. (2009). www.ncpgambling.org

National Survey on Drug Use and Health (NSDUH). (2007). www.oas.samhsa.gov/nsduh.htm (accessed on 5 July 2010).

O'Brien, C. P., & Kampman, K. M. (2004). Opioids: antagonists and partial agonists. In Galanter, M. & Kleber, H. D. *Textbook of substance abuse treatment* (3rd Ed.). Washington, DC: American Psychiatric Publishing, Inc.

Pbert, L., Ockene, J. K., & Reiff-Hekking, S. (2004). Tobacco. In Galanter, M. & Kleber, H.D. *Textbook of substance abuse treatment* (3rd Ed.). Washington, DC: American Psychiatric Publishing, Inc.

Prochaska, J., DiClemente, C., & Norcross, J. (1992). In search of how people change: Applications to addictive behaviors. *American Psychologist*, 47, 1102–1114.

Savage, S. R. (1993). Addiction in the treatment of pain: Significance, recognition and management. *Journal of Pain and Symptom Management*, 8 (5), 265–278.

Schottenfeld, R. S. (2004). Opioids: Maintenance treatmenr. In Galanter, M. & Kleber, H. D. *Textbook of substance abuse treatment* (3rd Ed.). Washington, DC: American Psychiatric Publishing, Inc.

Smoking Cessation Health Center. www.webmd.com/smoking-cessation (accessed on 5 July 2010).

Weissman, D. E., & Haddox, J. D. (1989). Opioid pseudoaddiction: an iatrogenic syndrome. *Pain*, 36, 363–366.

Williams, S. H. (2005). Medications for treating alcohol dependence. *American Family Physician*, 72(9), 1775–1780.

10 Chronic Pain in Medical and Psychiatric Illness

- Definitions
- Acute Pain
- Chronic Pain
- Psychosocial Functioning and Chronic Pain
- Assessment Issues
- Early Intervention
- Ethical Issues
- Treatment of Pain and Co-occurring Psychiatric and Addictive Disorders
- Suggestions for Primary Care Providers
- Conclusion
- References

Primary care is the entry point for most patients into the healthcare system and where most patients seeking relief from pain are seen. Pain has been described as the number one reason why people seek healthcare in the United States. Primary care providers serve patients with mental illness for their medical needs, including pain. Cross-culturally, the meaning of pain and people's responses to it vary, often in relation to its origin in the physical or psychic realm. For example, in some cultures people will seek out a traditional healer for psychosocial problems and "psychic" pain, but a "professional" practitioner for treatment of pain, say, from a fracture, while faith and spiritual solace are also very important for many suffering from pain.

Over the last several decades many studies have documented the increase in physical illness and higher mortality rates in people with mental illness. Corresponding with this increase in physical illness comes an increase in physical pain. Likewise, people with addictive disorders are also at risk for increased physical problems and therefore, an increased problem with pain. This chapter addresses the overlapping symptoms of pain and mental health problems, assessment strategies, and treatment options for co-morbid pain and mental health problems. Acute pain problems are addressed but the main focus is on the more complex and challenging chronic pain and mental health issues. The importance of identifying the psychiatric disorders that can modulate chronic pain and the role for primary care providers in caring for this population is emphasized.

Definitions

Pain is defined as "An unpleasant sensory and emotional experience associated with actual or potential tissue damage or described in terms of such damage. Pain is *always* subjective. Each individual learns the application of the word through experiences related to injury in early life. . . It is unquestionably a sensation in a part or parts of the body but it is always unpleasant and therefore an emotional experience" (APS, 1992). This definition is important in that it clearly underscores the fact that pain is always subjective and that the emotional experience of pain plays as important a role as the physical experience for each person. A useful definition for primary care providers is that pain is "whatever the experiencing person says it is, existing whenever s/he says it does" (McCaffery, 1968, p. 95). Pain may be classified as acute, cancer, or chronic nonmalignant pain (McCaffery & Pasero, 1999).

Suffering often accompanies pain but is a different entity. Cassell (1982) published the seminal work on suffering and described suffering in terms of an issue that transcends the bodily experience and threatens the intactness of the whole person. Cassell challenged physicians for not only failing to relieve suffering, but for also intensifying suffering at times. Ferrell & Coyle (2008) examined suffering in the context of the goals of nursing and stated "that most chronic and life-threatening diseases become whole-person experiences that inevitably include suffering" (Ferrell & Coyle, 2008, p. 9). Personal meaning of the experience of pain and/or illness is critical in understanding suffering. Nurses, as providers of the most intimate care for patients, play a major role in the relief of suffering, often by their presence and approaches with patients and families.

Additional definitions related to this discussion are listed in Chapter 9 and include the definitions of substance abuse, substance dependence, addiction, intoxication, cross-tolerance, and pseudo-addiction. The terms substance abuse, substance dependence, and addiction are often used interchangeably by healthcare providers, yet have very different meanings. The term pseudo-addiction is redefined here since it is of primary importance in the management of pain. Pseudo-addiction was defined in the 1980s as an iatrogenic syndrome created by the under-treatment of pain. It appears to be similar to addiction in the behaviors exhibited by patients, yet the behaviors resolve when adequate pain treatment is initiated (Weisman & Haddox, 1989).

Acute Pain

Acute pain is usually connected to an identifiable disease or injury, is time-limited, and resolves over hours to days in a way that relates to healing of the disease or injury. It may or may not be associated with observable, objective signs such as change in pulse, blood pressure, sweating, and/or pallor.

Acute pain typically is a crisis for patients and may result in an urgent appointment with a PCP, an emergency room visit, or hospitalization. Immediate assessment and treatment of pain while assessing for the cause of the pain is of utmost importance in the crisis. The effects of anxiety on pain are discussed further on, and are particularly important in acute pain situations. Untreated pain may limit the patient's ability to communicate with healthcare providers, thus affecting the diagnosis of the underlying problem. Untreated or under-treated pain can increase the suffering associated with the pain, and affect the patient–provider relationship. Also, a growing body of literature indicates that untreated acute pain may set the patient up for more complicated chronic pain conditions and subsequent difficulties in relieving pain.

CASE EXAMPLE: ACUTE PAIN AND ANXIETY

Jean is a 63-year-old single Caucasian female who came to the emergency room by taxi. She has had a severe headache for the past six hours and is quite frightened by this, as she rarely gets headaches and feared she was having a stroke. Jean is seen by the triage nurse who asks about her pain and then cuts Jean off when she tries to describe the pain, and focuses her questions on the timing of the headache and other medical history. Once she is settled in a room in the ER, Jean is seen by another nurse, and a physician, neither of whom even asked about the pain. After waiting another hour and a half without any further attention from staff, Jean, by now crying in pain and very upset, flags down a nurse and says "I don't think I can stand this pain anymore! Please get me something!!" When the nurse comes into Joan's room she is impatient with Jean and questions whether Jean is drug-seeking.

A patient in acute pain who presents at an emergency room for treatment is usually not known to the healthcare providers. Rapid assessment of the acute problem is the goal in this setting where the focus is on life-and-death issues. Pain may not be viewed by professionals as a life-and-death issue and therefore may not be the focus of intervention. Pain may be the patient's entire focus and the pain may be compounded by anxiety about the meaning of the pain and implications for danger to the patient's life. Lack of attention to the pain on the part of the professionals may also complicate the situation and confuse the patient and/or lead to more anxiety and suffering. This lack of attention may lead the patient to become more anxious, demanding, and emotional, as the case of Jean illustrates. Staff may respond to this behavior change as if the patient is a problem, rather than seeing that lack of attention to the patient's concern may have exacerbated the problem. Staff attitudes and labeling of patients as "drug-seeking" may obscure the underlying anxiety and suffering that patients experience, and result in distress for both the patient and the healthcare provider.

Chronic Pain

Chronic pain may be related to cancer or nonmalignant pain. Chronic pain may have neurological, vascular, visceral, joint, or muscular origins and may lack the observable, objective signs seen with acute pain. Chronic nonmalignant pain is defined as pain over six months in duration (McCaffery & Pasero, 1999).

A significant number of people who have chronic pain also have co-morbid psychiatric disorders. The most common of these conditions are mood disorders, anxiety, and somato-form disorders, maladaptive coping styles, as well as substance abuse problems (Fishbain, Cutler, & Solomon, 1998). Untreated pain in the presence of anxiety and depression can diminish the effectiveness of the treatment for anxiety and depression. Likewise, untreated depression and anxiety in the presence of pain can diminish the treatment response for pain. Under-treatment of either pain or psychiatric illness can have a serious impact on quality of life, and can worsen clinical outcomes and one's ability to function in work and social settings.

Chronic Pain and Depression

Depression has been identified in 30–54% of chronic pain patients with 37% of those having clinically significant depression (Bair, Robinson, Katon, & Kroenke, 2003). In fact, the two illnesses occur together so commonly that the terms depression-pain syndrome and depression-pain dyad have been developed (Bair, Robinson, Katon, & Kroenke, 2003).

Chronic pain patients may minimize their psychological symptoms out of fear that they will be labeled as "crazy" and/or have their pain ignored. Both pain and depression may have

a profound effect on an individual's functioning. Overlapping symptoms of sleep disturbance, appetite problems, fatigue, and lack of interest in normal activities may be present in
both pain and depression which can confuse clinicians and lead to inadequate assessment.
Assessment of the impact of pain on these symptoms and the individual's ability to function
in normal activities, and a separate assessment of depression and these same symptoms'
effect on individual functioning, should occur with patients who have chronic pain syndromes.

Although chronic pain is defined as existing after six months in duration, a patient's individual coping mechanisms may well be overwhelmed after a much shorter period of time.
When pain is severe or present for more than a brief period of time, patients should be
assessed not only for pain but also for symptoms of depression, as indicated above. It is likely
that there will be a change in function in the occupational and/or social life of the patient
when pain is complicated by depression. Coping abilities, self-esteem, and self-efficacy
issues may affect the person's ability to function, and therefore affect one's quality of life. A
thorough assessment of the patient's coping abilities may highlight non-pharmacological
interventions that may be indicated in the plan of care.

Depression should not be considered a normal part of the disease process when it is
associated with end-of-life and pain. Thorough assessment and treatment of major depression
at end-of-life may assist patients in achieving quality of life as they come to the end of their
lives (see Chapter 1 on palliative care).

Chronic Pain and Suicide

A connection between chronic pain and a high degree of suicidality has been established in
the literature. Fishbain (1999) reviewed 18 studies of chronic pain and suicide, including
suicidal ideation, attempts, and completion, and found that the risk in these studies ranged
from 17–66%. Suicide (ideation, attempts, or completion) was associated with longer duration of pain, higher intensity of pain and the presence of major depression in this review.

Patient comments such as "I can't take it anymore" or "I just want the pain to stop" are
cues that a suicide risk assessment is needed. The meaning and intent of these comments
should be explored by a provider who is able to sit and listen to the patient describe their
feelings. For patients who are not offering such comments, a routine screening question
included in the pain assessment such as "Has the pain ever been so bad that it made you think
about doing anything you could to stop it?" Follow-up questions of "What did you consider
doing?" and, "Do you feel that way now?" should be included if patients positively answer
the first question.

Thoughts of suicide must be taken seriously and the importance of evaluating pain patients
for depression and suicidal thoughts and plans cannot be emphasized enough. Evaluation
revealing serious suicidal thoughts is seen as a crisis by professionals; in the situation of
chronic pain it is an opportunity to reassess the entire treatment plan with the patient. The
response of the provider is important in conveying the idea that the suicidal thoughts are
taken very seriously. Listening to the patient is central, and determining the need to provide
additional supports or improved pain treatment, or further assistance from a psychiatric
provider, are key components of care in a patient who has suicidal thoughts (see Chapter 4
on suicidal and self-destructive persons).

Chronic Pain and Anxiety

It is considered "normal" to worry about pain and any threat to the body. Anxiety can exist
prior to the pain and also be the result of pain. Anxiety may also be a complicating factor in

the rehabilitation of patients with painful conditions in that anxiety around pain may prevent patients from actively engaging in movement, such as physical therapy, if pain from the movement is intense. Avoidant behavior as a result of pain may interfere with necessary participation in treatment with the goal of returning patients to their previous state of activity.

Anxiety and chronic pain commonly occur in tandem; patients with chronic pain have anxiety and patients with anxiety often have a higher incidence of pain complaints. Anxiety can occur prior to the development of a pain problem or following the development of pain. Chronic pain is common among patients experiencing posttraumatic stress, generalized anxiety, panic attacks, and those disorders such as obsessive-compulsive and adjustment problems, social phobia and agoraphobia. Additionally, patients with anxiety commonly abuse substances as a way of dealing with their anxiety.

Assessment of anxiety in the presence of pain should include questions such as "Does the pain change any of your physical problems? (i.e., pulse, blood pressure, sweating)." "Are you overwhelmed when you feel the pain and does this feeling affect your ability to do activities of daily living?" If anxiety interferes with healing or daily functioning, treatment of the pain-associated anxiety is essential for overall improvement of pain relief and quality of life.

Chronic Pain and Somatoform Disorders

The DSM-IV-TR (APA, 2000) classification of pain disorder is listed under the somatoform disorders section. Most somatoform disorders, including pain disorder, are often associated with medically unexplained symptoms that may present with a degree of distress and disability that are not consistent with medical findings. The diagnostic criteria of pain disorder includes pain that is the focus of the presentation, causes distress or impairment in functioning, the psychological factors associated with the pain that played a part in onset, severity, exacerbation, and maintenance of the pain, and the pain is not feigned (APA, 2000, p. 503). Of particular note, the authors state that most people have suffered with pain for many years before they come to the attention of mental health professionals (APA, 2000). Recent research is challenging the classification of somatoform disorders, suggesting that there is little reason to retain the somatoform disorder category and recommending greater integration of psychiatry into general medical practice (Mayou, Kirmayer, Simon, Kronenke, & Sharpe, 2005).

Chronic Pain and Psychological Coping Styles

Discussions about personality style, character traits, and personality disorders as they are related to pain have occurred over the last several decades with no causal relationships identified by research. Some studies have identified psychological factors or traits associated with adjustment to chronic pain conditions. Some of the factors associated with poor adjustment to pain, psychological distress, and physical disability include pain catastrophizing, pain-related anxiety/fear, and helplessness. Pain catastrophizing is described as "the tendency to focus on pain and negatively evaluate one's ability to deal with the pain" (Keefe, Rumble, Scipio, Giordano, & Perri, 2004, p.196). It is important to note that studies have indicated that psychosocial interventions can change catastrophizing over time (Keefe, Rumble, Scipio, Giordano, & Perri, 2004) (see Chapter 13).

Problems with pain-related anxiety and fear of pain can result in patients who are overcome with anxiety and engage in avoidant behaviors. The degree of pain-related anxiety and fear of pain are both considered predictors of how people will adjust to chronic pain conditions. Helplessness, a concept borrowed from learned helplessness theory, has been described in the chronic pain population. Patients with greater evidence of helplessness were more likely to discontinue attempts to manage their pain.

Factors associated with decreased pain, psychological distress and physical disability include issues such as "self-efficacy, pain coping strategies, readiness to change and acceptance of the pain" (Keefe, Rumble, Scipio, Giordano, & Perri, 2004, p. 196). Self-efficacy is defined as "a person's confidence in their ability to engage in a course of action sufficient to accomplish a desired outcome, such as control of his or her pain" (Bandura, 1997). Improvements in self-efficacy may result in improvements in pain coping and pain severity ratings, since confidence in one's ability to deal with the situation can improve the situation.

Chronic pain programs have utilized cognitive-behavioral therapy techniques to improve self-efficacy, and expand or increase individual coping strategies and acceptance of pain. With chronic pain, some patients become all consumed with unsuccessful efforts to manage their pain to the point where they neglect all other aspects of their lives. There are times when acceptance of the pain is an important requisite for the patient to reconnect with the neglected aspects of life, despite the pain.

Jerome Groopman, a physician and author, described his own problems following back surgery that left him in agony:

> My world fell apart. Because of the relentless pain, I couldn't work, I couldn't move, I could hardly think. And after two months, despite steroids and pain medication, there was no indication I would ever walk again free of pain . . . I became despondent. I wouldn't say depressed, because that's a clinical term. I was convinced that this would be my life, that I would spend the rest of my days incapacitated, in pain, unproductive. I began to lose hope . . .
>
> I still had my will. I still could decide which path to take. It was just an illusion that all choice in life had been taken from me . . . It took years, literally years . . . I relearned how to do simple things in ways that didn't set off pain . . . I had surrendered to bitterness and despair, believing I had lost my life. That doesn't have to be. Even in the most extreme circumstances, we can still make choices.
>
> (Groopman, 1997, pp. 189–191)

Chronic Pain and Addictive Disorders

Over the past two decades, the use of opioid treatment has become an accepted practice in pain management for those with chronic pain. For many patients, opioid treatment results in a lessening of pain and improvement in function. However, there are risks involved in long-term treatment with opioids including addiction, diversion, respiratory concerns, and loss of efficacy of the medications due to tolerance. Several studies have examined the problem of addiction and chronic pain, and screening tools have been developed to identify those with chronic pain who might be at risk of developing what has been referred to as "aberrant behaviors" (Compton, Darakjian, & Miotto, 1998; Passik, *et al.*, 2000). Issues such as selling drugs, prescription forgery, stealing, and injecting oral drugs are some of the behaviors that may predict a problem with addiction.

Pain is evident among patients who also have an existing addictive disorder. People with addictive disorders have more health problems, more psychiatric problems, and use more prescription and nonprescription drugs than their non-addicted counterparts.

Breitbart *et al.* (1997) compared people with a substance abuse problem with people without a substance abuse problem in a sample of HIV-infected patients. They found that those with a substance abuse problem had no significant differences in pain report, but that those with a substance abuse problem received significantly less pain medication for treatment of pain. The American Society of Pain Management Nurses (ASPMN) in a Position Statement on Pain Management in Patients with Addictive Disease stated "Too often a patient's request for more or different medications is erroneously assumed to be addiction, and the possibility of under-treated pain is not explored (2003, p. 2).

Psychosocial Functioning and Chronic Pain

Two additional issues that affect patients with chronic pain, and interventions for managing the pain, are sleep difficulties and post-traumatic stress disorder. Over 70% of chronic pain patients have reported sleep difficulties. The effects of sleep difficulties on quality of life and coping mechanisms can be severe. Sleep disruption among chronic pain patients can result in excessive daytime sleepiness, lack of concentration, drowsiness, and an inability to work and engage in other social activities (Argoff, 2007; NIH, 1996).

A meta-analysis of research related to childhood neglect, sexual or physical abuse history, and pain revealed that those who experienced neglect or abuse in childhood were more likely to experience pain as adults than those who were not abused or neglected (Davis, Luecken, & Zautra, 2005). Additionally, research revealed that patients with chronic pain are more likely to report a history of abuse than healthy individuals. The authors discussed the fact that a moderate relationship between childhood abuse and pain seems to exist but that there are many questions about the nature of the relationship. Age of abuse, gender, impact of any current distress, type of abuse or neglect, and reliance on self-report methods rather than documented abuse were presented as areas for further research (Davis, Luecken, & Zautra, 2005; Everett & Gallop, 2001). These studies highlight the additional support that may be needed when treating people with an abuse history and pain. Referral to a psychiatric provider for supportive therapy should be considered when caring for this population in a primary care setting.

Assessment Issues

Considering all the co-morbid psychiatric disorders that may coexist with chronic pain, the need for a thorough psychiatric evaluation is essential. Inpatient settings, particularly large teaching hospitals, may have a pain consultation service and/or psychiatric consultation, but smaller community hospitals and nursing homes rarely will have this kind of service readily available. Only since 2000 has JCAHO, the accrediting body for most U.S. hospitals, required documentation of pain assessment and reassessment. The need for assessment of the co-morbid psychiatric conditions is not currently a focus of the JCAHO review of pain assessment. Additionally, there have been few studies of the prevalence of pain in a population with chronic psychiatric problems.

With the increased co-morbid physical conditions among people with chronic mental illness, an examination of the problem of pain in this population becomes an important issue. Primary care providers should include a thorough pain assessment as part of the routine physical assessment. Assessment for the problems of depression, anxiety, and addictive disorders and sleep difficulties as related to chronic pain should be included as part of the physical assessment since these symptoms may not be related to the specific psychiatric disorder, but may occur in the context of the pain.

CASE EXAMPLE: PAIN AND COMPLEX MEDICAL AND PSYCHIATRIC ISSUES

Danielle is a 40-year-old divorced, Caucasian mother of three adult children, currently living with her lesbian partner of eight years. She presents for a physical exam with a new provider and has a chief complaint of insomnia, fatigue, and dyspnea on exertion (DOE). She has been sleeping two to three hours/night for the past seven to eight weeks; she was recently treated with antibiotics for an upper respiratory infection (URI).

PMH: COPD, obese, smokes despite recommendation to stop and requirement for oxygen (compliance questionable). Poorly controlled DM (has been referred to dietician), bilateral knee pain. Also has mental health issues—diagnoses include major depressive disorder, recurrent, severe with psychotic symptoms; poly-substance abuse, remission ×10 years; borderline personality disorder.

Medications:
  Effexor XR 150mg BID
  Invega 6mg daily
  Klonopin 0.5mg BID
  Wellbutrin 300mg daily
  Claritin 10mg daily
  Depo-provera 150mg q 3mths
  ASA 81mg daily
  Glucatrol 10mg daily
  Lipitor 80mg daily
  Nexium 40mg daily
  Novolin 70/30 q am and q 5pm
  Synthroid 137mcg daily
CPE—obese woman in respiratory distress, not wearing her 2L O2.
Random glucose 195 (2pm visit)
Moves slowly and purposefully
Alert and oriented ×3

Use of the CMHA tool described in Chapter 2 would provide a holistic functional assessment of Danielle. In the initial interview Danielle rates her physical health (item #1) as a 4 or poor, self-esteem (item #2) as a 4 or poor and problem solving ability (item #9) as a 4 or poor. Additionally she rates her comfort with her feelings (item #12) as 5 or always uncomfortable. She acknowledges a past history of physical and sexual abuse when item #13 is introduced but says that there has been no abuse in the last 20 years and that she has no contact with her abuser (item #19). She also acknowledges occasional thoughts of taking all of her medications at once when her pain is really bad, but says that she does not want to die and rates item #14 (self-harm or injury) as a 2 or mild risk. Her substance abuse is in the past and she has been sober for 10 years and she rates item #16 (substance use) as 1 or never. Finally, she rates item #5 (intimacy) as a 3, i.e., sometimes, indicating that she can sometimes rely on her partner when she is upset.

Danielle's problems demonstrate the interplay of medical and psychiatric issues and pain. She and her provider would agree that her physical health is poor. Her poor self-esteem and problem solving ability are evident in her difficulty managing her multiple physical problems such as her obesity, diabetes, and smoking despite her COPD. Her bilateral knee pain complicates her diabetes and depression in that her inability to walk and exercise may contribute to the course of both of these diseases, yet there is no indication that she is receiving any help with the pain. Her poor self-esteem also contributes to a sense of hopelessness that she can make changes in her life that might improve her general health.

The confounding issues of a history of poly-substance abuse and borderline personality disorder indicate ineffective or maladaptive coping mechanisms that also complicate care and may put her at risk for a relapse on substances and/or worsening depression if she does not receive some assistance in coping with the complex problems. A history of physical and sexual abuse is common in patients who have received a diagnosis of borderline personality disorder, and difficulty with feelings, family turmoil, and occupational problems are common. Often providers react negatively to people who have diagnoses of either substance abuse or borderline personality disorder and often do not do a thorough pain assessment and therefore do not treat pain appropriately, if at all. The stigma related to these particular diagnoses also often results in distancing on the part of providers and a lack of recognition or attention to patient complaints.

Danielle has a profound lack of sleep by her report (two to three hrs/night for seven to eight weeks) and has pain that she rated as a 7/8 on a 0–10 scale. She rated herself as a mild risk for self-harm, but careful questioning after review of her own CMHA scores reveal that at night, when she is unable to sleep and her pain is at its worst, she has more serious thoughts of taking all her medications. She also says that her partner is unaware of this even though she is usually willing to talk to her about her feelings when she feels this badly. The primary care provider is quite concerned at this point in the evaluation and is looking for some guidance in how to evaluate Danielle's risk for self-harm and/or suicide and is not even sure that she can provide physical care to someone with so many problems.

It can be very frustrating for any provider who is faced with a patient like Danielle with many co-morbid medical and psychiatric problems; even knowing where to begin the treatment is a challenge. Danielle's difficulty establishing a relationship with a provider, her history of non-adherence to treatment plans (i.e., weight loss, diabetes care, and smoking cessation) may seem to be insurmountable obstacles in this situation. The frustration that primary care providers feel may keep them from asking the appropriate questions to develop a full assessment of the problems and the care needed. Often patients like Danielle fall through the cracks, since the time to devote to the one patient is minimal in our current healthcare systems. Patients with this level of complex issues deserve compassionate, competent care. Collaboration between primary care and psychiatric providers in Danielle's care could provide both patient and providers with a way to make connections between her mental wellness and her physical wellness, including her pain, which would improve her overall health in the long term.

Early Intervention

Often patients who are referred for pain management and/or treatment of co-morbid psychiatric conditions have endured months or years of pain before they reach a pain specialist. This simple fact results in years of inadequate and at times maladaptive coping on the part of the patient. Studies have indicated that "early intervention has the potential to prevent the suffering and psychological distress associated with persistent pain (Keefe, Rumble, Scipio, Giordano, & Perri, 2004). These studies did not include people with a pre-existing psychiatric problem; when a primary care provider is caring for this population, referral to a psychiatric provider should be done early in the course of treatment. Cognitive behavioral interventions resulted in greater improvement in functioning and coping when it was delivered in those who had pain for less than six months (Keefe, Rumble, Scipio, Giordano, & Perri, 2004).

Encouraging active participation in treatment is important for the treatment of chronic pain; patients with pain need to develop coping skills that assist them over the lengthy course of their disease. A recovery model may assist in the development of a framework for treatment. Utilization of all of the patient's current coping skills and adding some new coping behaviors are necessary in the treatment of chronic pain. Letting patients know early in their care that treatment of chronic pain has to include all of our and their best efforts to achieve optimum relief is an important issue to discuss. Helping patients identify stressors that may lead to periods of increased pain is also necessary to prevent relapse of their pain condition.

Ethical Issues

All patients with pain deserve competent, compassionate pain management and respect for their individual, subjective experience. An attitude of respect for human dignity is part of the professional code of ethics for primary care providers. Seeking the perspective of the patient in pain, and advocating for that patient, is an outcome of this basic ethical duty towards patients. Patients with mental health and addictive disorders are more vulnerable to breaches of this ethical duty, and are in need of protection regarding the right to pain management.

Treatment of Pain and Co-occurring Psychiatric and Addictive Disorders

A respectful approach is of utmost concern when managing the pain of people with mental health issues and addictive disorders. Shoring up supports and resources will help enhance coping skills that improve the ability to include self-management strategies in the overall plan of care. A plan of care that spells out both provider responsibility as well as patient responsibility when managing chronic pain is the most promising. Patients engaged in their treatment rather than being passive recipients of care (most often in the form of medication, to alleviate pain), will fare better in terms of quality of life outcomes and effect on day-to-day function (see Chapter 2 on the service contract).

Lifestyle changes and alterations can include changes in activity, pacing of one's activities throughout the day, dietary changes, increased exercise or change in exercise, rest periods, utilization of massage therapy, and relaxation techniques should all be encouraged. Patient diaries charting periods of pain and activity level may assist patients in understanding what improves or worsens the pain they experience, so they can learn to include or exclude certain activities in their daily plans.

Pharmacological interventions are utilized in a manner similar to those without mental health issues in the management of pain. Use of analgesic medications, including opiates for moderate to severe pain may be indicated. Adjuvant medications such as tricyclic anti-depressant medication and anti-seizure medications may be very helpful in dealing with the depression, anxiety, and sleep difficulties that patients experience. Newer antidepressant medications have recently received FDA approval for use in diabetic neuropathy and fibromyalgia related pain syndromes and may be useful in other pain conditions as well (see Chapter 7 on depression).

For patients with addictive disorders there are additional recommendations determined by the patient's current relationship with substances. The development of a sound therapeutic relationship is the cornerstone of all treatment with this population. Honest dialogue about what can be provided is important; frank discussion about consequences of drug abuse during treatment must be included in a discussion about pain management. Development of realistic goals about pain relief is important; total relief of pain may not always be possible. A focus on pain relief to improve function in the patient's usual roles is a more realistic goal for pain management in this population. Use of toxicology screens and treatment contracts may be helpful and should be introduced in the initial discussion about pain management.

In acute pain situations where pain is expected (i.e. post-surgery) pain should be treated aggressively over the short-term period, taking into account that if the patient is addicted to opiates, tolerance for prescribed opiates will be high and dosages will need to be higher than what would be required by non-addicted patients. Opiate medication should be utilized for a specific short period of time post-operatively and tapered when the patient begins to recuperate. Patients who are in recovery from an addictive disorder should be consulted about their position on medically needed opiate medication, as many people in recovery believe that they must maintain a substance-free life even in the face of expected pain. Respect for and honoring of this decision is important in providing individualized care.

Management of chronic pain in people with addictive disorders should include a multi-disciplinary team and all of the various suggestions listed above. Use of long-acting opiates is suggested since the use of short-acting medications may provide more of a "rush" and trigger a relapse. The risk of relapse may increase in the presence of chronic pain, but untreated or under treated pain also increases the risk of relapse.

Patients who are maintained on opiate agonist therapy (OAT) such as methadone or buprenorphine maintenance will need the assistance of those providers in planning pain management care. Alford, Compton, & Samet (2006, p. 128) list four *misconceptions* that healthcare providers have about pain management and those receiving OAT:

1. The maintenance opioid agonist (methadone or buprenorphine) provides analgesia.
2. Use of opioids for analgesia may result in addiction relapse.
3. The additive effects of opioid analgesics and OAT may cause respiratory depression.
4. The pain complaint may be a manipulation to obtain opioid medications, or drug seeking, because of opioid addiction.

These misconceptions are shared by all professionals including nurses, and have the potential to negatively affect adequate pain management in those with addictive disorders.

Contact with providers who are prescribing OAT is important since routine drug screening is part of the care, and providers need to know about pain treatment. Guidelines for providing pain management to patients on methadone maintenance usually recommend that either another opiate is prescribed for managing pain, or additional methadone doses be provided for pain relief, since methadone is prescribed every six to eight hours when utilized for pain vs. once every 24 hours when utilized for opiate agonist therapy.

Pain management of patients receiving buprenorphine maintenance is more complicated and consultation with an addictionologist or psychiatrist is recommended. Alford, Compton, & Samet (2006. p. 131) have provided guidelines for treating short-term pain in this population and offer four treatment options:

1. Continue buprenorphine and add a short-acting opioid for pain.
2. Divide the doses of buprenorphine to take advantage of its analgesic effects (every 6–8 hour dosing).
3. If the patient is hospitalized discontinue buprenorphine and treat with opiates.
4. If the patient is hospitalized convert buprenorphine to methadone, and add other opiates for pain.

When the pain is resolved the methadone and opiate for pain can be discontinued and buprenorphine re-introduced. Since buprenorphine can precipitate opioid withdrawal, patients must be warned that they may experience mild withdrawal symptoms. Further research is needed regarding long-term management of pain when a patient is receiving buprenorphine maintenance therapy (see Chapter 9 on substance abuse).

Suggestions for Primary Care Providers

Patients who have chronic pain and co-morbid psychiatric conditions are best cared for by an interdisciplinary treatment team, including psychiatric advanced practice nurses (CNS/ NPs). Assessment of psychiatric disorders and help with enhancement of coping skills are areas where psychiatric CNS/NPs can play a vital role in the treatment of chronic pain. Advanced practice psychiatric nurses who manage patients whose illnesses affect the mind, body and spirit are in a unique position to identify, assess, and assist in the management of those with chronic pain and co-morbid psychiatric issues. Psychiatric nurses have initiated programs that address the wellness of chronic psychiatric patients; these programs could benefit from the inclusion of content related to pain management.

Conclusion

A number of psychiatric co-morbid conditions are associated with the adjustment to, and management of chronic painful conditions. Psychological interventions can decrease pain severity and improve functioning of those with chronic pain conditions. Early intervention in the course of the disease is an important issue in prevention of suffering and the development of inadequate or maladaptive coping behaviors. Primary care providers are in a unique position to address the intertwined medical and mental health facets of treating patients with acute or chronic pain. They can do this most effectively by establishing clear and stable interdisciplinary relationships with psychiatric professionals. Enhancing knowledge about the effect of co-morbid psychiatric disorders on pain treatment outcomes can facilitate the success of interdisciplinary care and treatment of those with complex co-occurring physical, psychiatric, addictive, and pain disorders.

References

Alford, D. P., Compton, P., & Samet, J. H. (2006). Acute pain management for patients receiving maintenance methadone or buprenorphine therapy. *Annals of Internal Medicine, 144*(2), 127–134.

American Pain Society (APS). (1992). *Principles of analgesic use in the treatment of acute and cancer pain* (Ed. 3). Glenview, IL: APS.

American Psychiatric Association (APA). (2000). *Diagnostic and statistical manual of mental disorders* (4th Ed.) text revision DSM-IV-TR. Washington, DC: American Psychiatric Association.

American Society of Pain Management Nurses. (2003). *ASPMN position statement: Pain management in patients with addictive disease.* Pensacola, FL: American Society of Pain Management Nurses.

Argoff, C. E. (2007). The coexistence of neuropathic pain, sleep, and psychiatric disorders: A novel treatment approach. *Clinical Journal of Pain, 23*(1), 15–22.

Bair, M. J., Robinson, R. L., Katon, W., & Kroneke, K. (2003). Depression and pain comorbidity: A literature review. *Archives of Internal Medicine, 163,* 2433–2445.

Bandura, A. (1997). *Self-efficacy: The exercise of control.* New York: W.H. Freeman.

Breitbart, W., Rosenfeld, B., Passik, S., Kaim, M., Funesti-Esch, J., & Stein, K. (1997). A comparison of pain report and adequacy of analgesic therapy in ambulatory AIDS patients with and without a history of substance abuse. *Pain, 72,* 235–243.

Cassell, E. J. (1982). The nature of suffering and the goals of medicine. *New England Journal of Medicine, 306,* 639–645.

Compton, P., Darakjian, J., Miotto, K. (1998). Screening for addiction in patients with chronic pain and "problematic" substance use: Evaluation of a pilot assessment tool. *Journal of Pain and Symptom Management, 16,* 355–363.

Davis, D. A., Luecken, L. J., & Zautra, A. J. (2005). Are reports of childhood abuse related to the experience of chronic pain in adulthood? A meta-analytic review of the literature. *Clinical Journal of Pain, 21*(5), 398–405.

Everett, B., & Gallop, R. (2001). *The link between childhood trauma and mental illness*. Thousand Oaks, CA: Sage.

Ferrell, B. R., & Coyle, N. (2008). *The nature of suffering and the goals of nursing*. Oxford: Oxford University Press.

Fishbain, D. A. (1999). The association of chronic pain and suicide. *Seminars in Clinical Neuropsychiatry*, 4(3), 221–227.

Fishbain, D., Cutler, R., & Solomon, H. (1998). Co-morbid psychiatric disorders in chronic pain patients with psychoactive substance abuse disorders. *Pain Clinics*, 11, 79–87.

Groopman, J. (1997). *The measure of our days: New beginnings at life's end*. New York: Viking.

Keefe, F. J., Rumble, M. E., Scipio, C. D., Giordano, L. A., & Perri, L. M. (2004). Psychological aspects of persistent pain: Current state of the science. *The Journal of Pain*, 5(4), 195–211.

Mayou, R., Kirmayer, L. J., Simon, G., Kronenke, K., & Sharpe, M. (2005). Somatoform disorders: Time for a new approach in DSM V. *American Journal of Psychiatry*, 162(5), 817 855.

McCaffery, M. (1968). *Nursing practice theories related to cognition, bodily pain, and environment interactions*. Los Angeles, CA: University of California at Los Angeles Students' Store.

McCaffery, M. & Pasero, C. (1999). *Pain: Clinical manual*. St. Louis, MO: Mosby.

National Institute of Health (NIH) (1996). NIH technology assessment panel on integration of behavioral and relaxation approaches into the treatment of chronic pain and insomnia. Integration of behavioral and relaxation approaches into the treatment of chronic pain and insomnia. *Journal of the American Medical Association*, 276, 313–318.

Passik, S. D., Kirsh, K. L., McDonald, M. V., Ahn, S., Russak, S. M., Martin, L., Rosenfeld,, B., Breitbart, W. S. & Portenoy, R. K. (2000). A pilot survey of aberrant drug-taking attitudes and behaviors in samples of cancer and AIDS patients. *Journal of Pain and Symptom Management*, 9(4), 274–286.

Weisman, D. E. & Haddox, J. D. (1989). Opioid pseudoaddiction: An iatrogenic syndrome. *Pain*, 36, 363–366.

11 Children, Adolescents, and Family Issues

With Valerie Grdisa

- Our Children: Primary Care and Mental Health
- DSM-IV Categories of Mental Disorders of Children
- Understanding Co-occurring Substance Use and Mental Disorders in Children and Youth
- Mental Health Assessment of Children in Primary Care
- Biology of the Brain: How It Relates to Thoughts, Feelings, and Behaviors
- Psychotropic Drug Treatment for Children
- Primary Care Integrating with Other Sectors
- Child Protection
- Summary
- References

The Committee is deeply concerned about the capability of the mental health system to respond to the needs of children and youth. Fragmentation, coupled with under-funding, a shortage of mental health professionals, and a failure to involve younger people, and their families in long-term treatment solutions, has resulted in delayed . . . treatment interventions. Simply put, this is unacceptable. A much greater investment in children's mental health is required if it is to shed its label as the "orphan's orphan" within the healthcare system.

(Kirby & Keon, 2006, p. 6.6).

This conclusion resonates around the world and requires strategic action; the mental health of our children represents the overall health and well-being of our society and its future. Although epidemiological research indicates that one in four or 25% of North American children (0–19 years) experience clinically significant mental illness or complex psychosocial issues (U.S. Department of Health and Human Services, 1999; Waddell, Hua, Garland, Peters, & McEwan, 2007), this chapter will demonstrate the importance of focusing on functional status as opposed to psychiatric diagnosis when responding to children's needs in primary care. It builds upon the principles introduced in Chapter 2 regarding multiple assessment approaches to identify individual and family strengths and promote optimal functioning. The leap to formulating a psychiatric diagnosis with psychopharmacological treatment (especially as primary intervention) for children should always be scrutinized regardless of practice specialty: primary care, pediatrics, or child psychiatry/mental health.

This chapter identifies strategies to meet the needs of children and their families affected by mental health concerns, psychosocial stress, or trauma. Opportunities for service integration with available pediatric or specialized mental health services are also explored. New conceptualizations will complement the four interactive perspectives of psychiatry: (1) disease, (2) dimensional, (3) behavioral, and (4) life story, to assist the PCP to assess and formulate why a child's psychological functioning is compromised or vulnerable (McHugh, 2001). The chapter summarizes common mental disorders of childhood and adolescence based on the DSM-IV.

Several mental health screening instruments for primary care are introduced and the benefits of combining the pediatric symptom checklist with the child screening checklist are demonstrated. The biology of the brain is reviewed in relation to emotional regulation and interactive factors affecting a child's level of functioning. The use of psychopharmacology for treatment is considered in relation to other therapeutic interventions. The integral role of parents in promoting child mental health is highlighted along with the devastating effects of childhood abuse, trauma, and neglect. Finally, you will meet two children with their stories, which are commonly faced by PCPs across North America, to illustrate how important your role is in promoting their overall health and well-being.

Our Children: Primary Care and Mental Health

Who typically assesses children when they are experiencing mental health or psychosocial problems that are affecting their overall functioning? Primary care practitioners (PCPs) such as family physicians (FPs) and family nurse practitioners (FNPs), or pediatric specialists such as pediatricians or pediatric nurse practitioners (PNPs), are the first points of contact for children, rather than mental health specialists such as psychiatrists, advanced practice psychiatric nurses, social workers, or psychologists. It is therefore imperative that PCPs, including pediatric specialists, screen for mental health or psychosocial protective and risk factors at every visit.

Child mental illness is a significant public health issue which threatens the overall health and well being of the next generation by causing lifelong distress and disability (McEwan, Waddell, & Barker, 2007). There are more than 150 million pediatric visits to PCPs in the United States and remarkably, these practitioners prescribe the majority of psychopharmacology and provide counseling to children and their families regarding mental illness, behavior and emotions, and related risk factors (U.S. Department of Health and Human Services, 2000). Furthermore, the direct costs for the treatment of child mental health problems (emotional and behavioral) in the United States are estimated to be approximately $11.75 billion or $173 per child (Sturm, *et al.*, 2000; Ringel & Sturm, 2001). This estimate includes only the cost of services provided by health and mental health professionals to treat mental illness and does not take into account the complex delivery of services in the education, child welfare, and juvenile justice sectors. Throughout all sectors of child service delivery, there is a plea to further examine the human and fiscal costs of current treatment approaches and ultimately, shift human resources towards prevention and early assessment strategies.

Previous research demonstrates "significant concerns about under recognition of mental health disorders in primary care settings and poor management of psychiatric disorders even when diagnosed" (Parikh, Lin, & Lesage, 1997, p. 933). Andreyeva and Sturm (2005) conclude that although utilization of mental health services among school-age children is increasing (up to five-fold), children with the highest need, predominantly black children and children in low-income families, are increasing utilization at a much lower rate than children overall. PCPs must make a difference by delivering mental healthcare focused on children with the highest needs rather than trying to increase the overall rates of service use.

DSM-IV Categories of Mental Disorders of Children

Mental health problems are the leading health problems that "children currently face after infancy—given the number of children affected, the associated distress and impairment, the burden of untreated disorders, and the lifelong consequences" (Waddell, McEwan, Shepherd, Offord, & Hua, 2005, p. 227). The limitations of *pathologizing* children's mental health and exclusively applying DSM-IV diagnostic criteria for assessment and treatment decisions were identified in Chapter 2 and it is imperative to reiterate this notion. The brains of children are even more pliable than their adult counterparts, which require all clinicians to be prudent when labeling children with psychiatric diagnoses based on subjective reports of symptoms at a moment in time.

However, it is equally important to understand multiple perspectives and review findings from the comprehensive review of children's mental health by the Surgeon General. Box 11.1 provides the Surgeon General's summary of mental health disorders that appear in DSM-IV. Although these disorders apply across the life span, this table represents commonly diagnosed conditions in childhood and adolescence. Busy PCPs may not have extensive knowledge regarding all mental health disorders or psychosocial morbidities but every inter-action should assess for overall functioning, physical health, and mental health.

Understanding Co-occurring Substance Use and Mental Disorders in Children and Youth

Although Chapter 9 provides a detailed overview of substance abuse, addiction, and mental health, it is important to highlight the rising trend and available resources for children and youth presenting with substance use disorders (SUDs). The National Survey on Drug Use study, reported by the SAMHSA, indicates that some children are already abusing drugs by age 12 or 13, which likely means that some may begin even earlier.

Early abuse includes such drugs as tobacco, alcohol, inhalants, marijuana, and psychother-apeutic drugs. If drug abuse persists into later adolescence, abusers typically become more involved with marijuana and then advance to other illegal drugs, while continuing their abuse of tobacco and alcohol. Early initiation of drug abuse is associated with greater drug

---

BOX 11.1   Common Mental Disorders of Childhood and Adolescence Based on the DSM-IV

- Anxiety Disorders
- Attention-Deficit and Disruptive Behavior Disorders
- Autism and Other Pervasive Developmental Disorders
- Eating Disorders (e.g. anorexia nervosa)
- Elimination Disorders (e.g. enuresis, encopresis)
- Learning and Communication Disorders
- Mood Disorders (e.g. Depressive Disorders)
- Schizophrenia (or early-onset psychosis)
- Tic Disorders

involvement, whether with the same or different drugs. The pattern of abuse is associated with levels of social disapproval, perceived risk, and the availability of drugs in the community, and therefore prevention programs are critical to decreasing the incidence of SUDs in children and youth (U.S. Department of Health & Human Services, 2003). Co-occurring substance use and mental disorders in children and youth requires careful attention by PCPs, family or caregivers, and the community because the short-term and long-term outcomes are poor.

As PCPs, your assessment and screening should include questions about substance use or abuse because SUDs frequently co-occur with mental health problems such as conduct, anxiety, and depressive disorders. PCPs often report that they glance over or "skip" these questions for fear of embarrassing youth (or selves?). The risk and protective factors that contribute to mental disorders also contribute to SUDs (Jessor, 1993). The key lesson for PCPs is to recognize the inherent complexity and reciprocal causality of factors, both contextual and individual, which contribute to co-occurring conditions and develop awareness of available resources. Box 11.2 provides you with web-based resources to direct parents or caregivers, youth, or community leaders to when a child or youth is presenting in your clinic and/or you identify a trend within your community.

Although there is a significant lack of high quality evidence regarding treatments for children and youth with co-occurring conditions, there is evidence supporting the use of multisystemic therapy, ecologically based family therapy, and functional family therapy, alone and with CBT. Therefore it is essential that PCPs collaborate with dual disorders, mental health, or addictions professionals or services to ensure that our children and youth get the best possible chance for recovering from the spiral of co-occurring substance use and mental disorders.

BOX 11.2 Web-based Resources

Al-Anon / Alateen
http://www.al-anon.alateen.org

Campaign for Tobacco-Free Kids
http://www.tobaccofreekids.org/

Drug Abuse Resistance Education (DARE)
http://www.dare-america.com/

Drug Abuse
http://www.druguse.com/

National Association for Children of Alcoholics (NACoA)
http://www.nacoa.net/

Partnership for a Drug-Free America
http://www.drugfreeamerica.org/

Substance Abuse and Mental Health Services Administration
http://www.samhsa.gov

Mental Health Assessment of Children in Primary Care

As noted above, clinicians are cautioned regarding psychiatric labeling with DSM-IV diagnoses and to shift clinical practice towards the assessment of functional status using assessment tools that capture the complexity of the interactive factors affecting mental health. However, PCPs should also be aware of research revealing that half of all lifetime cases of mental illness begins by age 14 (Kessler, Chiu, Demler, Merinkangas, & Walters, 2005)—highlighting the critical role of PCPs in primary and secondary prevention. Brown and Hoff (in Chapter 2) introduce several approaches to safety and mental health assessment for diagnostic formulation. They cite the plethora of symptom-specific scales while emphasizing the impracticality of research-oriented scales in busy primary care practices.

Jessor (1993) introduced a conceptual framework (see Figure 11.1) which identifies how risk and protective factors relate to risk behaviors and outcomes for adolescents. This conceptual framework represents the complexity of the interactive factors affecting mental health and captures the essence of McHugh's multi-dimensional perspectives for assessment and diagnosis. The key lesson for PCPs is to recognize the inherent complexity and reciprocal causality of factors, both contextual and individual, contributing to the mental health or psychosocial problems that children and their families experience.

*Factors Contributing to Youth Violence**

From coast to coast, American and Canadian cities have been struggling with crime that three decades ago might have been unthinkable. From gangland killings to the senseless beating of innocent passersby, youth and random violent crime appears to be escalating. These externalizing behaviors are an outcome of many of the risk factors identified above. In the United States, behavioral specialists assert that antisocial behavior by children should be viewed as a national emergency. For example, young children who bring weapons to school today may become future school dropouts, batterers, and rapists (Ellickson, Saner, & McGuigan, 1997; Webster, Vernick, Ludwig, & Lester, 1997).

Given the cultural norms, perhaps the most surprising thing is that there is not more violence. As a paradoxical commentary on the influence (or failure?) of the women's movement, many young girls and women use their newly found "freedom" to adopt the aggressive, bullying, and violent norms of men, including arming themselves in the illusion of self-protection (Wright, Wintemute, & Rivara, 1999). The incidence of violence by teenage girls is rising (one of every four juveniles arrested is female although female rates of homicide are far behind those for boys (Chesney-Lind, 1997). While some men are discovering the pleasures and growth potential of assuming the parenting and nurturing roles traditionally dominated by women, some women choose violence. They have yet to learn from the plight of battered women that violence begets more serious violence (Hoff, 1990). In their classic work, educators and youth workers Brendtro, Brokenleg, and Van Bockern (1990, pp. 6–7), drawing on non-violent child-rearing among Native Americans, trace the discouragement and alienation of youth at risk to four ecological hazards:

1. *destructive relationships*, as experienced by the rejected or unclaimed child, hungry for love but unable to trust, expecting to be hurt again;
2. *climate of futility*, as encountered by the insecure youngster, crippled by feelings of inadequacy and a fear of failure;
3. *learned irresponsibility*, as seen in the youth whose sense of powerlessness may be masked by indifference or defiant, rebellious behavior.

---

* This section is excerpted and edited from Hoff, Hallisey, & Hoff, 2009, Chapter 12.

A CONCEPTUAL FRAMEWORK FOR ADOLESCENT RISK BEHAVIOR
Risk and Protective Factors, Risk Behaviors, Risk Outcomes

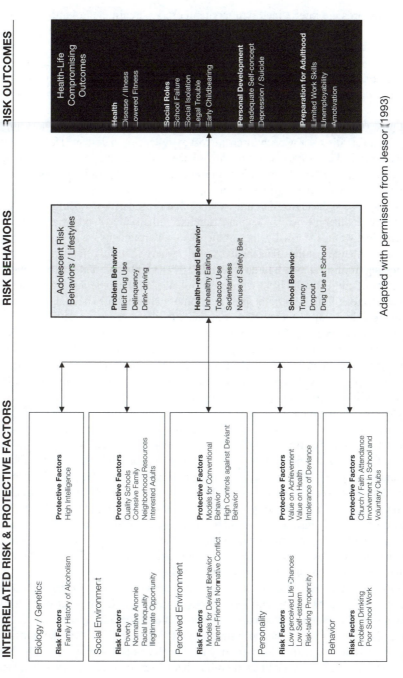

Figure 11.1 A Conceptual Framework for Adolescent Risk Behavior. Adapted with permission from Jessor (1993).

4. *loss of purpose*, as portrayed by a generation of self-centered youth, desperately searching for meaning in a world of confusing values and a culture of immediate gratification and individualism.

These hazards are intertwined with contemporary parenting and family life—among poor families, inadequate time and resources for effective parenting; among some privileged families, excessive material indulgence and permissiveness that leave a child with few boundaries and skills to control behavior, and a vacuum around life's larger meaning beyond consumerism. In the United States, in view of such factors as racism, the powerful gun lobby, and the plight of mothers who are raising children alone in an inequitable labor market, not only must "teachers, parents, and peers" (Walker, 1993, p. 23) influence antisocial children, but policymakers, church leaders, and all who care about the future of humanity must look "upstream" to discover why children are lost to violence and despair (Holinger, Offer, Barter, & Bell, 1994; West, 1994). In a study of violence and recurrent trauma among young African-American men, Rich and Grey (2005) present a model with positive prospects of interrupting the pathway to repeated injuries by violence.

In response to the crisis of youth violence that is primarily sociocultural in origin, will we invent yet another medicalized explanation like "urban stress syndrome" to excuse assailants and neglect victims? Or will we examine social environments we have created or allowed to fester as a plague that threatens the lives of all? Many youthful offenders have had no support in healing from childhood trauma (Mendel, 1994). Our homes and schools have many untold numbers of children who have witnessed violence. Will people make a connection between values (Eyre & Eyre, 1993), the proliferation of guns, and the shocking increase of children killing children—and others? This is not an either/or dichotomy. Mitigating circumstances must be considered in judging individual cases, but excusing violent action does nothing to facilitate the growth and resiliency that distressed people, including alienated youth, are capable of when supported through crisis. Previous victimization—by peers and/or parents— are strong predictors of youth violence. As in all cases of victimization and violence, we are *influenced* by our past, not *determined* by it!

Clearly, youth violence cuts across class, race, and gender boundaries. Despite continued disparity in educational and other resources between racial minority groups and the white majority, it is noteworthy that in the vast majority of recent school shooting tragedies, the assailants were white boys from a range of socioeconomic classes. These highly publicized instances of youth violence tend to obscure the statistical decline in youth crime rates, including school-based violence, over the past several years. But non-statistical examination of these dramatic examples of youth violence reveals the complexity of factors influencing each case; in many instances, social alienation, bullying and harassment by classmates, and mental health problems were evident but not attended to with preventive measures such as recognizing and responding to the meaning of supposedly "idle" verbal threats or unusual behaviors, and collaborating with pediatric PCPs.

Protective factors aiding in child resilience include extended family support networks, family connectedness, and family religious beliefs. Another protective factor is fostering a school and community that cares for and values all children, sets high expectations for all, and invites active school and community participation. Together, these factors can assist alienated youth to change the path they are on. But as frightening as youth aggression and violence can be, it is crucial to remember that *violence begets violence* (Carlsson-Paige & Levin, 2008). The greater challenge, then, is in the primary prevention domain of changing the socioeconomic and other factors—including a cultural climate glorifying violence— that severely shortchange young people, a nation's most precious resource. Youth violence is a widespread public health problem and research demonstrates that PCPs infrequently document any discussion of violence-related issues, specifically in youth who are demonstrating risk (Sigel, 2009). Practitioners need a better way to identify youth who are involved with violent behavior. Externalizing behaviors resulting in youth violence must be captured in mental health screening in primary care.

Importance of Relationship with Parents

PCPs including pediatric specialists need to recognize that they provide the bulk of child mental health services because parents or guardians prefer to bring their children to their *trusted* PCPs rather than mental health specialists. However, the sheer nature of PCPs' practice impedes the delivery of effective and age-appropriate mental healthcare, with the average length of a visit ranging between 11 and 15 minutes (U.S. Department of Health and Human Services, 2000). Another challenge is the disparity between parent and PCP's perceptions of emotional or behavioral problems. Box 11.3 includes a summary of interesting trends in primary care, which PCPs should monitor in relation to their own practice (U.S. Department of Health and Human Services, 2000).

PCPs have an opportunity to collaborate with parents and provide resources to assist children and parents coping with mental health concerns. Several strategies are recommended for PCPs and policymakers to address the identified trends, service gaps, and system barriers in Box 11.3. These efforts will address parental concerns as identified by lobbying group, Parents for Children's Mental Health (2008, p. 1): "Funding for children's mental health services is inadequate. There is no law that says children have the right to mental health services. There are long wait lists for services/supports. Families are overwhelmed/at the breaking point."

Since the PCP is often the preferred and most appropriate human health resource for children or their families to access, it is essential that PCPs have access to nationally recognized publications that provide accurate and evidence-based information for this susceptible population. The National Institute of Mental Health (2009) has recently published a question

---

BOX 11.3 Research Findings or Trends in Primary Care and Children's Mental Health

- Primary care physicians report that 19% of children have behavioral or emotional problems.
- Rates of recognition (48–57%) of these mental health problems remain low.
- Parents have significantly different perception of severity of behavioral or emotional problems.
- Girls (all ages) and younger children are less likely to be identified with mental health issues.
- Referral rates to specialty mental health services are similar for children of all ethnicities, however African and Hispanic American children have less accessibility to these services.
- African and Hispanic American children are less likely to be prescribed psychopharmacology.
- Primary care physicians primarily refer children with behavior problems to child psychologists.
- Average wait times from PCPs referral to specialty appointment is 3–4 months and approximately 60% children never visit the mental health specialist.
- Significant barriers to specialty services include: lack of available specialists, insurance restrictions, and lengthy wait times/lists.

and answer handbook regarding the Treatment of Children with Mental Illness which can be downloaded from the link: http://www.nimh.nih.gov/health/publications/treatment-of-children-with-mental-illness-fact-sheet/index.shtml (accessed on 17 July 2010). Also, the United States Department of Health and Human Services (USDHHS)—Substance Abuse and Mental Health Services Administration (SAMHSA) provides a comprehensive range of publications, quick fact sheets, and helpful clinical tools to assist PCPs in managing questions, problems orconcerns from children or their families at link: http://mentalhealth.samhsa.gov/publications/Publications_browse.asp?ID=14&Topic=Children+and+Families(accessed on July 6, 2010).

For example, a printable version of the *Twelve Questions Every Parent Should Ask* tool could be administered within your practice:

BOX 11.4 Twelve Questions Every Parent Should Ask

Does my child:

1. Often seem sad, tired, restless, or out of sorts?
2. Spend a lot of time alone?
3. Have low self-esteem?
4. Have trouble getting along with family, friends, and peers?
5. Have frequent outbursts of shouting, complaining, or crying?
6. Have trouble performing or behaving in school?
7. Show sudden changes in eating patterns?
8. Sleep too much or not enough?
9. Have trouble paying attention or concentrating on tasks like homework?
10. Seem to have lost interest in hobbies like music or sports?
11. Show signs of using drugs and/or alcohol?
12. Talk about death or suicide?

If you answered yes to four or more of these questions, and these behaviors last longer than two weeks, you should seek professional help for your child.

(Go to link: http://mentalhealth.samhsa.gov/publications/allpubs/fastfact1/default.asp (accessed on July 6, 2010), U.S. Department of Health & Human Services, 2008b).

Parents with Mental Illness and their Families

Tragic events involving parents or caregivers with mental illness inflicting violence upon their children is too often a frontline news story around the globe. Data from the National Comorbidity Survey (NCS) indicates that 65% of American women and 52% of American men diagnosed with mental illness are parents. Custody loss rates for parents with mental illness are astonishingly high at 70% to 80%. Two decades of research examining how parents with mental illness affect child outcomes demonstrates how risk and protective factors can enhance resilience or confer risk upon these children. SAMHSA has highlighted key findings:

- Rates of child psychiatric diagnosis among offspring range from 30–50% compared with an estimated rate of 20% among the general child population.

- Children may show developmental delays, lower academic competence, and difficulty with social relationships.
- Mediators or mechanisms relating parental mental illness to child outcomes include biopsychosocial risk factors such as illness characteristics, marital relationships, and family functioning.
- Moderators that can enhance or worsen child outcomes include socioeconomic stressors such as poverty, child characteristics, and therapeutic interventions.

(Nicholson, Biebel, Hinden, Henry, & Stier, 2001)

PCPs are uniquely positioned to assess and monitor the impact of parental mental illness on child functioning and to leverage the protective factors by regular mental health screening and collaborating with other associated providers.

Mental Health Screening in Primary Care

Although parents or guardians are central figures in their child's life and provide crucial insights regarding overall functioning, regular mental health screening from the child's perspective is fundamental to primary care/pediatric practice. Hoff, Hallisey, & Hoff (2009, pp. 104–105) have developed a Child Screening Checklist, which supplements the Comprehensive Mental Health Assessment Tool (CMHA) and focuses on the developmental concerns of children under seven domains: (1) family relationships; (2) school; (3) peer relationships (4) dissocial behavioral; (5) personal adjustment; (6) emotional; and (7) medical and developmental. Utilization of both tools provides PCPs with efficient, evidence-based assessment scales to capture the interactive factors contributing to the child's level of functioning.

The Keep Your Children/Yourself Safe and Secure (KySS) national program has the mandate "to promote the mental health of children and adolescents through the integration of mental health promotion, screening, and early evidence-based interventions" (NAPNP, 2008). NAPNP developed the KySS mental health guide which is an excellent resource for PCPs and PNPs to enhance their knowledge and skills to screen for and intervene early in the treatment of common mental health problems in children and teens (Melnyk & Moldenhauer, 2008). A myriad of diagnosis-specific scales exist in the field of child psychiatry (e.g. suicide, depression, and substance abuse scales) which require specialized training, and PCPs are encouraged to collaborate with mental health specialists or services to discern their appropriateness or applicability within primary care.

Since the average primary care or pediatric visit ranges between 11 and 15 minutes, there are additional noteworthy valid and reliable screening instruments to identify or monitor children who are at risk for mental health problems in primary care settings (see Table 11.1). All the table's screening instruments capture interactive factors contributing to level of functioning except for the Guidelines for Adolescent Preventative Services (GAPS) scales which specifically focus on screening for risk of depression or suicide. PCPs or interprofessional primary care teams are recommended to review available screening instruments for parents or children and determine their appropriateness or applicability within primary care practice. For example, the parent completes the Twelve Questions Every Parent Should Ask questionnaire and the child completes the Pediatric Symptom Checklist in the waiting room and these two tools are quickly reviewed by the PCP before initiating the mental health assessment. During the interview, the PCP uses the Child Screening Checklist to structure the interactive factors contributing to the child's level of functioning.

Table 11.1 Mental Health Screening Instruments for Primary Care

Instrument & Author	Scale Design	Practicability
Child & Adolescent Functional Assessment Scale (CAFAS) Hodges, 2008	24 items Age: 6–17 years Trained clinician uses scale	Scoring by provider takes 10 minutes Purchased via CAFAS website: http://www.cafas.com/
Child Screening Checklist Hoff, Hallisey, & Hoff, 2009	7 domains Age: 0–17 years Trained clinician uses scale	Scoring by provider takes <5 minutes Available via textbook: *People in crisis: Clinical and diversity perspectives* (Hoff, Hallisey, & Hoff, 2009)
Guidelines for Adolescent Preventative Services (GAPS) American Medical Association, 1994	Three sequential scales Age: 11–21 years Youth, parent or guardian forms	Practitioner administers via series of questions Free and public access via American Medical Association website: http://www.ama-assn.org/ama/pub/category/18112.html
Keep Your Children/ Yourself Safe and Secure (KySS) scales Melnyk, 2008	60 items 5-point scale Age: 10–20 years 13 items scale for youth/parents	Self-administered in <10 minutes Paper or e-version scale available Obtained through application with National Association of Pediatric Nurse Practitioners website: www.napnap.org
Parent Evaluation of Developmental Status (PEDS) Glascoe, 2008	10 items focused on < 8 years old Parent report	Self-administered in 2 minutes Paper or e-version scale available Purchased via PEDS website: http://www.pedstest.com/ Self-administered via internet for fee: http://www.forepath.org/
Pediatric symptom checklist (PSC) Jellinek, 2002	35 items 3-point scale Age: 4–16 years Parent report Youth self-report	Self-administered in <5 minutes Free and public access via website (Bright Futures) http://www.brightfutures.org/mentalhealth/pdf/professionals/ped_sympton_chklst.pdf

CASE EXAMPLE: MEET MICHELLE

Please read this case study and identify the interactive factors.

Michelle is a 13-year-old girl who is living in a small rural community and has just finished the seventh grade. Michelle has difficulty making friends and is often a victim of bullying or teasing. Michelle reports that she has been having difficulties for approximately two years (depressed mood, worries, decline in academic performance) and her greatest difficulty is low self-esteem. Michelle reports that she "worries all the time about": (1) people breaking into her house; (2) family members dying; (3) concerns about money; and (4) not performing well in school. Michelle has difficulty falling asleep due to these worries and she reports being very tired by the middle of the day. Michelle regularly meets with the district social worker (two years) related to coping with bullying and her low self-esteem.

Michelle denies history of substance or alcohol use and no addictions. Michelle's medical history is insignificant; she has presented with fine and gross motor incoordination. Due to Michelle's significant decline in academic functioning, she has been identified for a psychoeducational assessment to rule out a learning disorder. This is Michelle's first primary care assessment regarding her mental health status and overall functioning. Michelle completed the PSC scale and her score was 26, which indicates mild to moderate functional impairment.

There is a history of depression on maternal side of family, including maternal grandmother and mother (since age 21). Mother is currently prescribed anti-depressants and is on a leave of absence from accountant position for treatment of alcoholism (two-year history) at a local women's centre. Child Welfare has completed an in-home assessment due to mother's alcohol abuse and continues to monitor the family. Both Michelle and her mother describe father as highly anxious with an awkward presentation, but his psychiatric history is unknown. Michelle's parents are divorced and she lives with mother and brother (nine year old). Both Michelle and her mother concur that her brother is oblivious to the family stressors. Michelle visits with father every other weekend and her father is described as under employed (i.e. works as seasonal worker such as snow removal). Within past year, there have been three significant deaths on paternal side: paternal grandmother and two paternal aunts due to different cancers. Michelle reports being central to supporting her father through these losses and that these "adult" pressures were difficult to manage.

Responding to the Life Story of Michelle

Michelle represents a typical child that arrives at our practices with very complex worlds and intricate stories, which reveal their strengths and potential risks if prevention and early intervention is delayed. Regardless of the assessment tools used by the clinician, this case example reveals multiple interactive factors contributing to her decline in functioning. As a practitioner, how does one respond to this complex life story within the 15-minute *sound bite* that is typical of most practices?

Combining a self-administered screening tool such as the pediatric symptom checklist (PSC) with the Child Screening Checklist allows the PCPs to objectively verify the perspective of the youth or parent and combine these results with the seven domain framework (i.e. interactive factors). These tools enable the PCP to efficiently organize one's thoughts regarding the concerns, problems, and strengths presented by the child and/or parents, and to immediately intervene within the appointment with a summary of the interactive factors, observed strengths, and strategies in response to the child's concerns. This approach will address many of the dimensional, behavioral, and life story perspectives (McHugh, 2001) but how does the disease perspective get addressed? Within my practice, I have implemented a very quick and effective intervention that focuses on the biology of the brain as it relates to mental health: our thoughts, feelings and behaviors within the context of the child's story.

Biology of the Brain: How It Relates to Thoughts, Feelings, and Behaviors

Lewis (2008) demonstrates how the neural underpinnings of emotion in normal and clinically referred children are a biological aspect of the child that must be understood and incorporated into treatment planning. For every child and their respective family that access my care, the biology of the brain is reviewed as it relates to the interactive factors, which are affecting the child's level of functioning. This process involves the use of a whiteboard and four different color markers following the initial assessment and determination of the interactive factors and child's strengths.

The process flows in this sequence:

1. "Michelle and mom, did you know that how our brain manages our emotions and our thinking is very complex, especially when an individual is facing all of the challenges

you shared today. Let me show you how the brain communicates between different centers of the brain." The outer skull is drawn in *black marker* and then the brain stem or primitive brain is drawn with it extending to the lungs and heart. "Your primitive brain is the vital part of the brain that keeps the heart and lungs doing their job. As humans evolved, the next section of the brain is the one responsible for our drives."

2.   The limbic center or "emotion" center of the brain is drawn on top of the primitive brain in *red marker*. "Michelle, this is the part of your brain where all your feelings are managed, so when you are coping with big issues such as the loss of your grandmother and aunts, this part of your brain is trying to do its best to deal with this stress. Diagnostic imaging studies that record the brain's activity when there are changes in emotions like anger, grief or sadness show that this part of the brain is very active (i.e. color area with red) when a human is dealing with a lot of stress."

3.   The amygdala or "memory" center is drawn in *green marker* and we discuss how the amygdala attaches emotional significance to stimuli automatically based on memory and experience. "So when you are facing three deaths in the family in less than a year, your memory center communicates with your emotion center. Many of the worries that you are experiencing is your brain's reaction to so many challenges at once."

4.   The neo-cortex or "thinking" center of the brain is drawn in *blue marker* and the relationship between all three centers is summarized. Again, the concept of the emotion center being "red" and very active while the thinking center is "blue." "Remarkably, there is decreased activity in the thinking center of the brain when a human is experiencing strong emotions. The blue represents the cooling effect or less activity in the thinking center of the brain while the red represents the warming effect or increased activity in the emotion center of the brain. Undoubtedly, Michelle, you have been coping with lots of worries in your life because of concerns at school, home and losses; your brain is trying to find ways to work through all of these concerns."

Within this discussion arrows are drawn to indicate how the thinking-feeling-memory centers of the brain communicate and then finally, the cognitive-behavior therapy triangle is drawn on top of the image to make reference to building on existing strengths (which are identified) or developing new strategies to cope with the interactive factors. "Although you have experienced lots of stress including worrying about both parents, you have a good relationship with the school social worker, your mom is now 'taking care of herself' and in treatment, and you have been so amazingly supportive of your dad. What could we do to remove some of the adult pressures that you describe so that you can focus on school?" Undoubtedly, this approach generates an understanding of human thoughts, feelings and behaviors as they relate to interactive factors and individual strengths. Putting words to Michelle's experience and illustrating how her brain responds to stressors enabled Michelle to bring this new way of understanding the interactive factors back to her therapeutic relationship with the school social worker.

This approach ends with acknowledging that in some circumstances the brain chemistry and structures do not adjust accordingly to the interactive factors contributing to mental illness. Therefore, medication (combined with other therapies) is required to "treat" the brain and ultimately, improve level of functioning. Furthermore, PCPs are encouraged to rule out medical conditions that may be contributing to the decline in functioning. Hedaya (1996) introduces the following rules for identifying *medical mimics:*

1.   Never assume that an emotional symptom has a psychosocial cause until physical causes (or contributors) are fully investigated.

2.   Always have your patients get a very complete physical examination if they haven't had one since their symptoms began.

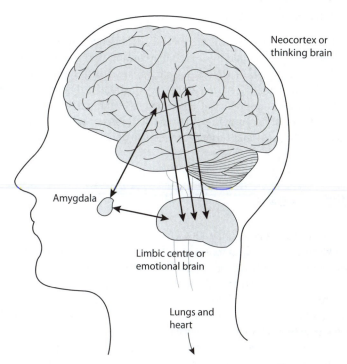

Figure 11.2 Biology of the Brain

3. Look for a history that doesn't fit.
4. Check personal and family history thoroughly.
5. Be suspicious if there is a history of recent onset of headaches, loss of function, unusual perceptions (tingling, dissociations, visual disturbances, paranormal experiences, or hallucinations—especially visual, olfactory, or tactile) or weight loss of a severe nature.
6. Drugs, drugs, drugs! Ask regarding over-the-counter or illicit substance use or abuse.

Hedaya (1996) introduces his personal mnemonic "THINC MED" which is a wonderful guide for primary care assessments of the biology of the brain. The screening assessment combined with a complete history and physical examination including pertinent laboratory tests should be performed on any child with debilitating symptoms or severe decline in functioning to rule out:

BOX 11.5 "THINC MED"

T = Tumors
H = Hormones
I = Infectious and Immune Disease
N = Nutrition
C = Central Nervous System
M = Miscellaneous
E = Electrolyte Abnormalities and Environmental Toxins
D = Drugs

The Impact of Death and Dying on Children's Mental Health

The case example with Michelle revealed that she has recently experienced the loss of several family members on the paternal side including a grandparent and two aunts. Severe life events such as death and dying (i.e. self or significant others) are precipitating factors for the diagnosis of mental illness (Duggal, *et al.*, 2000). Correspondingly, mental health assessment must carefully examine the impact of these severe events on a child's overall mental health and well-being. For children with palliative conditions or physical disability, PCPs should work collaboratively with other service providers to optimize available supports and services.

CASE EXAMPLE: MEET JEROME

Please read this case study and identify the interactive factors.

Jerome is a 14-year-old male in the eighth grade and lives in a suburban neighborhood. Jerome was discovered sending letters expressing suicidal intent to three school peers, and subsequently the principal recommended that Jerome be assessed. During Jerome's visit with his PCP provider, Jerome confirmed the following concerns: sending suicidal notes to school peers, decline in academic attendance and performance, limited peer relationships and social isolation, and escalating parental and family conflict.

Further exploration of issues with Jerome's mother reveal that two physical altercations have occurred between Jerome and his father which involved child welfare and the police. Jerome denies any substance use or alcohol use and no addictions. Jerome appeared obese and he reports a 10% weight gain in past year. No other significant developmental or medical history present except for diagnosis of ankyloglossia (i.e. tongue tie) that required a frenectomy at age five and subsequent speech therapy which was delayed to age ten (speech language deficits audible). Jerome completed the PSC scale and his score was 36, which indicates severe functional impairment that requires further evaluation by a qualified mental health practitioner.

Exploration of family psychiatric history reveals that one maternal aunt has a history of depression and a paternal cousin reportedly committed suicide due to depression. Otherwise the parents deny other psychiatric illness within family of significance. The family is of South Asian descent and immigrated from Trinidad six years ago. Initially, they moved to a small town but returned to a suburban environment due to racism as described by mother. Mother reports that they were the only South Asian family living within the small community and that both Jerome and his sister, Keera (17 years old.) were victims of bullying. Mother believes that the bullying and delay in speech therapy services was due to their ethnic background. The family practices Christian faith and have limited support networks or community involvement as most South Asians practice other faiths. Both parents are employed but mother reports that she is under-employed and her income is a common source of marital conflict.

Keera did not graduate from high school but works in the retail industry and recently discovered that she is four months pregnant. This news has contributed to increased family conflict. During the assessment, it was revealed that Jerome has had greater than 45 absences from school due to somatic complaints such as abdominal pain. The mother confirms that there is significant conflict in the family home and that the marital discord is severe and both parents are currently contemplating divorce. The mother describes that the marital discord is exacerbated by significant conflict with paternal grandmother and Keera, which Jerome regularly witnesses.

Responding to the Life Story of Jerome

In response to Jerome's story, the interactive factors and strengths are summarized in relation to the biology of the brain. However, the decline in Jerome's functional status is severe, which includes suicidal ideation, and the PSC scale verifies this. Furthermore, there are significant family relationship concerns that require immediate intervention to stabilize the family system. Within the 15 minute *soundbite,* it is important to directly emphasize with parents how these complex interactive factors may be contributing to their child's overall presentation. The assessment demonstrates that there was not an immediate concern regarding suicidal intent; however Jerome presents with several DSM-IV criteria for major depressive episode disorder.

What would you recommend at this point in the client visit? As discussed above, the NAPNP developed the KySS mental health guide for PCPs, which includes recommendations for service integration and interprofessional collaboration. Also, the AACAP provides clear guidelines to PCPS providers, pediatric specialists, psychiatrists, and non-physician mental health practitioners regarding when to access child and adolescent psychiatrists, go to: www.aacap.org/.

Undoubtedly, Jerome requires intervention, and current evidence indicates that the most effective interventions include: psychoeducation, family involvement, school involvement, cognitive behavior therapy (CBT) or interpersonal therapy (IPT), and potentially psychopharmacology (Birmaher & Brent, 2007). Although selective serotonin reuptake inhibitors (SSRIs) are recommended for children with severe depression, studies reveal that that there are no significant differences between placebo and SSRI response rate for children with mild to moderate depression (Birmaher & Brent, 2007). Other interventions such as CBT or IPT combined with family therapy and school involvement may be more effective for improving functional status. For other conditions such as anxiety disorders, both CBT and sertraline (i.e. SSRI) reduced the severity of anxiety in children and a combination of the two therapies had a superior response rate (Walkup, *et al.*, 2008).

Psychotropic Drug Treatment for Children

Every parent asks this question, "How do I know if medication is the right decision?" I answer this question with, "the prescription of medication for treating child mental illness should only occur when other treatment approaches have not resulted in an improvement in overall functioning or the child's functional status is severely limited or putting the child at increased risk of harm." It is important that PCPs conceptualize the treatment of children with psychopharmacotherapy as *a last resort.*

The mantra, "start low and go slow" applies to this population like no other because these medications were created and tested for an adult brain, not the pliable and less developed brain structure and chemistry of a child. Although there is burgeoning evidence, more data on efficacy and safety is still required. Finally, the family and child should be informed of the risks, benefits, possible side effects, or adverse effects of psychopharmacotherapy in relation to the other recommended treatment interventions.

The Federal Drug Administration Black Box Warning that accompanies SSRIs should be clearly communicated to child and family at an age-appropriate level. An explanation may include: "SSRIs are medications that adjust the brain chemistry with the goal to improve overall functioning, but during the adjustment phase (first four weeks of treatment), the antidepressants may increase the risk of suicidal thinking and behavior. Please let your PCP, mental health professionals, or providers know if you experience: worsening in depression, emergence of suicidal thinking or behavior, or unusual changes in behavior, such as sleeplessness, agitation, or withdrawal from normal social situations" (National Institute of Mental Health, 2010, p. 6). This black box warning has resulted in several comprehensive reviews of pediatric trials, and the evidence continues to demonstrate that with close monitoring, the benefits of SSRIs likely outweigh the risks, especially if combined with cognitive behavioral therapy (Bridge, *et al.*, 2007).

There are electronic practice guidelines available for PCPs from mental health specialty websites. For example, the AACAP has published 25 practice parameters that "are designed to assist clinicians in providing high quality assessment and treatment that is consistent with the best available scientific evidence and clinical consensus." (AACAP, 2008, p. 2). *As the PCP, your next step should be to collaborate with your local mental health practitioner or service to support Jerome to regain his optimal level of functioning.*

Primary Care Integrating with Other Sectors

Children's mental health concerns "permeate every aspect of development and functioning at home, at school, and in the community . . . The associated human and fiscal costs are enormous, arguably making psychiatric disorders the leading children's health problem today" (Waddell, Offord, Shepherd, Hua, & McEwan, 2002, p. 826). PCPs are central to effective and efficient service delivery as members of interprofessional teams and coordinators of intersectoral services. Furthermore, recent national and state government policy goals focus on service integration and collaboration to address fragmentation and lack of coordination. The Canadian Health Services Research Foundation (2003) warn that integration efforts for child and youth services are not necessarily driven by client needs, service utilization trends, or empirical research findings.

PCPs are encouraged to access continuing education opportunities and implement evidence-based screening and assessment approaches. Service integration strategies are highly recommended to improve collaboration between PCPs and mental health specialists or services (e.g. linking specialty services through consultation–liaison services, co-location with mental health services, or use of behavioral specialists) regarding specialized interventions for children such as psychopharmacology or psychotherapeutic interventions.

There are practical resources to assist PCPs and mental health specialists to collaborate, such as the previously mentioned NAPNP-developed KySS mental health guide for PCPs or the Collaboration Essentials for Pediatric and Child & Adolescent Psychiatry Residents project. The goal of this project is to promote collaboration between pediatricians and child psychiatrists to optimize care of children and their families and educate the next generation of pediatricians and child psychiatrists (Collaboration Essentials, 2008, p. 2). Finally, there are excellent electronic or text version drug information handbooks by publishers such as Lexi-Comp, which provide recommendations for dosing of psychopharmacology for children based on type of practitioner. These resources are essential to support medication monitoring when the child is discharged from the specialty practitioner or service back into the PCP's care.

Kelleher (U.S. Department of Health and Human Services, 2000) recommends the following policy goals to improve service integration between primary care and mental health specialists:

1. payment coordination to ensure reimbursement for behavioral services by primary care providers, care coordination, parallel incentives for managed behavioral health organizations, managed care organizations, and primary care practitioners;

2. data coordination through the Substance Abuse and Mental Health Administration (SAMHSA), Maternal and Child Health (MCH) Block grant requirements, Medicaid waiver requirements for sharing data, and state contract mandates, so that systems can track families and use reasonable case management across populations;
3. accountability standards for screens, referrals, and treatment;
4. expansion of the Early and Periodic Screening, Diagnosis, and Treatment (EPSDT) program.

Optimistically, government policy, professional motivation, and public participation will build momentum to remove barriers to commendable policy goals such as delivering services for children and youth that are coordinated, collaborative, and integrated at local, state, and federal levels. PCPs have a crucial role to play as advocates against goal displacement, to ensure the focus of policy goals remains the improvement of system, professional practice, and client outcomes.

Child Protection

The focus of this chapter has been child mental health and overall functioning. The incidence and prevalence of violence towards children around the world is staggering and within the past two decades there is burgeoning evidence of the biological effects of trauma, abuse, and neglect (Solomon & Heide, 2005). There are profound effects on several systems of brain function that include: hormonal, neural pathways, neurotransmitters, and even brain structure. Flaherty and Sege (2005) determined that 8–30% of physicians self-reported that they failed to report suspected child abuse at some time during their career.

Figure 11.3 charts the rate of child victims and children who received a disposition per 1,000 children in the national population during the years 2002–2006. The rate of all children who received a disposition increased from 43.8 per 1,000 children in 2002 to 47.8 per 1,000 children in 2006. The rate of victimization decreased from 12.3 per 1,000 children in 2002 to 12.1 per 1,000 children in 2006 (U.S. Department of Health & Human Services, 2008b). There is a direct link between trauma, abuse, and neglect in childhood and overall functioning, and therefore PCPs are uniquely positioned to identify and protect children from these devastating life experiences.

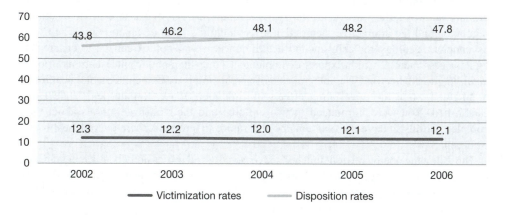

Figure 11.3 Child Disposition and Victimization Rates, 2002–2006

Source: Adapted from U.S. Department of Health & Human Services, 2008b

---

BOX 11.6 Resources for Child Protection

As busy PCPs, it is essential to access the resources that are available at your fingertips to ensure that children within your practices receive appropriate protection and advocacy:

Child Abuse and Neglect
www.childwelfare.gov/can

Defining Child Abuse and Neglect
www.childwelfare.gov/can/defining/

Laws and Policies
www.childwelfare.gov/systemwide/laws_policies/index.cfm

Preventing Child Abuse and Neglect
www.childwelfare.gov/preventing

Reporting Child Abuse and Neglect
www.childwelfare.gov/responding/reporting.cfm

Summary

This chapter identified strategies and available resources to meet the needs of children and their families affected by mental health concerns, psychosocial stress, youth violence, substance abuse, or trauma. The limitations of *pathologizing* children's mental health and exclusively applying DSM-IV diagnostic criteria for assessment and treatment decisions were reiterated, as was the importance of integrating services between primary care, pediatric, and specialty mental health services. With more than 150 million annual pediatric visits, PCPs have an opportunity to ensure that children struggling with mental health concerns, psychosocial issues, or child abuse and neglect receive appropriate screening, assessment, and treatment. Several mental health screening instruments for pediatrics in primary care were illustrated. The biology of the brain was reviewed as it relates to emotional regulation and the interactive factors that affect a child's level of functioning. The use of psychopharmacology for child mental health concerns was contextualized to ensure that PCPs access mental health experts or implement other therapeutic interventions prior to *defaulting* to medication. The integral role of parents in promoting child mental health was highlighted while the devastating effects of childhood abuse, trauma, and neglect was established. You were introduced to two children and their intricate stories about their complex worlds and your goal remains the same, to promote their overall health and well-being.

The following poem and quilt touched me personally and professionally as a mental health nurse practitioner working with children and adolescents—the faded figures within the groupings represent our children lost to suicide. May we collaborate together for our children to no longer be the "orphan's orphan" within the healthcare system.

We are children with mental illness
We have faces
We have names
We have hearts
We have feelings
We need your understandings
We need your support

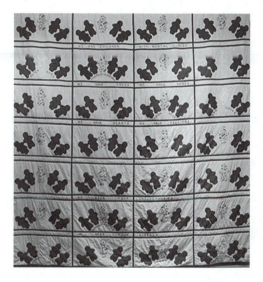

Figure 11.4 The Quilt of Honour

Source: Adapted, with permission by Parents for Children's Mental Health, 2005

References

American Academy of Child & Adolescent Psychiatry (AACAP). (2008). *Practice parameters*. http://www.aacap.org/cs/root/member_information/practice_information/practice_parameters/practice_parameters (accessed on October 5, 2008).

American Medical Association. (1994). Guidelines for Adolescent Preventative Services (GAPS). http://www.ama-assn.org/ama/pub/category/18112.html (accessed on October 2, 2008).

Andreyeva T., & Sturm R. (2005). *Changes in children's mental health care, 1997–2002* (abstract # 3160). Paper presented at meet of the Academy Health, Boston, MA.

Birmaher, B., & Brent, D. (2007). Practice parameter for the assessment and treatment of children and adolescents with depressive disorder. *Journal of the American Academy of Child & Adolescent Psychiatry*, 46(11), 1503–1526.

Brendtro, L. K., Brokenleg, M., & Van Bockern, S. (1990). *Reclaiming youth at risk: Our hope for the future*. Bloomington, IN: National Educational Service.

Bridge, J. A., Iyengar, S., Salary, C. B., Barbe, R. P., Birmaher, B., Pincus, H. A., Ren, L., & Brent, D. A. (2007). Clinical response and risk for reported suicidal ideation and suicide attempts in pediatric antidepressant treatment: A meta-analysis of randomized controlled trials. *Journal of the American Medical Association*, 297, 1683–1696.

Canadian Health Services Research Foundation. (2003) *The integration of health and social services for young children and their families*. Ottawa: Author.

Carlsson-Paige, N., & Levin, D. (2008). *Taking back childhood: Helping your kids thrive in a fast-paced, media-saturated, violence-filled world*. New York: Hudson Street Press.

Chesney-Lind, M. (1997). *The female offender: Girls, women, and crime*. Thousand Oaks, CA: Sage.

Collaboration Essentials. (2008). Collaboration Essentials for Pediatric & Child and Adolescent Psychiatry Residents: Overview. http://collaborationessentials.org/ce/index.html (accessed on October 6, 2008).

Duggal, S., Malkoff-Schwartz, S., Birmaher, B., Anderson, B. P., Matty, M. K., Houck, P. R., Bailey-Orr, M., Williamson, D. E., & Frank, E. (2000). Assessment of life stress in adolescents: Self-report versus interview methods. *Journal of the American Academy of Child & Adolescent Psychiatry*, 39(4), 445–452.

Ellickson, P., Saner, H., & McGuigan, K. A. (1997). Profiles of violent youth: Substance use and other concurrent problems. *American Journal of Public Health*, 57(6), 985–991.

Eyre, J., & Eyre, R. (1993). *Teaching your children values*. New York: Simon & Schuster.

Flaherty, E. G. & Sege, R. (2005). Barriers to physician identification and reporting of child abuse. *Pediatric Annals*, 34(5), 349–356.

Glascoe, F. P. (2008). *Parent Evaluation of Developmental Status (PEDS)*. Nolensville, TN: Ellsworth & Vandemeer Press. http://www.pedstest.com/ (accessed on October 5, 2008).

Hedaya, R. J. (1996). *Understanding biological psychiatry*. New York, NY: W.W. Norton & Company.

Hodges, K. (2008). *Child & Adolescent Functional Assessment Scale (CAFAS)*. Ann Arbor, MI: Functional Assessment Systems. www.cafas.com (accessed on October 3, 2008).

Hoff, L. A. (1990). *Battered women as survivors*. London: Routledge.

Hoff, L. A., Hallisey, B. J., & Hoff, M. (2009). *People in crisis: Clinical and diversity perspectives* (6th Ed.). New York and London: Routledge.

Holinger, P. C, Offer, D., Barter, J. T., & Bell, C. C. (1994). *Suicide and homicide among adolescents*. New York: Guilford Press.

Jellinek, M. (2002). Pediatric symptom checklist. In M. Jellinek, Ed. *Bright futures in practice: Mental health*. Georgetown University: The National Center for Education in Maternal & Child Health. http://www.brightfutures.org/mentalhealth/pdf/professionals/ped_sympton_chklst.pdf (accessed on October 5, 2008).

Jessor, R. (1993). Successful adolescent development among youth in high-risk settings. *American Psychologist*, 48(2), 117–126.

Kessler, R. C., Chiu, W. T., Demler, O., Merikangas, K. R., & Walters, E. E. (2005). Prevalence, severity, and co-morbidity of 12-month DSM-IV disorders in the National Comorbidity Survey Replication. *Archives of General Psychiatry*, 62(6), 617–627.

Kirby, M. J. L., & Keon, W. J. (2006). *Out of the shadows at last: Transforming mental health, mental illness and addiction services in Canada*. Ottawa, ON: Standing Senate Committee on Social Affairs, Science and Technology, www.parl.gc.ca/39/1/parlbus/commbus/senate/com-e/soci-e/rep-e/rep02may06-e.htm (accessed on October 5, 2005).

Lewis, M. (2008). *Change in brain activity marking successful treatment for children with behavior problems*. Paper presented at the meeting of the Provincial Centre of Excellence for Child & Youth Mental Health at CHEO on Made in Ontario: A showcase of leading practices in child & youth mental health, Mississauga, ON.

McEwan, K., Waddell, C., & Barker, J. (2007). Bringing children's mental health "out of the shadows". *Canadian Medical Association Journal*, 176(4), 471–472.

McHugh, P. R. (2001). Beyond DSM-IV: From appearances to essences. *Psychiatric Research Report*, 17(2), 1–5.

Melnyk, B., & Moldenhauer, Z. (2008). *The KySS^{SM} Guide to Child and Adolescent Mental Health Screening, Early Intervention and Health Promotion*. Cherry Hill, NJ: National Association of Pediatric Nurse Practitioners. www.napnap.org (accessed on October 1, 2008).

Mendel, M. P. (1994). *The male survivor*. Thousand Oaks, CA: Sage.

National Association of Pediatric Nurse Practitioners (NAPNP). (2008). *About KySS*. Cherry Hill, NJ: National Association of Pediatric Nurse Practitioners. www.napnap.org (accessed on October 1, 2008).

National Institute of Mental Health. (2009). Treatment of children with mental illness. http://www.nimh.nh.gov/health/publications/treatment-of-children-with-mental-illness-fact-sheet/nimh-treatment-children-mental-illness-faq.pdf (accessed on March 10, 2010).

National Institute of Mental Health (2010). Antidepressant medications for children and adolescents: Information for parents and caregivers. http://www.nimh.nih.gov/health/topics/child-and-adolescent-mental-health/antidepressant-medications-for-children-and-adolescents-information-for-parents-and-caregivers.shtml (accessed on March 1, 2010).

Nicholson, J., Biebel, K., Hinden, B., Henry, A., & Stier, L. (2001). Critical issues for parents with mental illness and their families. http://mentalhealth.samhsa.gov/publications/allpubs/KEN-01-0109/default.asp (accessed on March 10, 2010).

Parents for Children's Mental Health. (2008). The quilt of honour. http://www.parentsforchildrens mentalhealth.org/ (accessed on August 4, 2008).

Parikh, S. V., Lin, E., & Lesage, A. D. (1997). Mental health treatment in Ontario: Selected comparisons between the primary care and specialty sectors. *Canadian Journal of Psychiatry*, 42, 929–934.

Rich, J. A., & Grey, C. M. (2005). Pathways to recurrent trauma among young Black men: Traumatic stress, substance use, and the "Code of the Street." *American Journal of Public Health*, 95(5), 816–824.

Ringel, J. S., & Sturm, R. (2001). National estimates of mental health utilization and expenditures for children in 1998. *Journal of Behavioral Health Services Research*, 28(3), 319–333.

Sigel, E. (2009). Primary care practitioners detection of youth violence involvement. *Journal of Adolescent Health*, 44(2), S11–S12.

Solomon, E. P., & Heide, K. M. (2005). The biology of trauma: Implications for treatment. *Journal Interpersonal Violence*, 20(1), 51–60.

Sturm, R., Ringel, J., Bao, C., Stein, B., Kapur, K., Zhang, W., & Zeng, F. (2000). National estimates of mental health utilization and expenditures for children in 1998 (working Paper 205). Los Angeles, CA: Research Center on Managed Care for Psychiatric Disorders.

U.S. Department of Health and Human Services. (1999). *Mental health: A report of the Surgeon General*. Rockville, MD: U.S. Department of Health and Human Services, http://www.surgeon general.gov/library/mentalhealth/chapter3/sec1.html (accessed July 2008).

U.S. Department of Health and Human Services. (2000). *U.S. Public Health Service, Report of the Surgeon General's Conference on Children's Mental Health: A National Action Agenda*. http://www.surgeongeneral.gov/topics/cmh/childreport.htm (accessed July 2008).

U.S. Department of Health and Human Services. (2003). *Preventing drug use among children and adolescents: A research-based guide for parents, educators, and community leaders*. http://www.drugabuse.gov/pdf/prevention/redbook.pdf (accessed April 2010).

U.S. Department of Health and Human Services: Administration for Children and Families. (2008b). *Child disposition and victimization rates, 2002–2006*. http://www.acf.hhs.gov/programs/cb/pubs/cm06/figure3_1.htm (accessed August 2008).

Waddell C., Hua J. M., Garland O. M., Peters R. D., & McEwan K. (2007). Preventing mental disorders in children: A systematic review to inform policy-making. *Canadian Journal of Public Health*, 98(3), 166–173.

Waddell, C., McEwan, K., Shepherd, C. A., Offord, D. R., & Hua, J. M. (2005). A public health strategy to improve mental health of Canadian children. *Canadian Journal of Psychiatry*, 50(4), 226–233.

Waddell, C., Offord, D. R., Shepherd, C. A., Hua, J. M., & McEwan, K. (2002). Child psychiatric epidemiology and Canadian public policy-making: The state of the science and the art of the possible. *Canadian Journal of Psychiatry*, 47 (9), 825–832.

Walker, H. M. (1993). Anti-social behavior in school. *Journal of Emotional and Behavioral Problems*, 2(1), 20–24.

Walkup, J. T., Albano, A. M., Piacentini, J., Birmaher, B., Compton, S. N., Sherrill, J. T., Ginsburg, G. S., Rynn, M. A., McCracken, J., Waslick, B., Iyengar, S., March, J. S., & Kendall, P. C. (2008). Cognitive behavioral therapy, sertraline, or a combination in childhood anxiety. *New England Journal of Medicine*, 359 (26), 2753–2766.

Webster, D. W, Vernick, J. S., Ludwig, J., & Lester, K. J. (1997). Flawed gun policy research could endanger public safety. *American Journal of Public Health*, 87(6), 918–921.

Working Paper No. 205. In National Advisory Mental Health Council's Workgroup on Child and Adolescent Mental Health Intervention Development and Deployment (2001) (p. 93). *Blueprint for Change: Research on Child and Adolescent Mental Health*. Rockville, MD: National Institute of Mental Health. NIH Publication No. 01-4985.

Wright, M. A., Wintemute, G. J., & Rivara, E. P. (1999). Effectiveness of denial of handgun purchase to persons believed to be at high risk for firearm violence. *American Journal of Public Health*, 89(1), 88–90.

12 The Older Person, Preventive Mental Health, Cognitive Impairment, and End-of-Life Issues

- Growing Older: A Challenging Life Cycle Transition
- Rites of Passage: Community Support through Hazardous Change
- Major Themes and Issues of People Growing Older
- Older People who are Alive, Challenged, and Thriving
- Attitudes toward Seniors
- Primary Care and Holistic Services for Older People
- Vulnerability to Serious Age-related Cognitive Impairment
- Case Study: Interdisciplinary Assessment and Collaborative Treatment
- Friends as Family Standing by Beyond Death
- Attitudes toward Death, the Final Passage
- References

Gerontology and geriatric healthcare are burgeoning specialties answering the call for response to an array of issues and needs of a population group that will soon represent a majority in many societies. Aside from the shortage of gerontological health specialists needed by some older people, the reality is that primary care providers are front and center in their role with this population group whether by choice or client demand. Mirroring to some extent a society-wide pattern and a youth-focused culture, until recently, healthcare curricula have directed minimal attention to the needs of older people.

This chapter addresses key concepts and issues affecting the mental health of older clients served in primary care. The framework is role change and attendant stressors experienced during major life cycle transitions that typically include loss and challenges inherent in the next life phase. For older persons this often includes a decline in health status, cognitive impairment, and/or a serious illness. Readers are referred to specialty texts such as Melillo, & Houde (2005) for in-depth coverage of the psychiatric treatment and nursing care needed by some in this growing population group, e.g., dementia, or major depression with psychotic features. The focus here is on health promotion and preventive services. This includes the pivotal role of PCPs in monitoring drug treatments when interdisciplinary treatments are needed (e.g., orthopedic and vision services). When not carefully coordinated by a PCP, some injuries (e.g., confusion, accidental overdosing, and falling) can be traced to "polypharmacy" and dangerous interactive side effects from some drugs.

Growing Older: A Challenging Life Cycle Transition

What do the terms *transition*—or life cycle *passage*—mean for older people, their health, and happiness? For some it means relief from the demands of paid employment and the challenges of child-rearing, the end of worries about money, and time to "take it easy." Others face their later years with ill health, financial insecurity, loneliness, safety concerns, and fear of abandonment.

From a holistic perspective, it is a normal part of human life to grow and develop through childhood, adolescence, middle age, and old age to death (Doress & Siegal, 1987). Anthropologists and development psychologist Erikson (1963) have referred to these transition states as *life crises* (Kimball, 1960 [1909]). In anthropology, life crisis refers to a highly significant, expectable event or phase in the life cycle that marks one's passage to a new social status, with accompanying changes in rights and duties.

Such transition states are "critical" life phases, but not necessarily traumatic. For a person facing one's later years, this important transition has the *potential* for activating an *acute emotional upset* in the clinical sense (Hoff, *et al.*, 2009). As *turning points*, social and psychological processes involve the challenge to successfully complete developmental, social, and instrumental tasks—for example:

* changing one's image of self from young to middle aged, to old age, or from healthy to sick;
* downsizing from the family home to a smaller space needed when children are gone or one is widowed;
* finding a PCP who is sensitive to the healthcare issues of aging.

As turning points in the developmental process, these "life crises" (as Erikson defined them) fit the classic definition of crisis as a period of both *danger and opportunity*. Another connection between the anthropological and clinical definitions of crisis is the fact that individuals in acute emotional upset do not exist in a social vacuum; they are members of cultural communities. Across the lifecycle through particular developmental phases, people are influenced by social expectations of how to behave and by values guiding their interpretation of expected and unexpected life events, as in an expression such as "She's 65 years old and dresses like a teenager," or "He's old enough to know better."

Thus, if it is unclear *who* a person is, *what* the person is expected to do, or *how* the person fits into familiar social arrangements based on cultural values, status or role ambiguity is activated. Status and role ambiguity can create so much stress that a person with conflicting or changed roles may withdraw from social interaction or may try to change the social structure to redefine the anxiety-provoking statuses (Douglas, 1966). For example:

* If widowed people sense that they are a threat to social groups of married people, they may feel cut off from social support and thereby increase their risk of emotional crisis around traumatic events.
* If children of parents feuding about divorce are not allowed to see their grandparents, the deprived grandparent may ask, "What have I done wrong?"

Rites of Passage: Community Support through Hazardous Change

In his classic work, *Rites of Passage*, van Gennep (1909/1960, p. 11) distinguished three phases in the ceremonies associated with an individual's major life passages: rites of separation (prominent in funeral ceremonies), rites of transition (important in initiation and pregnancy), and rites of incorporation (prominent in marriage). A complete schema of rites of passage theoretically includes all three phases. For example, a widow is *separated* from her husband by death; she occupies a *liminal* (transitional) status for a time, and finally may be *reincorporated* into a new marriage relationship (Goody, 1962).

These rites protect the individual during the hazardous process of life passages, times considered potentially dangerous to the person if not supported by the community. Ritual thus makes public what is private, makes social what is personal, and gives the individual new knowledge and strength (LaFontaine, 1977). For example, instead of "fudging" about one's age, a person might host a retirement party and announce embarking on a venture to volunteer one's talent in a needy area. For some, however, financial constraints and/or emotional concerns lead one to a mental health counselor for help through this new life terrain. Indeed, in Kimball's (1960) introduction to the English translation of van Gennep's 1909 work, the "rituals" of individual and group psychotherapy serve as contemporary substitutes for traditional "rites of passage"—the "50 minute hour," the structure and expectations of group counseling sessions.

Major Themes and Issues of People Growing Older

It has been said that we are as old as we feel. However, the way we feel growing older is greatly influenced by psychological outlook, overall health status, social support, and economic security. For example:

- minority elders have lower incomes than white elders;
- three-fourths of elderly people below poverty level are female;
- older women earn much less than older men;
- low-income elders are much more likely to have limiting chronic conditions than high-income elders—often because of limited access to a healthy diet including fresh fruits and vegetables.

Among those wishing to remain in the workforce, some experience age discrimination (Yuan, 2007). Given the gender-based distribution of a society's paid and unpaid labor, women are the primary providers of home-based and institutional care needed by older people. Typically, those caring for impoverished and chronically ill women are underpaid, overworked, and overwhelmed.

These grim realities exist in concert with some lingering myths about old age; for example, old age is a disease, and old people are uniformly needy, dependent, and asexual. Let us consider these myths and realities in the lives of real people growing older, what we can learn from them, and where PCPs made (or might have made) a significant difference in these people's health status outcomes.

Older People who are Alive, Challenged, and Thriving

Vignettes and Learning Tips

Cheryl, age 70, and widowed since age 65, never acknowledges her age except on government documents and for her medical records. This is because everyone who has attempted to guess her age misses by at least ten years. Cheryl is open to finding a new life partner, and is keenly aware that most men her age prefer a "younger" woman. In her view, if any man she dates does not have the "social grace" of "never asking a woman over 40 her age," she cannot be bothered dating such men, preferring instead the good times she has with friends of both sexes. Her short blond hair is fashionably highlighted to enhance her youthful appearance. Cheryl, a law firm administrator, is 5'7", weighs 130 lbs, walks or rides her bike at least 20 minutes per day, works out at a gym twice weekly, and eats a "Mediterranean" type diet.

But Cheryl's health status was not always thus. When she was 45, she weighed 155 lbs and was diagnosed with adult-onset diabetes, controllable through diet and exercise. Both her mother and father, though never obese, had adult-onset diabetes. Laboratory tests also revealed that Cheryl was "borderline" for hypothyroidism—a condition apparent in her family history as well. During her "overweight" period, Cheryl injured her right knee from a fall off her bike, which was treated by physical therapy and a corticosteroid injection. Cheryl attributes the good health she enjoys today to her own efforts and the excellent care monitored by her PCP, which includes medication for hypothyroidism, and several supplements—calcium, a multi-vitamin, and fish oil. When she turns 75, Cheryl expects to reduce her paid job to part-time and treat herself to travel with her friends and sometimes, with her three children and eight grand-children.

Learning Tips

While keenly aware of but still camouflaging her age, Cheryl has a healthy self-image and takes advantage of modern technology to enhance her natural assets and avoid possible sleights emanating from both ageism and sexism. Although Cheryl might have avoided diabetes due to her being overweight in mid-life, because she works closely with her PCP, and has incorporated well-recognized healthy self-care and lifestyle habits into her daily life. Her example shows that it's never too late to discard unhealthy habits for healthy ones, given personal determination, a supportive social network, and stable connection with a PCP.

Raymond, age 68, is Cheryl's brother. He is 5'9", happily married, has three grown children and five grandchildren who live in neighboring communities. Raymond and his wife Anne work a small farm that supplies fresh produce to local restaurants, and keep bees for honey marketed to food specialty stores. Unlike Cheryl, Raymond has had a much bigger struggle controlling his weight, ballooning up to 210 lbs. At age 50 he was diagnosed with diabetes, was placed on insulin, and advised to modify his "meat and potatoes" diet. He now weighs 170 lbs and only occasionally "cheats" with sugary treats at family events. Raymond's elevated blood pressure is controlled with medi-cation, while recommended aerobic exercise is accomplished primarily by his vigorous farm and bee-keeping labor. At age 60, Raymond had cataract surgery on both eyes. While he held a valid driver's license, he observed on his own that his impaired vision made his driving hazardous. Raymond sought out an ophthalmologist who attributed the early cataracts to his years working outdoors and rarely protecting his eyes with sunglasses. Raymond says that farming is "in his blood" so "retirement" for him just means slowing down a bit in order to travel more and "see the world" beyond his rural but much-loved community.

Learning Tips

Available public knowledge about sunglasses for eye protection, or a recommendation from a PCP to wear sunglasses might have delayed early-onset cataract development. As with his sister, Cheryl—given his family history—diabetes might also have been avoided if Raymond had paid more attention to weight control. Regular contact with a PCP is something of a foregone conclusion in preventing some of Raymond's health problems.

Ted, age 81 and Betty, age 81, a childless couple, enjoyed 45 years together as home and work partners. Ted was a ship builder and avid sailor when he met Betty, a writer he fondly referred to as his "first mate" when she took breaks from her work as a journalist. Together, Ted and Betty enjoyed a wide circle of friends in the maritime community and through alumni events at the university where Betty had earned her journalism degree. Their friends included a physician who provided "informal" medical advice when needed. During one of her jaunts with Ted as "first mate," at age 60, Betty fell, and incurred a serious shoulder injury that was successfully treated after presenting in a local hospital emergency room. At age 65, Ted was treated for a cardiac arrhythmia and moderately elevated blood pressure, and prescribed medication for each condition. Aside from these medical incidents, Ted and Betty felt healthy and vigorous, and saw no need for regular physical examinations.

At age 80, Betty discovered a "red spot and lump" on her left breast. On examination and post-biopsy, Betty was diagnosed with Stage IV breast cancer that had metastasized to her lymph nodes. Following radical surgery, Betty underwent two rounds of chemotherapy. A year later following home care by Ted between treatments, Betty was placed in hospice care and died three weeks later. As it turned out, Betty had never had a mammogram, nor did she do regular self-examinations. Ted will never forget the special place of Betty in his life over their wonderful years together and keenly misses her companionship. Past immediate grieving, Ted is now looking for someone who might partner with him for travel and other interests over these later years of his life.

Learning Tips

While self-examination and mammograms are not guarantees of early breast cancer detection, both might have been done if Betty had regular visits with a PCP who could prescribe and monitor these screening and preventive measures. Although the special place of Betty in Ted's life can never be replaced, given his general good health and a vigorous 81 years, Ted says it's never too late to find love and new companionship for his growing *still older* together! Unlike some men his age, he does not rule out prospects of finding a woman in his own age bracket.

Jerry, age 70 and Bob, age 72 are a gay couple, with homes in cold New England and the Florida ocean front. Since retiring as university professors in the social sciences, they embarked on a "snow-bird" lifestyle, spending six of the "northern hard winter" months in Florida, and six months in their New England suburban home among friends and enjoying the great "summer" outdoors.

During a recent summer, Jerry fell, broke a hip and was prepared for hip replacement surgery, while Bob was being treated for end-stage renal disease at another hospital.

Over the course of six months, Jerry has successfully recuperated from hip surgery, but was acutely distressed about hospital policy allowing only a "spouse" and "immediate family" to visit Bob during his periodic hospitalizations, including dialysis. Only recently had Jerry and Bob "come out" with their gay identity, and while they had many friends outside the gay community, they did not take advantage of their state's legislation allowing "civil unions" between gay couples which includes hospital visitation and other rights common to straight couples. Between acute episodes of Bob's renal disease, the couple continued to travel between their Florida and New England homes. They made no special plans for home-based or long-term care in either their Florida or New England home, and seemed oblivious to the fact that they could not continue their six month travel and home re-location indefinitely. When Bob died during a summer in New England, Jerry was grief stricken, but very grateful for the emotional support and extraordinary assistance he received from friends, some of whom had challenging health problems of their own. Jerry resisted using available home-based social assistance, and insisted that he would continue to travel every six months back to Florida.

Learning Tips

Since each of us may harbor fantasies of "immortality," deep in our hearts we know that someday we may not be as vigorous and healthy as in our youth, and that eventually we will die. The major lesson from this example for everyone growing older is the price one can pay for denial and continuous delaying of realistic planning for one's later years—not to mention the toll of caretaker burden that can be alleviated with appropriate use of respite and other services. Primary care providers who observe such lack of planning associated with denial in medical records can be instrumental in advising their older clients about these important issues.

[Note: The following vignette—unlike other examples in this book—is undisguised and printed with permission of Margaret Ross]

Margaret Ross, now 68, was diagnosed with multiple myeloma at age 53. Her presenting symptom was back pain which led to cutting short an education and research trip to China. At the height of her career of teaching, research, and publication, Margaret was a distinguished professor of gerontological nursing at the University of Ottawa, Faculty of Health Sciences. Following medical leave from her teaching and research duties, and extensive diagnostic work-ups, she underwent an autogalous bone marrow transplant at the university hospital. Her sister Mary, also a nurse, acted as advocate through the grueling life-threatening procedure, during which Margaret was very close to death on two occasions over a three-month period. Margaret was and still is surrounded by a tight-knit and supportive extended family. Given the usually poor prognosis and life expectancy post-transplant surgery for this condition, all who have known Margaret refer to her as the "miracle patient." Soon after recovery from the acute stage, Margaret wrote a book entitled: *From the other side of the bed* (2000) recounting what she learned as a patient after all her years as a teacher of nursing. She also needed physical and occupational therapy, dialysis due to kidney damage post-transplant surgery, and extensive dental repair and "re-learning" how to eat.

During the first few years post-surgery, Margaret lived with her mother in a retirement community—each vigilant for the other's needs, with other family members close by. In 2005, Margaret's mother died after a brief stay in a nursing facility following surgery for a broken hip. Meanwhile, Margaret gradually recovered most of her lost weight, grew new curly hair, and has been able to travel across Canada and the U.S. for vacations—having arranged with local hospitals to provide her thrice-weekly kidney dialysis. She now lives with her sister, Penny, and plans social gatherings around her dialysis sessions, cooks regularly, hosts luncheons for friends, and enjoys a lifestyle not unlike her peers of the same age. Besides her contagious lust for life and fidelity to friends and family, Margaret is forever grateful for Canada's widely known comprehensive and tax-supported healthcare system covering all residents—a system in which primary care is highly valued, but includes advanced medical/surgical treatment without which she might not be alive today.

Learning Tips

All who have known Margaret have rejoiced in her recovery and learned from her undaunted spirit. Those of us who have treated and cared for people with very serious illnesses such as Margaret's have long been convinced of the intrinsic connections between body, mind, and spirit. Who can answer the question of how and why Margaret lives among us today, since most people with the diagnosis and similar treatment of multiple myeloma are not alive 15 years later? We do not know whether it was Margaret's determination to live and not die at such a young age of 53, the brilliance of the medical, surgical, and other members of the treatment team, the steadfast support of family and friends who stood by her through months of challenging recovery odds and could not easily imagine losing her, or a combination of these factors. But whatever the reasons, we are glad for her presence today, the inspiration of her indomitable spirit, and the message that life is worth living for whatever time we each have left. While we may never know the answers to how and why Margaret survived, it is timely to note one surgeon's comment: "If a patient tells me before surgery that he knows he will die, I won't operate, as it seems a foregone conclusion."

These lessons about self-care and necessary professional services for people growing older and/or are facing preventable illness and an early death are self-evident in these vignettes of people growing older. They also portray how PCPs can make such a remarkable difference to the outcomes of age-related illness and disability. The realities of successful transitions at this stage of the lifecycle require conscious planning with one's PCP and family for preventive self-care, end-of-life planning, and the smooth coordination of the inter-related health and social services needed for a healthier old age.

Attitudes toward Seniors

Despite increased political advocacy and advances in gerontological research, the vignettes attest that ageism and stereotypes about older people persist. Cultural values and the policies and practices flowing from them do not change rapidly. Old people are not as highly valued in mainstream North American society as they are, for example, in some native communities and most non-Western societies. Recent social emphasis on the small nuclear family has virtually displaced the extended family arrangement in most Western societies. Grandparents, aunts, and uncles are rarely integrated into a family home. Most children, therefore, routinely have only two adults (their parents) as role models and supporters. In cases of death, desertion, or divorce, children are even more deprived of adult models. Fortunately, this is changing with attempts to get children and old people together—for example, through nursing home visits by groups of children and other intergenerational volunteer programs in schools, and by organizing childcare and senior services in a single agency umbrella.

Health attitudes toward aging are also helped by books such as *The art of aging: A doctor's prescription for well-being* (Nuland, 2007). Through cross-cultural stories, Dr. Nuland cites the extraordinary rewards of growing old, especially by those with a keen sense of spirituality and life purpose, who nurture personal relationships, and who accept the fact that some goals may remain unaccomplished due to physical or mental infirmity.

Unfortunately, some older people experience even greater hardship than children do by their exclusion from the nuclear family. They feel—and often are—unwanted. They may feel treated as guests who have no significant role in matters of consequence in their children's families. If, because of health or other problems, an older person does live with their grown children, additional tensions may arise. Space is sometimes insufficient to give everyone some privacy, or the old person may seem demanding and unreasonable. This oft heard expression from someone facing old age is therefore unsurprising: "I don't want to be a burden to my children." Fortunately, housing developments in the U.S., Canada, and Europe catering to the special needs of older people in transition are a welcome respite from the prospect of social isolation and safety concerns many fear.

Primary Care and Holistic Services for Older People

When primary healthcare is closely integrated with available, necessary home-based services such as housekeeping, progress is possible toward the prized goal of "aging in place." This can help to prevent age-related health problems and avoid the institutionalization that many older people dread.

An older person living alone and who (for physical or psychological reasons) is unable to get out is particularly vulnerable to preventable healthcare problems and social isolation. In the U.S., Canada, and Western Europe "all inclusive care" housing developments, if used, provide a major source for keeping active physically, for establishing and maintaining social contacts, and for preventing emotional, mental, and physical deterioration. Financial and transportation assistance—plus counseling to accept help—are also negotiable through community-based senior centers in even the smallest town or rural communities. Visiting nurses are another key resource which PCPs and concerned family can contact to arrange services that help frail elderly people remain in their homes despite various age- and illness-related disabilities.

Vulnerability to Serious Age-related Cognitive Impairment

Despite self-care and primary prevention coordinated by PCPs, some older people will be visited by cognitive impairment, including vascular-related dementia, Parkinson's disease, delirium, and Alzheimer's disease.

Dementias, Delirium and Depression: Early Differential Diagnosis

Among the vulnerabilities to cognitive impairment among older people are various forms of dementia and the serious cognitive disturbance, delirium. These disorders (especially dementias) are increasingly apparent in affluent societies (or among elites in poorer nations) where financial means, informed self-care, ready access to preventive measures, social support, and acute care medical services have resulted in increased longevity of the population at large. The downside of these class-related advantages is the accompanying vulnerability to age-related disorders such as dementia and/or delirium.

The role of primary care providers in early detection, diagnosis, and treatment of these disorders cannot be overstated. This includes coordination with neuropsychology and gero-psychiatric specialists for in-depth testing of cognitive functioning and level of impairment. Our focus here is on the very important point of early recognition and differential diagnosis, effective referral to specialists, and collaborative follow-up as needed by both patient and family in primary care practice. It builds on the tertiary level of primary prevention discussed in Chapter 1.

Dementia, broadly defined, is a condition primarily affecting the brain, is most often observed in older adults, and encompasses Alzheimer's disease, cerebrovascular disorders, and related brain diseases. Dementia is not a disease per se, but rather, a syndrome—typically chronic and progressive—manifested in the impairment of cognitive functions and accompanied by the deteriorization of emotional control, language skills, social behavior, and functional ability (Remington, Gerdner, & Buckwalter, 2005; Sherrell & Iris, 2005). Generally, these disorders are considered irreversible, while their progression might be slowed by certain medications.

In contrast, delirium (while also seen mostly among elders) manifests itself primarily as an indicator of an underlying *physical illness* at any point along the healthcare continuum—emergency, community, long-term care, or end-of-life phase for patients with advanced cancers. Those with a pre-existing dementia are at further risk of delirium—an important factor in differential diagnosis. The main feature in delirium is confusion and inability to focus, with rapid fluctuations in level of consciousness, and accompanying restlessness, anxiety, agitation, hallucinations, or delusions. It is frequently seen in intensive care units and those with infectious diseases at any age. But most important for primary care providers is that —unlike dementias—delirium is *reversible* if it is recognized early on and its physiological precipitating causes are immediately addressed. These may include brain injuries or cerebral tumors, AIDS, acute alcohol poisoning, and chronic pulmonary disease (Dick & Morency, 2005, pp. 213–215; Milne, *et al.,* 2008). Also, because delirium can be life-threatening, it should be regarded as a medical emergency, with quick implementation of measures to prevent delirium in at-risk patients, e.g., vulnerable elders who have undergone hip fracture repair.

Dementia is typically more gradual in its manifestation to both family and providers, and hence must be considered in relation to a decline in a person's *normal* cognitive, emotional, and behavioral life functions. Another consideration in differential diagnosis is the presence or absence of *depression*, most often originating in major life changes or inadequate treatment following traumatic life events (van Gool, *et al.*, 2006). Also important is differentiating dementia from potentially reversible and treatable conditions such as psychotic-like reaction to corticosteroids, polypharmacotherapy, metabolic disorders, congestive heart failure, depression, and a psychiatric disorder like schizophrenia with paranoid delusions (Milne, *et al.*, 2008). In the early stages of Alzheimer's disease, for example, the patient may become depressed and fearful from conscious awareness of memory lapses (see Chapter 7). See Dick & Morency (2005, p. 222) for a more detailed comparison of clinical features of dementia, delirium and depression. Table 12.1 summarizes major features relevant to differential diagnosis of these disorders.

The Geriatric Depression Scale (GDS) is a widely used self-rated scale that may be helpful in detecting depression in older adults with co-occuring medical problems (Yesavage & Brink, 1983).

Table 12.1 Key Clinical Features in Comparative Perspective: Dementia, Delirium, Depression (adapted from Foreman, Fletcher, Mion, & Simon, 1996)

Clinical Features	Dementia	Delirium	Depression
Onset	Insidious, depending on cause	Acute or sub-acute	Associated with lifecycle changes and traumatic events
Progression	Slow	Rapid	Variable
Duration	Years, until death	A few hours to 3 to 4 weeks	A few weeks to years
Orientation	Depends on severity	Typically impaired	Normal
Memory	Impaired, especially for current events	Impaired for current events	Selective
Thinking	Generally impaired	Disorganized	Normal
Sleep–wake cycle	Variable	Very disturbed	Disturbed with early morning waking common

Mental Competency, Long-term Planning and Palliative Care

Regarding these disorders, the prevention, early intervention, and follow-up needs of both patient and affected family members cannot be over-emphasized. It is, after all, the primary care provider—not the neuropsychologist or psychiatrist—who typically (or least *ideally*) knows the "whole" patient, a person's early and subtle dementia symptoms of memory loss as a major symptom in relation to prior medical history, his or her lifestyle regarding independence, etc., and what she or he wishes regarding the need for home healthcare, assisted living, and end-of-life decisions regarding care. This includes, of course, coaching a patient (and/or family member or close friend) to have healthcare proxy documents in place in the event of a patient's decline in mental competence and ability to make decisions in accordance with one's values and decisions prior to brain disease-related incompetence. It also considers future palliative care needs as introduced in Chapters 1 and 2.

Advanced care planning and the ability to make decisions about treatment are very important in palliative care. People with mental illness or developmental disabilities may not have the capacity to participate in informed decision-making, or may be competent and refuse life-sustaining treatments. All competent persons have the right to make their own decisions even when that decision conflicts with what a majority would decide under similar circumstances. When the patient is a person who has schizophrenia or another mental illness, the ability to make decisions may be compromised by psychotic thought processes. However, having a diagnosis of a mental illness, even one with psychotic features, does not automatically mean that a person is mentally incompetent. When providers are not sure if the patient is competent to make decisions and there is no advanced directive about treatment wishes, then a psychiatric evaluation must be requested (Morgan, 2010).

Mental capacity indicates the ability to understand the problem and make decisions. A psychiatric provider makes an assessment of the patient's capacity to function in a specific area. "Competency" is a legal term and is decided by a court of law, and is often based on the capacity assessment by a psychiatric provider (Schouten & Brendel, 2004). Applebaum & Grisso (1988) outlined four criteria used to determine capacity to consent to treatment:

- patient expression of a preference;
- ability to understand the illness, the prognosis, with and without treatment, and the risks and benefits of the treatment (factual understanding);
- an appreciation of the significance of the facts (significance of facts);
- ability to use the information in a rational way to reach a decision in a logical manner (rationality of thought processes).

Intense pain, depression, delirium, dementia, and psychosis can affect competence. However, the existence of one of these conditions does not necessarily mean that a person is incompetent. Each patient must have a thorough assessment. A patient is not deemed "incompetent" until a court of law rules.

Medication Use in Older Adults with Delirium and Dementia

Care for older adults with a possible diagnosis of delirium or dementia is most often provided in a hospital setting. Identification of an underlying medical cause of delirium typically involves diagnostic testing and close monitoring of the patient's mental status. Providing for the patient's safety is of utmost importance during this period since behavior may be unpredictable and threaten the safety of the patient and others in the surrounding area. Environmental management that reduces stimulating factors in the surrounding area that make the confusion and misperceptions of delirium worse should be managed by the providers. This might include cueing of day and night changes in light (i.e., opening shades) and orientation to surroundings. Use of psychotropic medications is often the last resort in treatment of delirium since adding medications may increase confusion.

"Physical and chemical restraints should be avoided whenever possible and used only in situations where patients are at risk of injuring themselves or others, or when agitation or restlessness may interfere with necessary medical treatments" (Dick & Morency, 2005, p. 224). Low doses of antipsychotic medications such as haloperidol or droperidol may be utilized when psychotic symptoms and severe agitation are present. Use of benzodiazpines may be indicated for alcohol or sedative withdrawal (Dick & Morency, 2005), but should be avoided or used sparingly with older adults. The general approach to all medication use in a population of older adults is "Start low, go slow" and this approach is appropriate in the treatment of delirium and dementia as well.

Use of medications for treatment of dementia may be indicated and takes two forms: the symptomatic treatment of dementia and use of medications that either enhance cognitive function or slow the progression of dementia. The use of medications to manage symptoms such as depression, anxiety/agitation or psychosis and sleep difficulties are described in Chapters 6, 7, and 8.

Medications for the enhancement of cognitive function and slowing the progression of dementia are generally utilized for patients with mild to moderate cognitive problems and are utilized only following an extensive workup to rule out other causes before diagnosing dementia. Cholinesterase inhibitors are the medications used for this purpose and are listed in Box 12.1. FDA approval for tacrine, rivastigmine, glantamine, and donepezil for treatment of Alzheimer's disease has been achieved, yet tacrine is useful only for a few patients since it has been found to have hepatic toxicity resulting in a need for close follow-up of hepatic function (Milne, *et al.*, 2008). These medications can slow, but not stop, the progression of the disease and there are significant drug interactions with most of these medications.

BOX 12.1 Cholineterase Inhibitors

Donepezil (Aricept)

Tacrine (Cognex)

Galantamine (Reminyl)

Rivastigmine (Exelon)

Carnitine

Metrifonate (Selgiline)

Nicergoline (Sermion)

Physostigmine (Eserine)

CASE STUDY: INTERDISCIPLINARY ASSESSMENT AND COLLABORATIVE TREATMENT

Given the fact that both family and PCP may misinterpret early signs of memory loss as "just a normal part of growing older"—not to mention the near universal fear and *denial* that perhaps early Alzheimer's disease (AD) is what may be happening—it is paramount that PCPs interpret and follow up on any early signs of AD in the context of individual and family history. The widespread denial around the reality of this dreaded disease shortchanges what might be done to address it in the medical, nursing, and social domains available for living with the disease as pain-free as possible. The following case study dramatically illustrates even the life-threatening sequelae of relying simply on the patient's "ordinary" presentation in a primary care office visit—this, minus the data available from the later comprehensive home and family assessment of the client's situation.

Because of the genetic component now associated with AD—while not definitive without research evidence from brain autopsies of those afflicted—several preventive measures are indicated. One person with Alzheimer's disease evident in the genetic pool said: "If I had a choice of which disease might afflict me in older age, Alzheimer's would be at the bottom"—this, not only because of the anticipatory anxiety of losing one's ordinary self-care and daily life management ability, but mostly because this disease gradually destroys one's sense of self and who one is as a unique individual in a family and community context.

This case study also illustrates the pivotal role of one's PCP in early diagnosis and possible drug treatment to slow the progression of this devastating disease. Besides early recognition of symptoms, the example reveals the necessity of *interdisciplinary collaboration for comprehensive treatment and supportive holistic care* once the PCP makes a preliminary diagnosis and keeps close track of what happens between visits to the PCP office. It also highlights the life-threatening implications of breakdown in communication between a PCP and neuro-psychiatric specialists for people with cognitive impairments presenting by older people—not to mention the person's family and friends left to "pick up the pieces" of such breakdown.

This point cannot be overemphasized, as it is the PCP who knows the whole person and his or her social circumstances that have such a major impact on the long-term health compromises for a patient afflicted with Alzheimer's disease. While well aware of the specialty education and care-taking skills needed by those attending a person with Alzheimer's, the focus here is the PCP's role in making the services needed more readily available through early referral. We also focus attention on the morbidity issues presenting to PCPs by family members that can be traced to the daily and often unmitigated stress of living with and caring for a spouse with Alzheimer's disease (Melillo & Houde, 2005).

A Woman with Memory Problems: Early Symptoms

Rose Jefferson is a 65-year-old African-American woman, twice divorced, whose parents immigrated from a Caribbean island 60 years ago. Rose is familiar with mental health issues not only from her work, but also through her former husband, a psychiatrist. She presents to the office of a new primary care provider found for her by Susan, a close friend. Susan briefly explained the following history and reasons for seeking a new primary care provider for Rose.

Susan and other friends noticed a definite problem with Rose's memory. A year earlier, on their urging, Rose saw her "family doctor" whom she also knew through professional circles. Presentation on this visit was not remarkably different from other medical visits over several years. Results of the overdue physical examination and laboratory tests were also within normal limits. Rose confided to her doctor her concerns about memory, but denied any other health or social problems. To reassure her, this physician recommended a neuro-psychiatric consultation which Rose vehemently protested. Rose also decided "I'll never see that doctor again!" Over the next 18 months, Susan and other friends noted a marked increase in memory problems, plus the following observations when visiting Rose at home: She often forgot appointments, was very behind on paying bills, and had trouble with putting together a lunch as she had done so easily and routinely in the past, and sometimes even forgot to eat. Although Rose's home had always been impeccable, a build-up of clutter was noted, and lately, was downright unkept and unclean. Friends also noticed an over-crowded refrigerator and on one occasion, food that was rotting in a container in the dining room.

Rose's friends finally convinced her to follow through on the recommendation for a neuro-psychological battery of tests, after repeated cancelled appointments. Results suggested Alzheimer's disease. Although the consulting psychologist shared the findings with her, Rose could not remember the outcome and insisted on another opinion. However, she accepted a recommendation for weekly "psychotherapy" sessions, several of which she attended with reminders from friends. One of Rose's friends from counseling circles advised that "psychotherapy" was contraindicated in that Rose could not remember from one session to the next what was discussed. Susan finally persuaded Rose to see a new PCP, while Susan's nurse-friend strongly indicated the need for a comprehensive "home-based" assessment which could only happen if prescribed and directed by a PCP. Prior to the appointment with the new PCP, a gerontology nurse practitioner, Susan called with this information, noting that she was accompanying Rose to the appointment.

Susan expressed grave concern regarding Rose's mental status and her increasing memory problem. Susan further warned the nurse practitioner, "Please do not be fooled by what Rose might tell you . . . she isn't doing well at all." Susan also expressed concerns about the relationship between Rose and her daughter Jessica, believing that Jessica (who had a serious drug problem) takes money from Rose to support her habit without Rose's knowledge. Susan noted that this has happened many times in the past when Rose had confided in her, but questions whether Rose would be aware if the stealing was still going on.

The nurse practitioner requests a meeting with Rose, her children (son, age 37, daughter, age 35) and friend Susan. At this meeting the NP conducts a comprehensive mental health examination with Rose, accompanied by friend Susan. Her children were unable to attend.

Presenting Situation and Initial Assessment Results

Rose is a highly educated woman with a PhD in applied sociology, focusing on business administration. Her most immediate family includes only her two children, and a grandson who lives nearby, with distant relatives in far-away states. Rose had a very successful career and speaks proudly of her last position before retirement as the executive director of a social service agency. She presents very well groomed, clean, and dressed appropriate for the weather. Rose is articulate and engaging. When told of her friends' call and concerns, Rose chuckles "They just worry too much . . . I'm fine and I have plenty of help if I need it from my daughter and my grandson."

The physical exam revealed a physically healthy, postmenopausal woman who appears younger than her stated age. Her memory appears intact when reviewing her past history but notably she changed the subject every time the nurse practitioner attempted to discuss current events. She was oriented to person, place, and time. Her weight is within normal limits but is down 20 pounds from last exam 1.5 years prior. The nurse practitioner orders a chemistry panel, TSH level, and a CBC, all of which (except TSH) come back within normal limits and are consistent with her borderline hypothyroidism. She is currently on no medication except 60mcg. of Levoxyl for hypothyroidism.

Rose Jefferson is an accomplished, African-American, twice divorced, 65-year-old female who agrees with some hesitation to a comprehensive mental health examination. While cooperative and polite during interview, she denies need for help. She reluctantly allowed the nurse practitioner to also meet with her daughter and friend, stating, "I know it looks like I am hiding something if I don't let you talk with my family. I know how it works." Rose was accompanied to this assessment session by her friend Susan.

Mental Health Functioning and Stress Levels

Results of assessment using the CMHA tool as guide included the following items with ratings of 3 or above (moderate to high stress), with supporting comments by Rose, her friend Susan, and the nurse practitioner:

Item 2: Self-acceptance/Self-esteem: *I failed two marriages. Yes, I was successful in my career but I always wanted to be truly loved by a man . . . I don't like to be alone.*

Item 6: Residential/Housing: Susan (exasperated and suspicious of Rose's daughter Jessica) had requested a home health evaluation be done to assess the situation. Rose loves her beautiful home. Susan has arranged for homecare for Rose in the past but when the people show up she will not let them in. Rose admits she sometimes forgets to eat and that going to the grocery store is tiring but states, *Jessica could help me more, but I know she's got problems of her own.*

Item 7: Financial Security: Nurse Practitioner notes possible financial exploitation to be explored, based on Susan's suspicion of Rose's daughter, most likely with Adult Protective Services.

Item 8: Decision-making/Cognitive Functioning: Rose became angry during discussion about her ability to make decisions for herself. She has always been independent and is offended by the suggestion that she is losing her mind. But she acknowledged her daughter's concerns about forgetfulness and her capacity to make decisions for herself. Friend Susan echoed this sentiment.

Item 9: Problem-solving Ability: Rose admits to feeling more frustrated with regular life. As the interview progressed, Susan spoke about rotten food in the refrigerator, spoiled milk, no fresh fruit or vegetables, the mess in the house, Rose forgetting to pay bills, eat, and wash her clothes.

Item 10: Life Goals/Spiritual Values: Rose said *My life has been wonderful and difficult. I've succeeded professionally and failed personally. Now it looks like the people I love want to put me out to pasture!*

Item 11: Leisure Time/Community Involvement: Rose said *I have to admit I don't do much anymore. I'm not sure why.* Apparently unable to connect reduced social engagement to cognitive decline and struggle with ADL.

Item 12: Feelings/Anxiety: *Sometimes I'm afraid to be alone now.* Friend Susan had described calling Rose *and she picks up the phone in tears, crying about her daughter and failed marriages.*

Item 14: Injury to Self: No history of suicidal ideation or attempts. Potential for danger of accidental injury secondary to inability to care for self and maintain safety independently.

Item 15: Danger to Others: No history of violence toward others, although she expresses some anger about her current situation and the people trying to "control" her life.

Item 18: Agency Use: Susan feels grateful for meeting today and being included. She and Rose's other close friends feel desperate for assistance. They are worried for her safety and are hopeful this meeting will be the beginning of a collaborative effort to assist Rose. Previous primary care provider had obtained a neurological assessment. Rose does not recall this examination or its results suggesting early Alzheimer's.

When asked about any other concerns she had or wish to see a counselor, Rose stated emphatically, *I don't really need any help right now. . . No, I do not think I need a counselor*, while Susan said *I just want to make sure we can work together.*

Mini-Mental State Examination Score: 13. She had difficulty with naming and could name a pencil but not a watch, was unable to do serial 7s, and no 3-minute recall. She was oriented but lost a point on location of office building. [A score of 23 or less can indicate cognitive impairment in someone at Rose's level of education—Folstein, 1983.]

Summary of Functional Assessment:

1. Risk for injury related to forgetfulness and as evidenced by spoiled food, cluttered/unkempt home, and living alone.
2. Impaired memory as evidenced by forgetting to eat, bathe, and pay bills, and poor recall during MMSE.
3. Altered nutrition, risk for less than body requirements, as evidenced by 20 lbs weight loss and lack of nutritional food in home as well as assistance to prepare meals.
4. Social isolation related to retirement and change in mental status and as evidenced by self-report, "I don't do as much."
5. Bathing/hygiene self-care deficit as evidenced by patient not bathing for four to five days.
6. Family coping, potential for growth, as evidenced by patient's allegiance to children but questionable practices of daughter.
7. Knowledge deficit related to Alzheimer's disease.
8. Fear related to loss of memory, loss of career as evidenced by self-report and sadness.

Diagnostic and Statistical Manual Diagnoses (DSM)

Axis I	Dementia of the Alzheimer's = Type, early onset
Axis II	Deferred (pending further evaluation)
Axis III	Hypothyroidism
Axis IV	Living alone
Axis V	Inadequate home care services
	GAF = 38

From this intake and follow-up sessions, the nurse practitioner enacted a service plan for Rose, including home-based assistance with ADL, regular appointments to assess daily functioning and medication regimens, and linkages with Adult Protective Services—depending on assessment and reports of her concerned friends.

Analysis, Guardianship, Final Years

Rose's case is both typical and atypical of the progression and final stages of Alzheimer's leading to death. Given Rose's intelligence and academic credentials, perhaps the strong denial following initial diagnosis was exacerbated by her outstanding personal and professional accomplishments, social status in her community, and her ability to "cover" and compensate for memory deficits so obvious to those who knew her well over time.

Losing one's ability to self-care and manage activities of daily living, while also being aware in the early stages that it is happening and is beyond one's control, can be a truly terrifying and sometimes life-threatening experience. At one point over dinner with Susan and two other friends who were supporting her during and well beyond diagnostic workups, Rose began weeping and said: "I feel like I'm losing my soul." At a later point when dealing with her anger at having an appointed guardian to manage her affairs, she said: "I want to kill him and then myself." While Rose's life was in danger from wandering off in front of running cars, etc., by this phase in development of the disease, she in fact would have been incapable of the planning, etc. necessary for committing either murder or suicide.

During this challenging two-year period for Rose and her friends (her de facto "family") the problems and obstacles in implementing a coordinated service plan for Rose were more egregious, given her history as a patient in a multi-disciplinary treatment facility with medical school teaching affiliations. Of particular note in this case and for this chapter is that the comprehensive treatment, protection, and personal service plan for Rose finally occurred only following a letter by her three friends to the judge who had declared her mentally "competent" (copied to various players in this case) asking whether they would be reading in the newspaper about their friend's demise on the street for lack of the services and protection she needed. Also of note is that two of Rose's three friends who made this final appeal to the judge were experienced health and social service professionals. This leaves us wondering what happens to others who lack such informed advocates.

In response to this letter, a year later, as the disease progressed and Rose could no longer be left alone, through advocacy by the legal guardian, friends, and Adult Protective Services, Rose was admitted to a nursing facility with a specialized unit for persons with Alzheimer's. She continued to mourn her losses, needing more and more assistance with grooming, hygiene, and nourishment, remaining mostly in her room except when receiving visitors. Before final decline when she could no longer recognize or identify her friends and family members, Rose never lost the core of her gracious personality in interaction with visitors and the caring and devoted nursing facility staff. Her death followed complications from Alzheimer's, and her funeral was attended by family and friends from afar.

For primary care providers, Rose's painful saga and her friends' struggles to get Rose the treatment and care needed, offer several lessons for prevention and intervention on behalf of others:

1. Easy and early access to a gerontological specialist by a PCP might temper the tendency to denial, alleviate some of the delays in early treatment, and help slow the progression of symptoms from cognitive impairment.
2. "Boundary" issues, in this case the overlapping "personal/professional" relationship between the "family doctor" and client, might have delayed delivering the needed

"straightforward" message about prospects of Alzheimer's disease earlier than occurred in Rose's case.

3. The incorporation of "home assessment" and functioning is a *critical part of comprehensive assessment* as soon as memory loss and other symptoms suggest the onset of Alzheimer's disease.

4. While geropsychiatric specialists are integral to differential diagnosis and treatment (including emotional and material support), the patient's PCP should recognize that "psychotherapy" is not appropriate for someone with serious memory loss.

5. When legal guardianship issues emerge, PCPs can be influential with court proceedings that include information beyond what the cognitively impaired patient may present; for example, in early stages of Rose's illness when Adult Protective Services were engaged, the judge ordered everyone out of the courtroom except Rose. This action served to reinforce Rose's denial, as she was able—in a short time space—to convincingly present her case to a judge who apparently had no knowledge about Alzheimer's disease when evidence from "home assessment" and daily functioning was absent, and who agreed with Rose's plea that she did not need a legal guardian.

6. The lack of coordination and interdisciplinary collaboration in this case most likely cannot be attributed to race discrimination, but rather as a "symptom" of the U.S. healthcare system that sometimes fails to serve people in a smoothly coordinated system of care regardless of race, class, gender, or other disadvantaged social status.

7. One of Rose's friends, as a result of what she learned about "denial" from this case, asked her PCP to note in her medical record something like the following: "If at some point you observe and suspect that I have early signs of AD, you recommend neuropsychiatric and other tests, and in the event I'm in denial and resist early treatment as my friend Rose did, please review for me that on this day I asked you to remind me that my symptoms are *part of the disease*—not a sign that I'm crazy."

Friends as Family Standing by Beyond Death

Rose's case reveals the powerful impact of Alzheimer's and other cognitive impairments not only on the patient, but the entire social network. The emotional responses to the diagnosis of dementia, especially AD, include: the fear of stigma and devaluation; mourning associated with actual and anticipated losses; and a sense of increased vulnerability of self.

Recent advances in diagnostic accuracy have resulted in earlier detection and prospects of slowing the process with medications. This has created a unique opportunity for (a) research to recruit people with dementia early in the course of the disease who are still capable of reflecting on and verbalizing their subjective experiences and service needs; (b) supportive interventions to maximize adaptive coping and quality of life outcomes; and (c) raising public awareness about the disease and subjective experiences of people with dementia in an attempt to dispel myths and stigmas attached to the disease, and empathize with people affected by it. Ideally, emotional support and other interventions should begin in the diagnostic phase (Aminzadeh, Byszewski, Molnar, & Eisner, 2007).

Families of persons with AD should avail themselves of the many support and technical sources needed in some cases over years. If available and affordable, a professional geriatric care manager can provide assistance with the complex legal, medical, and nursing care required (Melillo & Houde, 2005). Comparable specialty assistance is available through publicly funded sources, with information about access to services readily available in PCP offices. Without such support, family caretakers are vulnerable to fall among the ranks of the increasing morbidity and mortality rates of family caretakers of a spouse with AD or other dementias (Liken, 2001).

Attitudes toward Death, the Final Passage

Death has been a favorite topic of philosophers, poets, psychologists, physicians, and anthropologists for centuries. Volumes have been written by authors such as Aries (1974), Bertman (1991), and Mitford (1963). There is even a science of *thanatology* (study of death and dying). Yet death is still a taboo topic for many people, which is unfortunate because it means the loss of death as a "friendly companion" to remind us that our lives are finite. Such denial is the root of the complex situations cited in some of the vignettes above. As vast and important as the subject of death is, consideration of it here is limited to its implications for PCPs and their pivotal role in assuring the coordination of services and palliative care needed by those growing older and facing death.

As Tolstoy (1960 [1886]) wrote so eloquently in *The death of Ivan Ilyich*, the real agony of death is the final realization that we have not really lived our life, the regret that we did not do what we wanted to do, that we did not realize in and for ourselves what we most dearly desired. Such issues were borne out in Goodman's (1981) research in which she compared top performing artists' and scientists' attitudes toward death with a group who were not performing artists or scientists but were similar in other respects. She found significant evidence that the performing artists and scientists were less fearful of death, more accepting of death, and much less inclined to want to return to earth after their death if they had a chance. Having led full and satisfying lives, they were able to anticipate their deaths with peace and acceptance. They had "won the race with death."

Noted writer and humorist Art Buchwald decided not to let death have the last word. He held court with friends and others and planned his funeral during his final months in hospice. There, in effect, death waited for him to invite his children and various well-known people like Carly Simon and Tom Brokaw to write eulogies that he included in his last book, *Too soon to say goodbye* (2006). Here he treats death with his famed sense of humor and offers the living inspiring ways to face life's final loss.

The denial of death, so common in U.S. society, is a far greater enemy than death itself. It allows us to live our lives less fully than we might with an awareness and acceptance of death's inevitability. Through works like those of Buchwald, Sherwin Nuland, and many others, we have made progress in dealing with death openly. However, some health professionals and families still are reluctant to discuss the subject openly with a dying person (see Christakis & Asch, 1995; Ross, Fisher, & MacLean, 2000).

This is changing through the promotion of living wills, advance directives regarding the use of extraordinary treatment, and the public debate about physician-assisted suicide. For many, the assisted-suicide issue is primarily one of maintaining control over one's last days and not suffering unnecessary pain. As Dubler (1993) notes, the culture of medical institutions must change to accommodate the notion of negotiated death. The Patient Self-Determination Act passed by the U.S. Congress in 1990 facilitated such change by requiring healthcare institutions to inform patients of their rights to make advance medical directives. The act encourages people to think about what treatment they wish if terminally ill. It also ensures compliance with their wishes for the kind of death they envision. See Haynor (1998) for detailed information on how PCPs can empower patients and assist them in decision making around advance directive requirements and palliative care (Connor, 2009).

Yet, examples of avoidance cited in Kübler-Ross's classic book, *On death and dying* (1969), still occur unless the staff has had extensive sensitization to the needs of dying patients. Family members and everyone working with the dying will recognize the phases of dying (from denial, etc. to acceptance) described by Kübler-Ross from her interviews with over two hundred dying patients. All people do not necessarily experience all the stages, nor do these stages occur in a fixed, orderly sequence. But Kübler-Ross's work sensitizes health and hospice workers to some of the major issues and problems faced by the dying. For example, a quiet presence, communicating one's caring by a touch or a look, and assuring that the person's wishes such as advance directives are respected.

How we die by physician Nuland (1994) is another attempt to break through denial by his blunt account of the physiological process of ending life. Death can be viewed as a prototype of all life transitions in that each phase of the lifecycle requires leaving something behind—a loss—in order to make way for challenges and joys of the next phase. Coping with the biggest loss of all—death—is aided by success in handling various "mini-deaths" over one's lifetime, and the good fortune of social support from family, friends, and caretakers who must carry on.

Much of this supportive process by PCPs and others depends heavily on how comfortable one is with the topic of death and one's own mortality. For a PCP this includes the knowledge and courage to inform family when hospice care is indicated and should be initiated, since medical assessment reveals when death is imminent. When the person's wishes have not been made explicit through documents such as "Healthcare Proxy" that should be part of everyone's medical record, and family members are not emotionally prepared to "let go," this is a moment when high technology may be inappropriately applied to add a few more hours or days to the dying person's life—potentially adding additional and unnecessary pain of losing a loved one. (See Temel, *et al.*, 2010.)

As the final stage of growth and transition, death is the most powerful reminder that we have only one life to live and that to waste it would be folly. In this vein, one woman's conversation with her ancestors and mantra for purposeful living is: "Mother, may I never disappoint you . . . Death, may I be ready to greet you." Certainly one of life's final blessings is to maintain one's sense of self and feel ready to let go of life—grateful for what one has done for family and community, while un-bitter about relinquishing some unfinished tasks due to physical or cognitive infirmity. In that respect, Rose had neither choice nor cognitive awareness of her final moments. Many say their greatest fear is not death itself, but dying alone—a testament to our essential membership in community. To all appearances, Rose did not know in the end whether or not she was alone. But the universal value of respecting the living, those dying, and the dead was evident in Rose's community of friends and caretakers who did not let her die alone.

References

Aminzadeh, F., Byszewski, A., Molnar, F. J., & Eisner, M. (2007). Emotional impact of dementia diagnosis: Exploring persons with dementia and caregivers' perspectives. *Aging & Mental Health*, 11(3), 281–290.

Applebaum, P. S., & Grisso, T. (1988). Assessing patients' capacities to consent to treatment. *New England Journal of Medicine*, 319, 1635–1638.

Aries, P. (1974). *Western attitudes toward death from the middle ages to the present*. Baltimore, MD: Johns Hopkins University Press.

Bertman, S. L. (1991). *Facing death: Images, insights, and interventions*. Bristol, PA: Hemisphere.

Buchwald, A. (2006). *Too soon to die*. New York: Random House.

Christakis, N. A., & Asch, D. A. (1995). Physician characteristics associated with decisions to withdraw life support. *American Journal of Public Health*, 85(3), 367–372.

Connor, S. R. (2009). *Hospice and palliative care: The essential guide* (2nd Ed.). New York and London: Routledge.

Dick, K., & Morency, C. R. (2005). Delirium. In K. D. Melillo & S. C. Houde (Eds.), *Geropsychiatric and mental health nursing* (pp. 213–230). Boston: Jones & Bartlett.

Doress, P. B., & Siegal, D. L. (1987). *Ourselves, growing older*. New York: Simon & Schuster.

Douglas, M. (1966). *Purity and danger*. London: Routledge.

Dubler, N. N. (1993). Commentary: Balancing life and death—proceed with caution. *American Journal of Public Health*, 83(1), 23–25.

Erikson, E. (1963). *Childhood and society* (2nd ed.). New York: Norton.

Folstein, M. F. (1983). The mini-mental state exam. In T. Crook, S. H. Ferris, & R. Bartus (Eds.). *Assessment in geriatric psychpharmacology* (pp. 47–51). New Canaan, CT: Mark Powley.

Foreman, M., Fletcher, K., Mion, L., & Simon, L. (1996). Assessing cognitive function. *Geriatric Nursing*, 17(5), p. 229.

Goodman, L. M. (1981). *Death and the creative life*. New York: Springer.

Goody, J. (1962). *Death, property, and the ancestors*. London: Tavistock.

Haynor, P. M. (1998). Meeting the challenge of advance directives. *American Journal of Nursing*, 98(3), 26–32.

Hoff, L. A., Hallisey, B. J., & Hoff, M. (2009). *People in crisis: Clinical and diversity perspectives* (6th Ed.). New York and London: Routledge.

Kimball, S. T. (1960 [1909]). Introduction. In A. van Gennep, *Rites of passage*. Chicago, IL: University of Chicago Press. *Rites of passage* (A. van Gennep, Trans.). Chicago, IL: University of Chicago Press.

Kübler-Ross, E. (1969). *On death and dying*. NewYork: Macmillan.

LaFontaine, J. (1977). The power of rights. *Man*, 12, 421–437.

Liken, M. (2001). Caregivers in crisis. *Clinical Nursing Research*, 10(1), 52–68.

Melillo, K. D., & Houde, S. C. (2005). *Geropsychiatric and mental health nursing*. Boston, MA: Jones & Bartlett.

Milne, A.,Culverwell A., Guss, R., Tuppen, J., Whelton, R., (2008). Screening for dementia in primary care: A review of theuse, efficacy and quality of measures, *International Psychogeriatric*, 20(5), 911–926.

Mitford, J. (1963). *The American way of death*. New York: Simon & Schuster.

Morgan, B. (2010). End of life care for patients with mental illness and personality disorders. In B. Ferrell & N. Coyle (Eds.), *Oxford textbook of palliative nursing* (pp. 757–766). New York: Oxford University Press.

Nuland, S. B. (2007). *The art of aging*. New York: Random House.

Nuland , S. B. (1994). *How we die: Reflections on life's final chapter*. New York: Random House.

Remington, R., Gerdner, L. A., & Buckwalter, K. C. (2005). Nursing management of clients experiencing dementias of late life: Care environments, clients, and caregivers. In K. D. Melillo & S. C. Houde (Eds.), *Geropsychiatric and mental health nursing* (pp. 252–266). Boston: Jones & Bartlett.

Ross, M. (2000). *The other side of the bed*. Self-published.

Ross, M. M., Fisher, R., & MacLean, M. J. (2000). Toward optimal care for seniors who are dying: An approach to care. *Mature Medicine Canada*, 127–130.

Schouten, R., & Brendel, R.W. (2004). Legal aspects of consultation. In T. A. Stern, G. L. Fricchione, H. N. Cassem; M. S. Jellinek, & J. F. Rosenbaum, (Eds.), Massachusetts General Hospital handbook of general hospital psychiatry. 5th Ed. (pp. 349–364). Philadelphia, PA: Mosby.

Sherell, K., & Iris, M. (2005). Nursing assessment of clients with dementias of late life: Screening, diagnosis, and communication. In K. D. Melillo & S. C. Houde (Eds.), *Geropsychiatric and mental health nursing* (pp. 231–249). Boston: Jones & Bartlett.

Temel, J. S., Greer, J. A., Muzikansky, M. A., *et al.* (2010). Early palliative care for patients with metastatic non-small-cell lung cancer. *New England Journal of Medicine*, 363(8), 733–742.

Tolstoy, L. (1960 [1886]). *The death of Ivan Ilyich*. New York: New American Library.

Van Gennep, A. (1960 [1909]). *Rites of passage*. Chicago, IL: University of Chicago Press.

van Gool, C. H., Kempen, G. I. J. M., Bosma, H., van Boxtel, M. P. J., Jolles, J., & van Eijk, J. T. M. (2006). Associations between lifestyle and depressed mood: Longitudinal results from the Maastricht Aging Study. *American Journal of Public Health*, 97(5), 887–894.

Yesavage, J. A., & Brink, T. L. (1983). Development and validation of a geriatric depression scale: A preliminary report. *Journal of Psychiatric Research*, 17, 37–49.

Yuan, A. S. V. (2007). Perceived age discrimination and mental health. *Social Forces Volume*, 86 (1), 291–311.

13 Complementary and Alternative Treatments-CAM

Healing Body, Mind, and Spirit

with Jane Bindley

- Theoretical Overview
- Diet, Exercise, Self-Care, and Self-esteem: Inter-relationships
- Collaboration between Primary Care and Alternative Therapy Practitioners
- References

"It's like a miracle . . . What is it that you did for me? I can barely believe that maybe you're saving me from the back surgery the orthopedic surgeon said I might need."

This is the response of Carol, a client and hospice care nurse herself, referred by a nurse practitioner to physical therapy. Carol's story inspired us to write this chapter for the benefit of other clients and their primary care providers. Clearly, the therapy received was not at all miraculous. Rather, it is based on principles of Eastern medicine and increasingly popular manual therapy (touch, e.g., massage) as alternatives to pharmacological and surgical responses to various ailments and scientifically diagnosed conditions like Carol's—spinal stenosis.

This chapter presents the trend toward collaboration among Western and Eastern healing traditions, as millions of people seek natural healing alternatives to the treatment of chronic pain and other conditions. In the United States, this group comprises about one-third of adults in a population of over 300 million (CAM, 2005). The alternative therapies discussed are those offered by licensed professionals. Thus, for example, anyone can practice yoga simply by reading a book on the topic, although certain yoga positions (e.g., the head or shoulder stand) are contraindicated for someone with spinal stenosis. In contrast, zero balancing cannot be practiced without special training, and typically this includes already licensed practitioners such as physical therapists, registered nurses, and massage therapists.

Theoretical Overview

To address as well as contain the wide array of complementary and alternative therapies (CAM) practiced by licensed professionals and the general public, it is important to understand the basic premises of CAM, what it encompasses, and how it is related to conventional medical practice, including safety issues.

Complementary and Alternative Medicine (CAM): Definition and Categories

This chapter draws on the following definition of CAM cited by the U.S. Institute of Medicine, the Committee on the Use of Complementary and Alternative Medicine by the American Public, Board on Health Promotion and Disease Prevention (2005):

> Complementary and alternative medicine (CAM)—also known as "integrative medicine") is a broad domain of resources that encompasses health systems, modalities, and practices and their accompanying theories and beliefs, other than those intrinsic to the dominant health system of a particular society in a given historical period. CAM includes such resources provided by their users as associated with positive health outcomes. Boundaries within the CAM and between the CAM domain and the domain of the dominant system are not always fixed.
>
> (CAM, 2005, p. 19).

Broadly, this definition encompasses the five CAM categories adopted by the National Center for Complementary and Alternative Medicine (NCCAM) of the U.S. National Institutes of Health:

1. alternative medical systems;
2. mind-body interventions;
3. biologically based treatments;
4. manipulative (manual) and body-based methods;
5. energy therapies.

Primary care providers as well as their clients should be familiar with these key features of CAM for best possible outcomes around health and mental health issues:

- They are safe and effective.
- Collaboration among interdisciplinary healthcare providers is needed.
- Compassion and caring are recognized as important.
- Medical practice is continuously shaped by larger socio-economic, cultural, and political forces.
- Integrative medicine requires openness to diverse meanings of health, illness, and healing.
- Effective practice in integrative medicine requires inclusion of its key concepts in the standard curriculum preparing healthcare professionals.

The CAM definition and categories complement two major themes of this book: They are patient-centered and they resonate with the cross-cultural diversity of mental health and illness maladies, as well as the different *meanings* people attach to what they are suffering and how they can find relief. Some first see a "professional," others find a traditional healer, still others seek and find comfort in religious rituals, and/or meditation, exercise, and relaxation. Central here is the element of patient choice, safety, and what works—either alone, or in combination with conventional treatment such as surgery or prescribed medication.

While the therapies addressed here may be unfamiliar to some primary care providers, they happen to coincide with some of the most basic principles of healthy living and self-care widely advocated by government agencies concerned with the nation's health and the growing epidemic of diabetes, for example, and other preventable diseases. Following is a summary of three alternative therapies; how they differ from and complement mainstream

Western medicine; self-care fundamentals like diet and exercise; and an analysis of why such widely available and often repeated information (in print and other media) is not more readily translated into daily self-care practice. The examples illustrate how continued pain and/or dysfunction in everyday life from various medical conditions—if not relieved—can lead to depression or even suicide among clients seeking pain relief.

Published volumes on alternative therapies based on Eastern and other healing theories are legion. They are widely available in bookstore "self-help" sections and at pharmacy and some supermarket check-out displays. A comprehensive coverage here is therefore both unnecessary for primary care providers, and beyond the scope of this book. Our aims instead are (1) to show how Eastern and Western treatment strategies complement rather than contradict each other—that is, a both/and *not* an either/or approach; and (2) to invite PCPs to consider alternative therapies as supplements to scientifically supported treatment strategies already mastered. We focus our attention especially on those alternative and natural healing therapies that may apply to clients who are either disappointed with pharmacological and surgical outcomes, and/or are skeptical of their application for particular health problems. Since for some this topic is viewed skeptically, we steer clear of any already discredited "therapies" that are untested for their effectiveness—such as laetrile, garlic cures, and foreign cancer spas—while also recognizing from scientific medicine's clinical trials the "placebo effect" as evidence of mind-body connections.

Eastern and Western Medicine: Complementary Aspects and Differences

Our discussion and case illustrations are deeply influenced by the works of several healers trained in both Western and Eastern (or "integrated") medicine, especially: Fritz Frederick Smith, *Inner bridges* (1994); Andrew Weil, *Natural health, natural medicine* (2004); Dr. Smith's student, John Hamwee, *Zero balancing* (1999); and surgeon Bernie Siegel's *Peace, love and healing* (1990). Dr. Smith persuasively shows how his immersion in the empirically based medical model had shortchanged him. He had accepted this model without question, but later learned that the intuitive and experiential side of life encompasses the broader topic of health, wholeness, and human potential. His analysis brings us full circle to a major premise of this book presented in Chapter 1—that is, the ancient wisdom of Hippocrates, the father of medicine who recognized the vital connections between body, mind, and spirit.

The title of Dr. Smith's book underscores his hope of building bridges between Western medicine and the range of alternative therapies that are increasingly embraced by more and more people—with or without the approval of licensed physicians. His thoughtful analysis also lays a solid foundation for distinguishing between potentially dangerous self-help remedies and those therapies that may lack empirically tested evidence of their effectiveness (as in randomized clinical trials), but nevertheless have resulted in reports of healing and the subjective experience of improved health and sense of well-being as revealed in reduced pain and increased functioning in activities of daily living, e.g., walking, uplifted mood, etc.

However, trained medical professionals may well question the wisdom and safety of some non-prescription remedies that patients use without the advice or approval of their primary care provider. While many of these therapies lack measureable efficacy from controlled trials, patients may choose them as an alternative to treatment that is scientifically supported but which often entails serious or very unpleasant side-effects (as in powerful chemotherapeutic agents for cancer treatment). Such choices are based on the person's subjective "evidence" of their value, ranging from personal experience of pain relief, for example, the advice of family or friends, to the recommendation of a PCP based on early results of scientific research on these alternative therapies. On the other hand, while the Institute of Medicine has included

CAM under its scientific umbrella, it is timely to note the daunting parameters and formal requirements of randomized controlled trials to ascertain the efficacy of various self-help remedies adopted as a personal choice by many millions of people. In contrast to such free choice, as a research participant in controlled trials, the formal agreement between the researcher and participant requires, for example, informed consent, adherence to a prescribed regimen, freedom to drop out, etc.

Dr. Smith credits these East/West links to the past few decades of introduction and translation of Eastern philosophy and therapies such as acupuncture, herbology, meditation, and the martial arts—including the basic principle of *ch'i,* the vital life force, or *energy* moving in the physical body. As evidence of this energy he cites common everyday expressions related to our energy fields: "I'm running out of steam," "I'm at a low ebb," "I feel high" (or "really low"), plus our "conscious awareness of the struggles and joys of the life process itself" (Smith, 1994, pp. 22–23). The body's skeletal system constitutes the major integrating flow connecting us to nature, while energy in human communication and listening fields bring us together socially. Dr. Smith notes, for example, that the "best communication begins by energetically responding to another person," for instance in the rituals of shaking hands, hugging, and sincere greetings that lessen tension and facilitate resonance and harmony between people (p. 43).

Currents within the energy model are organized through three layers, with the deepest layer flowing through the skeletal system that is accentuated by walking and other physical activity; while the middle layer flows through the soft tissue which is closely associated with our physiological, mental, emotional, and spiritual functions. The seven major energy centers, or chakras in Eastern yoga philosophy, correspond to the human skeletal system and the laws of physics. In this Hindu system, the seventh chakra is associated with the top of the skull and signifies the belief in a Universal Soul with which an individual's soul can unite. As attested by the variety of yoga books and classes attended by many people in the West, there are various paths and approaches to the practice of yoga. However, common to all is developing mental and physical purity through thought and breath control and quieting the mind, which resembles the body–mind–spirit triad common in Western culture (Smith, 1994, pp. 47–59), and in the widely cited work of Dr. Herbert Benson and colleagues regarding the "relaxation response."

Dr. Smith wisely notes the potential for physical, mental, and spiritual discord in our fast-paced high-technology driven society. If the chakra ladder leads from competition to cooperation to wisdom, and is used in a healthy and creative way, we may discover that cooperatively merging our high-tech society with ancient systems of knowledge "is truly a catalyst for creating a better world" (p. 73). This would seem to apply especially to stressed out people in American society who notably have less vacation time than individuals in other modern countries and many of whom, when they do go on holiday, remain tethered to the electronic devices that keep them constantly wired to work sites. A hopeful sign of the detrimental health effects of constant connection to work is this recent remark by a book editor who responded thus to a question about his availability through his "blackberry" while out of office: "No, I will not be tied to that 'ball and chain' while away!" The similar refrain, "It's really crazy how hard we work," heard from many of late, may signal a growing awareness of the benefits of a less technologically driven lifestyle that shortchanges these vital connections between mind, body, spirit, and life's meaning.

The differences between the Western medical model and alternative healing are reflected in the different perspectives of health and illness and can be summarized thus: In the Western medical model, illness is typically considered as an event or conditions such as diabetes or heart disease that require lifelong medication. In the natural healing perspective, illness is viewed as part of a person's broader life process reflecting an underlying stress or energy imbalance; for example, hypertension may evolve to a normal rate in relation to relief of stressful events in the person's life (Smith, 1994, p. 149).

Zero Balancing

Much of Dr. Smith's analysis of "inner bridges" is taken from the structural acupressure system known as "Zero Balancing" which is explicated by one of his trainees, John Hamwee, in a short book by the same name (1999), and to which there is a dedicated following by many alternative healing practitioners. The most basic proposition of energy balancing is touching the energy and structure of the bone and joints.

Hamwee points out that one can choose to work only with structure, as do osteopaths and orthopedic surgeons, or only with energy, as do most acupuncturists and Reiki practitioners. But Hamwee suggests, for example in treating people suffering back pain, that by working with structure and energy together, structure work may re-establish flows of *energy*, and energy work may re-establish *re-alignment of structure*—in effect, bringing them "back to Zero" in order to once again enjoy life and undertake things previously thought too difficult, given the constraints of painful symptoms (p. 38). In effect, instead of focusing simply on symptoms or "what is wrong with me," Zero Balancing directs attention to getting back to "who you are" as the whole human being you were before, rather than simply on defining a client as just another body identified by the illness, i.e., "what you've got" (p. 53).

Building on the established principle of medicine to "Do no harm," the most fundamental technique of Zero Balancing is the concept of the "fulcrum" or balance point, which incorporates the accepted holistic principle that the client is in charge of what happens. The American Heritage Dictionary defines fulcrum as "A position, element, or agency through, around, or by means of which vital powers are exercised." Applied to Zero Balancing, the fulcrum or balance point is created through direct pressure on tissue and bone points to "get in touch" with the client's energy body (Smith, p. 80). Different body parts are associated with different emotions and the relation of body parts to each other: For example, a person is urged to "stand up for himself" (personality assertiveness), or in considering aspects of a psychological or ethical dilemma one says "I have a 'gut' reaction that this is just not right," or "It just doesn't feel right."

However, from centuries of success of the scientific method in demonstrating "cause and effect" relationships, and unhelpful fall-out from the Cartesian separation of mind and body ("I think and therefore I am"), it is tempting to discount the effects of the Zero Balancing technique because its energy treatments are outside the Western paradigm. Yet, most Western practitioners accept the common observation that people whose immune systems are compromised or debilitated, and those experiencing extraordinary social stressors or problems tend to become physically ill more easily and recover more slowly. As Hamwee states: "You cannot see an emotion through a microscope; equally, you cannot know the chemical composition of an amino acid by sheer intuition. So, although there may be no scientific proof that a mental state or an emotion is lodged in a particular part of the body, it may still be true" (p. 73). Thus, for example, drooping shoulders may signal hopelessness. Or, as psychiatric practitioners have long observed, the lifting of a "depressed facies," more lively gait, and renewed social engagement suggest improvement from treatment for depression.

The "Touching" Principle, Trauma Histories, and Healing

Since Zero Balancing treatment is enacted primarily through touch of the body's energy in the bone, some discussion of the *potential of such touching for both healing or trauma* is in order. A principle from Western medicine about touching is: Always touch the person "where it hurts." Thus, while touching is pivotal in some diagnoses, it can also re-traumatize a person whose history includes abuse—especially sexual assault—if not sensitively addressed with the patient. The following example supports this principle, and also has economic implications regarding the cost of certain diagnostic procedures that might have been unnecessary if the "touch" principle had been applied.

CASE EXAMPLE: DIAGNOSTIC TOUCH

A woman, age 55, returned from a normal early evening walk, noticed some knee discomfort, sat down to dinner, and could barely stand up again because of excruciating pain in her knee. After resting in her chair for a while with no pain relief, she called a taxi and went to the closest emergency department. On arrival, she needed a wheel chair to get to the examining room. There she was examined first by a physician assistant and then by an orthopedic surgeon, given a strong pain medication and discharged with instructions to see her primary care provider (PCP) the next day for further evaluation. The PCP ordered an MRI to establish a diagnosis of "Baker's cyst" which the patient herself could then clearly palpate on back of the knee. Physical therapy sessions were prescribed which included a series of exercises and eventual abatement of symptoms. Of note in this case is that none of the three prac- titioners within a 24-hour period of examining the patient ever touched the back of her knee. It is plausible to suggest that, had they done so, a $1000 fee for the MRI diagnosis might have been spared. Another facet of this case is the orthopedist's instructions to the patient to "avoid using stairs" but failing to note that this restriction applied only during the acute healing phase of whatever caused the initial painful episode presumably from an inner knee stressor. Consequently, two years later another practitioner noted the woman's "flabby thighs" attributed to continued avoidance of stairs and no strengthening exercises.

While Zero Balancing touch is done with the client fully clothed, knowledge of a client's medical history is critical before embarking on any touching—just as critical as ruling out severe pathology such as a fractured hip when applying energy techniques. This is because the client's history may include deeply imprinted trauma lodged in the body and psyche from inappropriate touching, childhood sexual abuse, and/or rape—an indication of the deep mind–body connections in healing from trauma that may surface in later treatment. In the absence of healing for such trauma, touching—even when therapeutically intended—can re-activate the emotional trauma from such abuse and violence.

This caution coincides with medicine's "do no harm" principle and the skills that all practitioners (Western and Eastern) have in the ground rules of the therapeutic relationship. It also underscores for PCPs the importance of incorporating victimization assessment and treatment strategies in primary care protocols as discussed in Chapter 5 of this book (see also Hoff, Hallisey, & Hoff, 2009; Hoff, 2010; Levine, 1997). And when PCPs consider referring clients for physical therapy or alternative treatment such as Zero Balancing, they should include abuse histories if already disclosed, and/or initial impression of possible unresolved psychological vulnerabilities. That said, given these precautions and other facets of Zero Balancing therapy, healing touch can be safe, and its potential for *healing* is great for address- ing the traumas of inappropriate touch and psychic scars from violence (Hamwee, 1999, p. 131).

Communication, then, with the client, and between collaborating professionals, is a key ingredient of observing these safety issues and holistic, client-centered therapy in both Eastern and Western healing traditions. The internet site is www.zerobalancing.com. This website includes information about therapists licensed to practice Zero Balancing across a wide array of communities in the United States and internationally.

BioSynchronistics®

This therapeutic modality draws on traditional physical therapy techniques, and is enhanced by a holistic approach based on both the force of gravity and the body's inherent ability to heal itself. BioSynchronistics combines manual techniques that balance, sequentially, all of a body's systems. When learned in full, it is quickly usable, complies with current HMO requirements, and treatment is accepted by most insurances.

As a form of manual physical therapy, BioSynchronistics is effective in treating the common neuromusculoskeletal conditions experienced by non-athletes and athletes alike. Earmarks of modern life, such as too much sitting, repetitive motions, pushing yourself too far/too soon in athletics, emotional stress, etc., can cause one's body to deviate from its natural biomechanical equilibrium into malalignment, thus changing the body's center of gravity from its normal position. This change is felt as unwanted, uncomfortable, tiring, painful, awkward tightness, strain, or functional limitation in daily activities.

Actually, these are only symptoms resulting from the body's compensation for its malalignment. Our body is working to remain upright and functioning. Muscles tighten, sometimes even spasm, to help deal with any malalignment. Merely removing this tightness will only bring temporary relief from symptoms. But BioSynchronistics-trained therapists view the body as a whole and take fully into account a client's lifestyle and the body's working arrangements. BioSynchronistics treatment systematically corrects one's underlying malalignment and restores biomechanical equilibrium within the body. Successful treatment is evident when the body can let go of its difficult and even painful compensations, thus providing lasting relief: "You *feel* better because you *are* better!" Patients report much satisfaction with Biosychronistics.

Clinical Acupressure (CA)

Clinical Acupressure utilizes fundamental acupressure methods to support the body's own balancing and healing processes. All parts of a human being, and nature itself, are interconnected and dependent on each other. Teachings about this perspective can be traced back thousands of years. The Chinese mapped predictable energy pathways (meridians) throughout the body nearly 4,000 years ago, and have been using them as a health reference ever since. Ancient teachings from India inform us about major energy centers in the body (chakras). These traditions address the vital energies of the body, to facilitate balance, rejuvenation, and wellness.

Clinical Acupressure addresses many common physical symptoms including back problems, headaches, respiratory, digestive and systemic problems as well as colds, flu, allergies, and healing from injuries. Hands-on work with the fully clothed body releases and strengthens the body's energy systems—meridians and chakras. This form of acupressure is especially helpful with stress-related conditions, including post-traumatic stress.

What makes Clinical Acupressure so effective? Often described as "acupuncture without needles," Clinical Acupressure promotes balance, rejuvenation, and wellness by accessing and addressing the vital energies of the body. Clinical Acupressure promotes better health and renewed energy by actively involving the client in his or her own healing and growth process. See: internet site www.soullightening.com/train_clinical.php.

Together, creatively applied and with careful attention to medical history, we believe primary care providers may find these alternatives to Western medicine as valuable adjuncts to some of their clients' healthcare needs.

Diet, Exercise, Self-Care, and Self-Esteem: Inter-relationships

Before illustrating some Eastern techniques with case examples, a review of the most basic elements of wellness and the prevention of various illnesses provides a foundation for more effective treatment outcomes—either from Eastern medicine or Western medical and surgical interventions. Eastern-inspired techniques are built on the perspective of treating the whole person, not just symptom relief; or a combination from both traditions. These lifestyle and wellness principles may indeed be the foundation for a client's positive attitude toward considering alternative and natural healing remedies for various afflictions.

The Power of a "Take-Charge" Attitude toward Health and Wellness

Before addressing the issue of attitude, a caveat is in order. Over the years many pages have been written suggesting, for example, that if nurses would only maintain a positive upbeat "attitude" they could avoid the abusive behavior that has been directed toward them over the entire history of nursing. Put another way, while a particular individual's attitude may be a component in achieving desired outcomes of problems faced by staff, a fundamental principle of successful conflict resolution is the alignment of strategies with the nature of the problem. Thus, if the problem can be traced to policies that support unequal power and benefits in the workplace (i.e., a socio-political source), the "attitude" of an individual will have little impact on effecting needed change; in fact, a cheerful attitude or tacit acceptance of the status quo may aid, abet, and contribute to entrenchment of harmful policies. On the other hand, a hopeful proactive attitude and belief in oneself aligned with like-minded others, combined with knowledge and skills in social change, is more likely to achieve positive outcomes. For example, a problem like the obesity epidemic requires both individual and socio-economic strategies to bring about change.

Applied to the health provider/client scenario, PCPs' recommendations to individual clients regarding diet and exercise are likely to be received and followed with greater care if delivered with knowledge and compassion about the serious social and financial obstacles some clients face in trying to take care of themselves. An individual's attitude and willingness to engage in a healthier lifestyle is necessary, but may not be sufficient for someone facing daily survival challenges. For example, it has not escaped the notice of many that there is serious inequality based on financial means affecting access to the fresh fruits and vegetables so central to a healthy diet.

Many poor people in inner cities have limited availability of supermarkets in their neighborhood, as is common in affluent suburbs and where virtually everyone owns a car. One result of such inequality is that some must carry heavy grocery bags by as many as three public transportation routes to feed their families healthier and obtain less expensive fare than that offered at the corner "convenience" store usually highly stocked with "junk" food. These social and public policy issues need to be kept in mind by all if the national epidemic of obesity and diabetes is to be addressed in addition to the role of public education and self-care in response to the epidemic.

That said, whether or not alternative therapies are even chosen—as stand-alone techniques or as complements to Western medical regimens, not to mention their effectiveness—may indeed depend on the attitudes and self-care practices of clients themselves. It is now widely recognized in the United States that clients are increasingly expected to "take charge" of navigating their healthcare through the increasing complexities of one or several healthcare agencies, including the intricate and demanding bureaucracy of the insurance and pharmaceutical industries affecting their care. Even highly educated clients and healthcare professionals themselves can be overwhelmed with a time-consuming and exasperating process such as obtaining a consultation appointment, or correcting a minor error in a prescription or financial statement. It is therefore daunting to consider what a very sick person, a client not fluent in English, or with financial and other disadvantages might suffer in attempts to get needed help.

At the same time, it is also very challenging for dedicated PCPs to do all they possibly can for clients, yet observe that some fail to follow the most basic guidelines for health and well-being. Of course the point here is not "blaming the victim," as it has already been noted how social factors like poverty and racism can negatively affect one's best self-care efforts. A young medical student's decision about her future practice aptly illustrates this point in respect to her dilemma regarding personal self-care and professional responsibility.

This student was very observant about healthy eating, exercise, etc. in her own life. During her medical school rotations, she was keenly set on primary care as her future practice arena, wanting to help alleviate the shortage of primary care physicians. Yet she ended up choosing pathology—the other end of the medical spectrum! A stunned friend inquired how she came to this decision, to which the young doctor replied along these lines: "During more than one rotation I kept noticing how many patients didn't eat right, wouldn't exercise, smoked, drank too much and other things that it seems like everybody by now should know about how to stay healthy. I felt helpless a lot of times—and sometimes angry—working with these patients, and when I thought about it for future practice I could see myself maybe getting very impatient . . . yet we're taught to be objective, not judgmental. So I decided it was best to just focus on pathology where I wouldn't have to deal with the frustration of trying to treat people who don't take care of themselves."

Addressing this self-care scenario is the case of Carol which includes a foundation or "infrastructure" for the prospects of Eastern medicine techniques complementing the best of Western medicine. As it turns out, Carol is a recent avid follower of Dr. Andrew Weil who, after graduating from Harvard Medical School, went on to found the Arizona Center for Integrative Medicine at the University of Arizona in Tucson. Many already know Dr. Weil for his work on natural healing which is featured in widely read magazines and other media. While many medical schools publish regular health newsletters, Dr. Weil's self-healing work is particularly valuable for the "both/and" approach he takes to many well-known as well as emerging questions about professional healthcare and self-care. We cite his work for his "balanced" (no pun intended) views on issues that encompass Western and Eastern approaches. In a non-preachy manner, he answers questions about "popular" new therapies and non-prescription supplements, and carefully critiques all for their status as either "quack" or insufficiently tested using scientific and clinical trial criteria. But as we see, Carol struggled long and hard on her own before being strongly affirmed by the integrative facets of Eastern and Western medicine.

CASE EXAMPLE: CAROL HAYES AND CAM

Carol, age 71, 5'7" and weighing 128 pounds, was referred to physical therapy with the diagnosis of spinal stenosis. Overall, Carol is a healthy and socially engaged person who appears much younger than her biological age. She is a registered nurse with a Masters degree who worked in acute care, followed by several years in a bariatric surgery unit until her retirement six years ago. Currently she works part-time as a hospice nurse which she finds much less stressful than the intensity of hospital nursing. Carol's family history includes diabetes and hypothyroidism on both maternal and paternal sides, an aunt with diabetic blindness, and a grandmother who had a leg amputation due to uncontrolled diabetes. Her father died at age 80 of complications from diabetes and emphysema after 40 years of smoking, and her mother's death at age 82 followed a diagnosis of Alzheimer's. A computer-based genealogical analysis of her extended family revealed her ethnic group as one with high rates of Alzheimer's.

Well before her parents' deaths, on physical examination required for admission to nursing school, Carol was advised of her vulnerability to diabetes if she failed to keep her weight under control. As a teenager, Carol was a "double dessert" kind of girl, finishing leftover pie, etc., but she seriously considered the physician's warning, resolved she would "never be fat," weaned herself off excess sweets, and embarked on what today is generally known as the "Mediterranean diet." Still, she struggled greatly to control her weight until she found and stuck to an exercise regimen of twice weekly gym aerobic exercise, daily walking between 20 and 30 minutes, and daily yoga interspersed with stretching exercises. Since many people have remarked on Carol's physical fitness and weight control—seemingly "without effort"— we also wanted to note for this chapter what she sees as the secret to her success.

Her symptoms began five years earlier with what she thought might be "restless leg syndrome" increasing to the point of right leg pain that awakened her at night, but quickly disappeared by the time she walked down the stairs from her bedroom. When the pain caus-ing nighttime wakening spread to Carol's left leg, circulatory and/or neurological causation was explored and ruled out. A few months later Carol began to experience difficulty with normal activities mastered with ease before, such as carrying groceries only a few blocks. Anxiously, she exclaimed to her PCP: "It feels a bit like I've become an old woman in just a few months!" Her PCP then ordered X-rays and an MRI, the results of which indicated spinal stenosis. On follow-up consultation with an orthopedic surgeon, three options were presented: (1) Keep moving as much as possible. This coincided with Carol's experience of leg pain relief as soon as she was up and walking, plus her already active walking life. (2) A corticosteroid injection into the spinal column which might result in temporary pain relief up to several months, and the option of two more injections. This resulted in nighttime pain relief for one week, and very unpleasant side-effects. (3) Spinal surgery which the surgeon explained was "minimally invasive" with an incision of only about one square inch, and with plausible success rates.

Despite the surgeon's reputation, Carol's response to the surgery option included high anxiety and memories from her nursing years of patients' horror stories following back sur-gery. She resolved to do everything possible—including physical therapy—as an alternative before deciding on surgery. Her PCP, a nurse practitioner, agreed, which is how Carol was introduced to Zero Balancing.

Carol was treated with two therapies, Zero Balancing and BioSynchronistics. Over a course of bi-weekly sessions for several months, her symptoms gradually decreased. Carol also asked her therapist to evaluate her daily yoga and stretching regimen for the possibility that some of the exercises may be exacerbating her symptoms. The yoga shoulder stand and "plough" were ruled out, and three other strengthening exercises demonstrated to replace them. The therapist also advised to stop loading her shoulders as though she was a "pack horse" and instead, use a rolling cart or back pack for grocery shopping. In two months time and significant symptom relief, Carol's anxiety level about any imminent need of surgery also subsided. Nighttime awakening from right leg pain continues intermittently, but Carol has learned to simulate "walking motions" in the bed which usually relieves the pain. Her PCP also prescribed a half dose of Ambien which Carol takes PRN, depending on cumulative sleep deprivation and the time of night awakening from leg pain. Carol does not want to become dependent on Ambien, and continues with intermittent Zero Balancing treatment. She may reconsider having spinal surgery at some future point when it would entail least interruption with her work life and travel plans.

We do not suggest with Carol's story that her example applies to all. But given her family history, our inspiration from her struggles to avoid diabetes, her obvious vitality in later years, and her openness to alternative therapies, we asked her to share with our readers the secrets to her success with diet and self-care. Here is what she shared.

- Nutrition: (1) Don't ever go on a diet, vs. just eating right as part of lifestyle. "Dieting" doesn't work because it "fools" the body into temporarily lowering one's metabolism rate and eventually re-gaining whatever temporary weight gain was achieved. (2) Don't deprive yourself of anything you truly love, but have it occasionally and in small amounts. After an "ice cream" binge and cholesterol "surge" for a couple of years, Carol discovered the same pleasure from two ounces of gourmet ice cream as from an oversized cone that resulted in skipping a balanced meal later. When Carol came on financial hard times, she discovered the joys of home cooking which not only benefited her pocket book, but eliminated heartburn that often followed a restaurant meal. Carol also took a lesson from a colleague who told her she "never cooks a real meal except for company," interpreted this behavior as a manifestation of low self-esteem, and said to herself: "I deserve a healthy good meal, even if I have to eat it alone." (3) Don't munch all day, eat on the road, or over the sink. An incentive for keeping to this rule is remembering the connection between oral and general health: If there's no chance to brush teeth, don't let microbes fester all day long from snacking.
- Exercise: (1) Don't let yourself off the hook by saying "I don't have time." Saying this may signal low self-esteem and that everything else on your agenda is more important than taking care of yourself. (2) To assure that it becomes part of your lifestyle, write in your appointment book whatever your exercise of choice is, which puts it on par with going to work, playing with the children, putting them to bed, and reading to them. (3) When exercise seems like a burden, try to remember the rewards and what your body feels like after a gym workout, swimming, a brisk walk, how the mind clears and "new ideas" just seem to emerge with some healthy down time, and how bad it feels after gorging on a box of cookies, two pieces of pie, or a double ice cream cone.
- Self-Esteem and Self-Care: Treat yourself to what you deserve and love to do alone and with friends. And if stress or unexpected burdens are truly troubling and dragging you down from achieving your life goals, consult a counselor who can help you work things through to a happier, healthier life with yourself and others.
- Meditation: Take at least ten minutes a day for complete quiet to just let go—whether it's meditation or just sitting quietly in a beautiful nature setting or a prayer space to signify that "This is *my* time."

Carol is reconciled to some of the ailments and slowdowns she attributes in part to her age, but Zero Balancing has encouraged her to delay or refuse outright the prospects of spinal surgery, depending on possible symptom exacerbation and life goals. She also hopes that through her self-care regimen, and by remaining socially and intellectually active, she may escape or at least delay the ravages of Alzheimer's disease which she had discovered in mid-life was a risk factor in her family gene pool.

CASE ILLUSTRATIONS: ZERO BALANCING, BIOSYNCHRONISTICS ® AND CLINICAL ACUPRESSURE

Jim Bennet: Orthopedics

Jim was 28 years old and in excellent health except for his bladder problem. He was a runner and stretched daily. Jim reported he had frequency of urination for many years. As the condition worsened, he found himself very tense and high-strung, and reduced his social engagements to save himself from any embarrassment. At a loss for any further treatment, his urologist referred him to physical therapy with the diagnosis of pelvic floor restriction. Evaluation by the physical therapist revealed restriction in his hamstrings, lateral abdominals with no space between his ilium and ribs, and the muscles of the pelvic floor. BioSynchronistics and appropriate home stretching changed the restriction and improved bladder function. Jim had difficulty relaxing. He had a job with daily deadlines and high expectations for himself. He was beginning to doubt his successful work performance, and had seen a psychiatrist for several sessions, but with no symptom relief. The physical therapist added Zero Balancing to his treatment. He experienced deep relaxation, and said this was a new experience for him and his body. He had weekly Zero Balancing treatments for one month. On a return visit to his urologist after these treatments, his bladder function was normal. He reported he had been able to hold on to the new experience of relaxation.

John Parks: Parkinson's Disease

John, age 53, was referred to physical therapy with the diagnosis of atypical Parkinson's disease. He reports experiencing loss of strength and coordination of his right lower extremity and his right hand. This was his third exacerbation of symptoms. The first two he had overcome with diet change and rest followed by exercise. He had been unable to work for the past year due to his symptoms. He had begun to take a low dose of Sinamet but had no change in symptoms. He had foot drop, ambulated with a cane, and fatigued quickly with ambulation.

John reported he had been physically abused as a child by a sibling babysitter. He suffered a fractured cervical vertebra and a concussion. His mother and father never acknowledged the acts of abuse. Over the years John had many psychotherapy sessions which helped him understand the aftermath of childhood abuse, but with no relief of his chronic neck and upper trapezius pain. He was treated with BioSynchronistics first to address spinal imbalance and fascial restriction. This brought temporary relief. He was then treated with Zero Balancing. John began to feel change in his energy level and his symptoms. His gait is normal some days, and he is hopeful he will continue to improve.

Katherine Meyer: History of Sexual Abuse

Katherine is a 64 year old with a history of neck and low back pain referred by an orthopedic physician for treatment. After treating Katherine for several weeks, she shared a history of sexual abuse by her former husband. Initially Katherine had resisted the touch of BioSynchronistics, but relaxed over time and began to experience pain relief. She reached a plateau and was then treated with Zero Balancing. She experienced a deep relaxation during these treatments which carried over to her everyday life. She had lasting relief from her back and neck pain. Katherine began to feel she had control over her body and her residual trauma-related pain.

Mari Rodrigues: Torture Victim and Witness to Violence

Mari is a 28-year-old Central American woman. She was referred by her primary care physician after seeing many specialists for her constant migraine headache and seizures. She was accompanied to her weekly appointments by her husband (and interpreter) and two sons, six and eight years old. She was treated with Clinical Acupressure. Mari had relief from her headache for two or three days after treatment and then it would return. During her treatment, her sons played in the room with our department toys, and her older son would come to the table and embrace and kiss his mother. In the eighth week, I asked her husband if she had ever witnessed violence. He said, yes. She had seen her family tortured and killed. She was the lone survivor. I held her head in my hands and said to her "You are safe now, you are safe." She softly cried and then experienced deep relaxation as the acupressure continued. Her headache was gone after the next two sessions as well as her seizures.

Walter Reed Army Medical Center: Care of the Caretakers

Working with traumatized patients in traditional or alternative therapies can take a toll on caretakers themselves—now typically referred to as "vicarious traumatization." This issue is gaining increased attention among providers, some of whom are "wounded healers" themselves (Hoff, 2010, pp. 199–204). Without support around this issue, "compassion fatigue" or burnout is the predictable result. The following examples illustrate an approach to this caretaker need, including the use of modalities presented in this chapter.

A non-profit group, CrossingsHealingworks, features practitioners who are volunteering to treat those who care for veterans. Their special concern is for members of the military, their families, and their caretakers. In 2005 the group began by setting up a free clinic for nurses at Walter Reed Army Medical Center in Washington, DC during National Nurses Week. They identified a need they could respond to and expanded the clinic to all staff at the hospital and a weekly clinic in 2007.

The clinic, Restore and Renew Wellness, is staffed by six volunteers offering acupuncture, Clinical Acupressure, and Zero Balancing. They believe reducing stress in any aspect of the hospital affects all others, including patients' families, caregivers, and administrators. In six months they have found the immediate effects of treatment reported as follows:

- more relaxed—99%
- mind at ease—95%
- less stress—94%
- more energy—79%
- less pain—74%—"better than aspirin."

Longer term effects were also cited:

- aware of need for self-care—96%
- improved mood—94%
- more ease in relationships with co-workers—83%
- more compassion with patients— 81%
- better sleep—79%
- more pleasure in personal relationships—78%.

Many of the hospital staff reporting these results had served in Iraq (Duncan, 2008).

We Care Vets, based in Northhampton, MA and San Diego, CA, is another organization whose volunteers treat veterans. In Boston in September 2008, a group of massage therapists and physical therapists had a day of treating Iraqi Veterans Against the War (Bindley, 2008).

Collaboration between Primary Care and Alternative Therapy Practitioners

These examples illustrate the profound effects of considering not just "what is wrong" with the client, as in medical diagnostic terms, but rather the whole person, the integrally connected "body, mind, and spirit" in active collaboration with the suffering client. We believe with the natural healers we have cited that the sharp distinctions between body, mind, and spirit cannot be maintained, since they are integral aspects of the whole person. Our final illustration of the both/and approach suggests further promise and growth on the horizon of combining the best of Eastern and Western traditions of healing, and portends enormous cultural change in medicine and holistic healthcare (Hamwee, 1999, p. 129; Edmands, Hoff, Kaylor, Mower, & Sorrell, 1999). The following correspondence between three physicians regarding treatment by a physical therapist using manual therapy underscores the promise of collaboration among diverse practitioners. This exchange is a testament for primary care providers to seriously examine alternative therapies on behalf of their clients and colleagues. The letter is printed with permission of the author, and edited to protect privacy.

Illustration: Physician and Physical Therapist Referral and Collaboration

Dear Paul and Barry,

I hope you both are well.

I wanted to update you both about my back, and in doing so, bring your attention to a very skilled physical therapist, Jennifer, on the hospital staff (I'm copying her on this message). As you both know, when I first saw Larry [orthopaedic surgeon] in the beginning of the year my low back pain was so intense that I was basically asking for a surgery. Larry wisely pointed out that such an intervention was not only not indicated, but may be counterproductive. We tried a course of steroids, which helped for a while, but ultimately my pain returned. At that time, I went to meet with Anton [orthopaedic surgeon], who again was very helpful. He put me on Lidoderm patches, which actually provided great relief, told me we could consider a TENS unit, and sent me to physical therapy.

I specifically requested to work with Jennifer, primarily because I know her personally and had some sense of her approach to her work. I had also sent her patients in the past who had done very well. After four sessions with Jennifer, my pain is 80% better. I still have some stiffness on some days when I get up from sitting, and my back still hurts sometimes when I sneeze, but I never expected that I could feel this well again. I stopped using the Lidoderm two weeks ago. I'm really grateful for my improvement.

I'm e-mailing you two because I actually think you both should consider chatting with Jennifer about her approach to therapy. You both must see an awful lot of patients with acute or chronic low back pain, and I'm sure all three of us refer many of these folks for physical therapy. But in my practice, I'm indiscriminate in my referral. I just write the prescription and tell my patients to go someplace near their workplace or home. But I now realize that this would be akin to arguing that all neurosurgeons, physiatrists, or internists are equal, and we three know that's not true. I clearly need to more closely interrogate the centers to whom I refer my patients.

I don't know enough about Jennifer's technique to represent it to you, but at our first meeting she told me that I had significant muscular dysfunction which likely contributed to skeletal misalignment. She didn't disregard the diskogenic component of my pain, but she told me that if she could get my muscles and bones right and decompress the vertebrae, I may feel an awful lot better. So I went with that. And the results thus far have been really good.

So, gents, I'm writing you to update you on what's been going on, to THANK YOU both for your help, and to encourage you to get in touch with and chat with Jennifer. She only works part-time, so I don't know how many patients she wants to take on, but she's definitely broadened my understanding of my own practice.

Be well.

Jason

Follow-up Referrals

In the two weeks following the letter from Jason, he referred seven of his patients to Jennifer for PT treatment. Here is what Jennifer shared about these referrals: BioSynchronistics was used for evaluation and treatment, while searching for the cause of the ailment. For example, muscle tightness in the pelvic floor may be the cause of neck pain; the psoas muscle and the continuation of its fascia may be the cause of chronic knee pain; abdominal scarring from 20-year-old appendectomy surgery may be the cause of right hip and knee pain; a ten-year-old hysterectomy scar frequently is the cause of low back pain. With two of these patients, there was an emotional component associated with their pain. One was in shock from a traumatic injury and the second a family death coincided with the injury. Zero Balancing or Clinical Acupressure will be used for treatment. If they do not respond to treatment, Jennifer may recommend that they might benefit from psychotherapy in addition to physical therapy.

Jennifer said: "Sometimes I am wrong with what was initially identified as the cause of the problem. Therein lies the challenge and fascination with the work. You never stop learning, there is always something new."

To conclude, the wide array of self-help and alternative therapies suggests a cautionary note to providers as well as clients. Since research on the effectiveness of some widely used alternative practices is only in beginning phases, further study and education about these modalities is paramount for enhancing client safety. If patients do not voluntarily disclose to their primary care provider the health, wellness, and alternative activities they embrace, the PCP should inquire with a view to ascertaining any adverse interactions that may occur, for example, as the result of mixing "home remedies" with prescribed medications. Such inquiry is aided by the fact that many medical history intake forms now require a list of all non-prescription supplements the patient is taking, including dosage and frequency.

If the patient does disclose various "new self-help" tactics unfamiliar to the PCP, in an interested but neutral tone the provider should ask questions like these: "What effect did this have for you? How has this treatment changed your symptoms or quality of life? I've not heard about that treatment . . . What kind of license does the practitioner hold?" For example, "magnet therapy" requires no license. The basic principles are client safety and effectiveness, and special training requirements by those licensed to practice alternative therapies such as Zero Balancing and Acupuncture. Primary care providers seeking further information are recommended to this source from the Federation of State Medical Boards of the United States: *Model Guidelines for the Use of Complementary and Alternative Therapies in Medical Practice*, cited in the CAM internet site.

References

Bindley, J. (2008). Personal communication.

CAM (2005). Retrieved from www.National Institutes of Health U.S.. March 12, 2010. National Center for Complementary and Alternative Medicine (NCCAM). National Academies Press.

Duncan, A. (2008). Restore & Renew Wellness Clinic: A Systems Approach to Tending Traumatic Stress in Military Hospitals. Presentation at Force Health Protection Conference (August 2008). Albuquerque, NM: aduncan@crossingshealingworks.org.

Edmands, M. S., Hoff, L. A., Kaylor, L., Mower, L., & Sorrell, S. (1999). Bridging gaps between mind, body, spirit: Healing the whole person. *Journal of Psychosocial Nursing*, 37(10), 35–41.

Hamwee, J. (1999). *Zero balancing: Touching the energy of bone*. Berkeley, CA: North Atlantic Books.

Hoff, L. A. (2010). *Violence and abuse issues: Cross-cultural perspectives for health and social services*. London: Routledge.

Hoff, L. A., Hallisey, B. J., & Hoff, M. (2009). *People in crisis: Clinical and diversity perspectives* (6th Ed.). New York: Routledge.

Levine, P. (1997). *Waking the tiger: Healing trauma*. Berkeley, CA: North Atlantic Books.

Seigal, B. S. (1990). *Peace, love and healing*. London: Arrow.

Smith, F. F. (1994). *Inner bridges: A guide to energy movement and body structure*. Atlanta, GA: Humanics New Age.

Weil, A. (2004). *Natural health, natural medicine: The complete guide to wellness*. Boston, MA: Houghton Mifflin.

Epilogue: Do No Harm

We were "in press" and too late for citing the current book: *Anatomy of an epidemic: Magic bullets, psychiatric drugs, and the astonishing rise of mental illness in America* (2010) by Robert Whitaker (New York: Crown). This work shows from long-term outcome studies the importance of a cautious approach to the use of psychotropic drugs. Whitaker exhaustively documents from national and international research cited in professional journals, NIMH, WHO, etc. the iatrogenesis of chronic mental illness and lifetime disability (physical and mental health decline) traceable to the overuse of psychotropic medications as revealed in randomized clinical trials.

The author's major point from extensive peer-reviewed articles and other sources is the "cautious and selective" use of psychotropic medications. While addressing this issue throughout our book, we did not have the benefit of examining Whitaker's work before manuscript delivery. Whitaker describes the influence of the powerful pharmaceutical industry and the "disease" model vs. a broader psychosocial and psychodynamic approach to psychiatric treatment. His work parallels the increasing attention to this issue in the mainstream press.

We recognize from our own clinical experience, and the testimony of patients, both the benefit and potential dangers of psychotropic drugs. Long-established research findings indicate that psychotropic drugs are most efficacious when used in combination with psychosocial and related therapies. Primary care providers are in strategic positions to advocate for this kind of holistic care through their relationships with patients and collaboration with mental health providers for specialized treatment.

Lee Ann Hoff and Betty D. Morgan

Index